S0-AYY-331

Nutrition

for a Healthy Pregnancy

ALSO BY ELIZABETH SOMER

Food and Mood:
The Complete Guide to Eating Well and Feeling Your Best

Nutrition for Women: The Complete Guide

The Essential Guide to Vitamins and Minerals

Nutrition
for a Healthy Pregnancy

The Complete Guide to
Eating Before, During, and
After Your Pregnancy

Elizabeth Somer, M.A., R.D.

An Owl Book
Henry Holt and Company • New York

3 9354 00131834 0

Henry Holt and Company, Inc.
Publishers since 1866
115 West 18th Street
New York, New York 10011

Henry Holt® is a registered
trademark of Henry Holt and Company, Inc.

Copyright © 1995 by Elizabeth Somer
All rights reserved.
Published in Canada by Fitzhenry & Whiteside Ltd.,
195 Allstate Parkway, Markham, Ontario L3R 4T8.

Library of Congress Cataloging-in-Publication Data
Somer, Elizabeth.
Nutrition for a healthy pregnancy: the complete guide to eating
before, during, and after your pregnancy / Elizabeth Somer.
p.   cm.
Includes bibliographical references and index.
1. Pregnancy—Nutritional aspects.   2. Pregnant women—Nutrition.
I. Title.
RG559.S66   1995   94-42167
618.2'4—dc20   CIP

ISBN 0-8050-3775-6 (An Owl Book: pbk.)

Henry Holt books are available for special
promotions and premiums. For details contact:
Director, Special Markets.

First Edition—1995

DESIGNED BY PAULA R. SZAFRANSKI

Printed in the United States of America
All first editions are printed on acid-free paper. ∞

5   7   9   10   8   6   4

Grateful acknowledgment is made for permission to reprint from *Nutrition During Pregnancy and Lactation: An Implementation Guide*, copyright
© 1992 by the National Academy of Sciences, courtesy of the National
Academy Press, Washington, D.C.

To my two sweet children, Lauren and William,
who have taught me so much about life,
love, wonder, joy, and purpose.

The nutritional and health information presented in this book is based on an in-depth review of the current scientific literature. It is intended only as an informative resource guide to help you make informed decisions; it is not meant to replace the advice of a physician or to serve as a guide to self-treatment. Always seek competent medical help for any health condition or if there is any question about the appropriateness of a procedure or health recommendation.

Contents

Foreword

Congratulations on your decision to have a baby! There will be some exciting times ahead of you. Eating properly is an everyday event that can have a profound influence on both you and your developing baby. Helping you to build the best baby you possibly can is the goal of *Nutrition for a Healthy Pregnancy.* In this book you will find recommendations for eating good food rich in nutrients and a commonsense approach to eating healthfully during this most critical period in your and your baby's life. Much of what you choose to do, or not do, will leave a legacy for your child that will last a lifetime.

Elizabeth Somer has done all the homework for you! Over six hundred scientific articles support the information she has packed between these two covers. She has covered pregnancy from "thinking about it" through postpartum, giving you the nuts and bolts of why proper nutrition is so important. *Nutrition for a Healthy Pregnancy* makes it easy to eat right, without overspending at the supermarket or living in the kitchen. Step by step, the menus provided deliver those critical nutrients that will take your baby from a few tiny cells to a whopping eight pounds (we hope!) within nine short months.

In these pages you will find a comprehensive view of the links between nutrition and pregnancy. This is the first book of its kind to present sound dietary guidelines on all aspects of pregnancy, including high-risk pregnancies such as teen pregnancy, multiple births, over-forty pregnancy, and HIV-positive pregnancy. Keeping up with the latest scientific data by reading hundreds of studies each month enables Elizabeth to consistently present the most current information available.

I hope you enjoy this insider's look at the growth and development of your soon-to-be new child. When you stop and consider how amazing life really is, the Baby-wise Diet makes all the sense in the world. Use this guide throughout your pregnancy—from the planning stages through your recovery—and good luck in working toward having the healthiest possible baby!

MIRIAM ERICK, M.S., R.D.
Department of Nutrition,
Brigham and Women's Hospital, Boston,
and author of *No More Morning Sickness*

Preface

For many women, nutrition becomes an important issue after the pregnancy test comes back positive. They know that what they eat during the next nine months will affect the outcome of their pregnancies and the health of their babies, possibly for life. However, many women don't realize that what they eat prior to and following pregnancy may be just as important for their health and their babies' well-being. In addition, women pregnant for the second or third time have their own unique set of dietary considerations and may be at even higher nutritional risk than first-time mothers.

Why I Wrote This Book

I entered pregnancy a bit naïve. Granted, I knew a lot about nutrition, having been a registered dietitian for years. But I wasn't nutrition-wise about the hurdles to eating well during pregnancy, from morning sickness to heartburn. I also wanted the very best for myself and my baby during this time. Adequate wasn't good enough. I wanted to know what researchers were finding out about zinc or folic acid and birth defects. Could I get everything I needed from diet alone or would I need supplements and, if so, which ones were the best? What about nutrient interactions? If I took an iron supplement, how would that affect my zinc or copper status and, more important, the health of my baby? What tests should I have to make sure I was eating enough iron-rich foods? What nutrients were most important during different stages of pregnancy? How could I make sure I left pregnancy and nursing in optimal nutritional status? As a nursing mother, would I need more calcium, vitamin D, or vitamin B6 and how could I get these extra doses from my diet? What nutritional challenges would I encounter as I geared up for my next pregnancy?

I scoured the bookstores and the library, but couldn't find any books that answered all my questions. So I became my own health advocate, read the scientific literature, and learned about medical tests. When I complained of fatigue and was told by my physician that feeling tired was "normal," I ordered my own serum ferritin test and found that I was iron deficient, even though I wasn't anemic. When I was given a prescription prenatal supplement, I compared it to the wealth of research on vitamin and mineral needs of a pregnant woman. I threw out the prenatal pills and designed my own supplement program.

By the time I was ready for a second pregnancy, I was well aware of how important nutrition was for the months and year prior to pregnancy. I again reviewed all of the available books and found that none of them took this critical period seriously, despite a growing body of scientific evidence showing that prepregnancy nutrition is as, if not more, important than diet during pregnancy. I wondered why all of this research wasn't appearing in the popular press. Then I decided to write this book.

For Women Who Want Optimal, Not Just Adequate

This book is a reliable reference source for nutrition prior to, during, and following pregnancy. It is for women who want more than just a "how to eat" guide. Although *Nutrition for a Healthy Pregnancy* includes the Baby-wise Diet and daily menus and recipes for each of the stages of pregnancy, from the preconception months through the years after your baby is born, it also provides a detailed review of the current scientific research on nutrition for pregnancy. The information in the following pages is a thorough review and summary of state-of-the-art findings on everything from how nutrition can improve fertility and prevent birth defects to how diet can help you avoid postpartum depression and strengthen the mother-child bond. Included in the following pages is the latest research on:

- Old wives' tales, folklore, and facts regarding fertility foods
- The role vitamins and minerals play in pregnancy outcome
- What foods to avoid during pregnancy and why
- Who needs extra nutrients and how to choose the best supplement
- Optimal, not just adequate, nutrition during pregnancy
- Dietary guidelines for the pregnant woman over 35
- How diet can help prevent common problems, from morning sickness and food cravings to heartburn and muscle cramps
- How what you eat can affect your labor and delivery
- What foods and nutrients can speed your recovery after the baby is born
- How to regain your figure and maintain your health after the baby is born
- How Dad's diet affects when, and if, you conceive, as well as the health of your baby

Nutrition and Love

The dietary and nutrition guidelines in this book can help you design a personal and realistic dietary plan. They are not intended to add further stress, higher expectations, or more guilt when not followed. Keep in mind that the most important job you have in life is to produce, nurse, and raise a healthy child. That goal always should head a parent's priorities list. Nutrition plays a key role in that process, both for you and your baby, but it is valuable only if combined with love, dedication, and respect.

I have always considered myself a contented person. But now every time I look at, snuggle with, or hug my two sweet children, I am in awe of a newfound and deeper happiness, and I wonder what I was so happy about before I had children. Having and raising an emotionally and physically healthy child is one of the— if not *the* most—important accomplishments of your life. I hope that the information in this book contributes, even if in a small way, to that wonder-filled life experience.

Acknowledgments

Writing a book is much like having a baby. It takes months of hard work, patience, dedication, and a few sleepless nights. Those months are filled with thrills, joys, crises, frustration, and wonder. And each book has a personality of its own; some are easy to write, some are difficult.

As with pregnancy, writing a book requires support and help from others. I especially want to thank Andrea Larson, M.D., for her help in reviewing and providing feedback on the medical content of this book and Janet Haley for reading every word. This book is another shared labor of love with my editor and friend Paula Kakalecik. I also want to thank Kathy Schwab, Betsy Horton-LaForge, Kimberlee Livengood, and Sue West for sharing their pregnancy experiences with me. Finally, this endeavor was completed because of the support, expertise, and help of many researchers and scientists, including:

Lindsay Allen, Ph.D., Professor of Nutrition at University of California, Davis

Carol Archie, M.D., Assistant Professor in the Department of Obstetrics and Gynecology at UCLA Medical Center

Steven Blair, P.E.D., Director of Epidemiology at the Cooper Institute for Aerobics Research in Dallas

Jeffrey Blumberg, Ph.D., Professor of Nutrition at Tufts University

Larry Christensen, Ph.D., Chairman of Psychology at the University of South Alabama

William Connor, M.D., Professor of Medicine and Clinical Nutrition at Oregon Health Sciences University in Portland

Andrew Czeizel, M.D., Director of the Department of Human Genetics and Teratology at the National Institute of Hygiene in Budapest

Bess Dawson-Hughes, M.D., Chief of Calcium and Bone Metabolism Laboratory at USDA Human Nutrition Research Center at Tufts University in Boston

Stephen DeFelice, M.D., Chairman of the Foundation for Innovation in Medicine in New York

Johanna Dwyer, D.Sc., R.D., Professor at Tufts University School of Medicine and the Director of the Nutrition Center at the New England Medical Center in Boston

Miriam Erick, M.S., R.D., Obstetrical Clinical Dietitian at Brigham and Women's Hospital in Boston

Brenda Eskenazi, Ph.D., Associate Professor of Maternal and Child Health in the School of Public Health at the University of California, Berkeley

Robert P. Heaney, M.D., a calcium expert at Creighton University in Omaha, Nebraska

Douglas Heimburger, M.D., Associate Professor and Director of the Division of Clinical Nutrition at the University of Alabama at Birmingham

Janet King, Ph.D., R.D., Professor in the Department of Nutritional Sciences at University of California, Berkeley

Ralph LaForge, M.S., Director of Health Promotion at the San Diego Cardiac Center and Medical Group

Sarah Leibowitz, Ph.D., Professor of Neurobiology at Rockefeller University in New York

Paul Mills, Ph.D., Research Epidemiologist at the National Institute for Occupational Safety and Health in Cincinnati

Robert Sack, Ph.D., Professor of Psychiatry and Director of Adult Sleep Disorder Medicine at the Oregon Health Sciences University in Portland

David Williamson, Ph.D., at the Division of Nutrition at the Center for Disease Control and Prevention in Atlanta

Walter Willett, M.D., Dr.P.H., Chairman of the Nutrition Department at Harvard

Bonnie Worthington-Roberts, Ph.D., Professor of Nutritional Science at the University of Washington in Seattle

Gary Zammit, Ph.D., Director of the Sleep Disorders Institute at St. Luke's Hospital in New York

INTRODUCTION

Eating for Baby and Me

Baby making is the most miraculous experience of a woman's life. Entering into pregnancy is like walking through a door into a new chapter of your life, one filled with surprises, intense feelings, purpose, devotion, and love like you never have experienced before. While some women call it work, other women are so moved by the awe of life that they describe pregnancy and becoming a mother as an adventure into life's richer meanings. You will never be the same again, but if you are ready to commit yourself to the responsibility of parenthood, pregnancy will be the start of the richest and most joyous experience of your life.

If you are pregnant or thinking about becoming pregnant, you probably have spent many moments pondering the new baby and how your life will change. What will the baby look like, what funny little mannerisms will she or he have? You probably are filled with hopes, dreams, and expectations. Will the baby have your red hair or daddy's green eyes? Will she or he inherit granddad's wit or grandma's gentleness? At the end of each daydream, however, is this first and foremost wish: please, just let my baby be healthy.

Many factors influence the health of your baby and your pregnancy experience. For one, your genetic blueprint and your partner's, handed down from one generation to another, will determine many physical and personality traits, from eye color to temperament. Every genetic blueprint has a flaw or two that may or may not become part of your baby's legacy. For example, diabetes or heart disease are prevalent in some families, partly because of the genetic blueprint. On the other hand, your baby may have a genetic blueprint for longevity if your parents and other family members have lived to ripe and healthy old ages. You can't change the genetics, but you do make choices every day that can increase or decrease the chances that those weak spots in your blueprint will have serious consequences for your baby. He or she might inherit a risk for developing high blood pressure, but with a healthy beginning and a lifetime of exercise and good diet, that weakness might never develop or might result in only minor increases in blood pressure.

Nutrition and Birthing Babies: What We Knew Then, What We Know Now

Science and medicine have come a long way during the past hundred years. In our great-grandparents' time, dietary beliefs often were fashioned by the emotional and mystical aura surrounding pregnancy. For example, a pregnant woman might be forbidden to eat salty, acidic, or sour foods for fear the baby would be born with a "cranky" disposition. These superstitions have, for the most part, disappeared; however, many cultural beliefs still persist. For example, some Korean-American women report avoiding blemished fruit because of the traditional belief that it might produce an infant with a skin disease or an unpleasant face.

Dietary recommendations also reflected the economic conditions in our great-grandparents' day. Women and children often worked long hours with limited exposure to sunlight. Coupled with poor diets throughout life, this lifestyle encouraged vitamin D deficiency. Rickets was a common nutritional disorder that interfered with normal bone formation during the growing years and caused malformation of the pelvic bones. A woman with a vitamin D–induced contracted pelvis had difficulty delivering a full-size baby, and complications during the birthing process often resulted in maternal or infant death.

In the 1880s, a German physician named M. O. Prochownick advocated a fluid-restricted, low-carbohydrate, high-protein diet to retard infant growth for women with contracted pelvises. These low-birth-weight infants were easier to deliver and fewer complications were experienced during the birthing process. Although the Prochownick diet met a temporary need, it soon became the standard diet for all pregnant women, even after the original reason for its use no longer applied. Unfortunately, remnants of this diet linger today, even though it could seriously jeopardize the development of a healthy baby.

Another misconception that shaped dietary advice until recent generations was the concept that the baby was the "perfect parasite." Regardless of the mother's nutritional status prior to conception or her dietary habits during pregnancy, the baby would draw all necessary nutrients from the mother's nutrient "stores." It didn't matter if the mother's diet was protein poor; the baby would steal protein from her tissues. Her diet could be iron depleted, and the baby still would obtain ample iron by draining iron "reserves" somewhere in the mother's body. The mother should, but didn't have to, drink milk because the baby would siphon calcium from the mother's bones and teeth—thus the old wives' tale that you lose a tooth for each child. This myth perpetuated a generally careless attitude toward the pregnant woman's diet, her weight gain, and how nutrition affected the baby's development.

Most of these superstitions and misconceptions have been replaced by sound, well-documented information on the role of diet in the baby-making process. The famines and food restrictions imposed on the people of Leningrad and occupied Holland during World War II proved that the mother's diet was critical to both conception and pregnancy outcome. There, women who had given birth to healthy, robust babies prior to the war when food was abundant then delivered small, low-birth-weight babies and experienced more spontaneous abortions, stillbirths, and congenital disfigurements as a direct result of poor diets. In Great Britain, however, pregnant women received special-priority ration cards for better nutrition, and the infant death rate dropped between 1940 and 1945, despite the ravages of war. The association was clear: the baby is a product of the mother's diet prior to and during pregnancy. If her diet is poor or she gains less than 25 pounds during her pregnancy, then conception, infant development, and delivery might be seriously affected. The likelihood of having a healthy baby increases if the mother's diet and weight gain are good. In essence, the health of the baby is directly related to what the mother eats prior to and during her pregnancy.

What You Eat = Your Baby

If you have been pregnant, are pregnant, or have talked to pregnant friends, you know there is no life experience as miraculous as producing a baby. Whether you have danced through life insensitive to your body's signals or have closely cared for your body, the changes that occur as a result of pregnancy cannot be ignored.

You feel different, you look different, you might be more emotional or insecure, you might feel more loving or irritable. You cry over commercials or become angry at things that never bothered you before. Your sleep is affected or you experience heartburn for the first time. All your physical and mental signals might be scrambled, so you don't know what to expect from yourself from one moment to another.

On top of that, your body is changing and growing to nurture the developing human being inside you. And of course, the baby is growing from two cells to a highly diversified and complex miracle of life. It is no wonder your dietary needs change and your nutrient requirements are greater than at any other time in your adult life.

Coupled with your body's increasing demands for nutrients is your baby's absolute dependence on you during the next nine months for all the vitamins, minerals, protein, calories, and other food factors necessary to produce life. You are your baby's sole source of nutrition during the most critical period of development. Every choice you make, from the cereal you select to the supplements you take to whether or not you drink coffee, directly affects your baby. Every gram of protein, every microgram of folic acid, every drop of water, every trace of copper comes from you.

Some essential nutrients come from the limited stores you have stockpiled in your tissues if your diet was optimal prior to pregnancy. Other nutrients are not stored in your body or are stored in such limited amounts that your diet is virtually the only place your baby can get what is needed. Consequently, your baby is a product of what you have eaten before and during pregnancy. If this is your second or third child, this baby also is a product of what you have eaten since your last pregnancy to replenish lost stores. A baby grown on a diet composed mostly of refined, processed foods or inadequate calories is very different from a baby nourished on a variety of wholesome, nutritious foods.

Granted, some of the differences are subtle and a baby grown on a diet of chocolate bars and soda pop may arrive on the scheduled due date and appear fine. However, how much healthier could that baby have been if the mother had snacked on carrots and milk instead? What long-term consequences will result? How will the baby's memory, concentration, IQ, health in later years, or even his or her own children be affected? Why take the risk when eating right is so easy?

Your Diet and the Growing Process

Why is your diet so important to the growth and health of your baby? For one, developing from two cells into a human being is a complicated process that requires a wide array of nutrients in varying amounts at different times. Your diet determines if those nutritional building blocks will be there when they are needed.

Growth is not just getting bigger. From conception to birth and beyond, all your baby's organs and tissues form, grow, and mature at different speeds, rates, and times—each with its own characteristic pattern. Three general growth levels are operating simultaneously during the baby-making process: (1) the entire body is growing; (2) the organs and tissues are forming and increasing in size; and (3) the cells within each organ and tissue are differentiating, increasing in number, and expanding in size. This symphony of growth processes is different every day, week, month, and trimester of your pregnancy.

Not to Mention Personality and Preferences

We know that from an infant's earliest impressions of the world, he or she forms attitudes that affect behavior into adulthood. For example, if food and love are there when the baby cries, that baby grows into an adult who views the world as a safe and trustworthy place to live. It is possible that these attitudes begin even earlier, before a baby is born. Small babies born to malnourished mothers smile less and are more drowsy and passive compared to babies born to well-nourished mothers. And the effects last into childhood, where children who were malnourished during development also perform less well in school.

Nutritious, wholesome food throughout pregnancy and the first years of life fuels more than just the physical health of your baby. It also nurtures trust, autonomy, feelings of safety and security, and fulfills other psychological and social needs. Before your baby can cry out for food, she or he must trust you to supply all the essential nutrients when they are needed, to help realize the hopes and dreams of health you have for your child.

Nutrition: Here, Now, and Always

One normally thinks of the effects of nutrition in terms of the present. We feel good in the afternoon because we ate a nutritious breakfast, but a friend is sleepy or irritable because she skipped breakfast and opted for a cup of coffee. However, the effects of today's diet are long term and also can influence your health for years to come. In fact, the best way to ensure good health when you are old is to eat well and maintain a desirable weight when you are young. Your eating habits today as well as yesterday are a major determinant of whether or not you will develop cardiovascular disease, cancer, diabetes, high blood pressure, obesity, or another degenerative disease later in life.

But at no time in life are the effects of nutrition on future health more dramatic than while a person is in the womb. Even the dietary habits of your mother during her pregnancy with you might have effects on *your* baby's lifelong health. Dr. D. P. Barker at Southampton General Hospital in England compiled a review of the research that showed that malnutrition during pregnancy might program the newborn for cardiovascular disease later in life.

For example, the nutritional health of the uterus at the time of conception is critical to whether the fertilized egg successfully implants in the uterine wall and begins to develop. During the first few weeks following fertilization—called the implantation stage—the egg cell divides into many cells and these rudimentary cells sort themselves into three layers: the outer, middle, and inner layers. Diet is critical at this stage to ensure a healthy beginning, while inadequate nutrient intake can result in failure of the fertilized egg to implant in the uterine wall or in other conditions that result in the loss of the egg.

Also, nutrient needs during pregnancy reflect the rapid and dramatic growth that occurs in each of the three trimesters. You need more protein, calcium, phosphorus, and magnesium for the rapidly dividing cells and for bone formation. You need more iron, vitamin B12, copper, and vitamin B6 to produce hemoglobin in red blood cells for your rapidly expanding blood volume. You need twice as much folic acid for each of the billions of new cells to divide properly. Your nutritional state prior to becoming pregnant will determine how "packed" your vitamin and mineral stores are, and your diet during every stage of pregnancy will determine whether or not you have the nutritional "what it takes" to build every cell, tissue, and organ that makes up your child.

Not only are you nourishing your baby to be born healthy, you are also setting the stage for your baby's health throughout life. A dramatic example of this is a baby born to a mother who abused alcohol while she was pregnant. Her baby may be permanently damaged physically and mentally. The baby could have a smaller brain size, some degree of mental retardation, and certain facial characteristics such as a low, broad nose bridge; a long convex upper lip; and large eye folds. This child might never achieve normal growth and his or her IQ might not improve with age.

A mother whose diet is low in zinc might feel fine during pregnancy, with no overt symptoms of malnutrition and adequate zinc stores for her own body needs, but her baby could be born with a cleft palate and an abnormal heart caused by inadequate available zinc during cell growth and development. Inadequate intake of vitamin D and calcium during pregnancy increases the child's risk for later dental and bone disorders. Low folic acid intake is associated with increased risk for birth defects, in particular neural tube defects, which will be discussed in detail in chapter 1.

Your diet is the nutritional legacy that your baby will live with forever.

What You Eat = Your Pregnancy, Delivery, and Recovery

In addition to affecting your baby's immediate and lifelong health, what you eat before and during your pregnancy could be one of the most important considerations for your health and happiness during those months. Fortunately, most women do not develop serious complications during pregnancy; it is the minor nuisances that might turn a wonderful nine months into an ordeal. Fatigue, morning sickness, constipation, hemorrhoids, varicose veins, tooth and gum problems, leg cramps, nose bleeds, skin problems, colds and infections, mild depression, and mood swings are only a few of the nutritionally related side effects of pregnancy that might be avoided or at least lessened by proper diet.

For example, a diet and supplement program that guarantees optimal iron intake reduces your likelihood of experiencing fatigue, irritability, and mood swings. Ample intake of protein, carbohydrate, and vitamin B6 can reduce some of the discomfort of morning sickness. Including a variety of fibrous foods in the daily fare reduces your risk for developing constipation and hemorrhoids.

What you eat prior to and during pregnancy also can affect your childbirth experience. For one, an optimal diet helps prevent the onset of premature labor. Second, you will need all the strength and endurance you can muster to help bring that baby into the world, and a well-nourished body is the foundation and source of that energy and resiliency. A well-nourished woman won't necessarily have a pain-free, one-hour labor, but she will be more able to cope and draw on her well-stocked energy reserves for any labor experience, as compared to a woman whose body enters labor already fatigued and depleted of essential nutrients.

Think of yourself as a highly trained competition athlete entering a marathon. You are most likely to run your best, experience minimal fatigue and damage to your body, and have the fortitude and reserves to push your hardest during the final stretch if your body is fueled for the event. In contrast, you are more likely to injure yourself, experience exhaustion, or run out of energy if you have not made the effort to nourish your body ahead of time.

The physical and emotional stresses of childbirth are enormous, regardless of whether your labor is three hours or thirty hours, whether you have a planned cesarean or a long labor ending in cesarean. Your body will require optimal fuel and resources to mend and revitalize itself. There are stretches, tears, incisions, sutures, blood loss, lost sleep, and numerous other physical tolls on your body that must be tended to. Nutrition is important in this mending process. In addition, your diet is essential for the health of your baby if you plan to breast-feed.

The Bottom Line

Never before have babies had better chances of being born alive and well. In the past, little was known about "birthing babies," and the survival of both the mother and the baby was mostly left to chance. Today, having a healthy baby is mostly up to you. You can minimize the risks and maximize the likelihood of having a healthy baby, a smooth and enjoyable pregnancy, an uncomplicated delivery, and a quick recovery to your "old" (or an even-better) self if you take the time to eat well for you and the precious little person growing inside you.

I.

Before Pregnancy

CHAPTER ONE

Preparing for Pregnancy

Three months to one year prior to conception:

1. Follow the guidelines outlined in the Baby-wise Diet (see chapter 2).
2. If you are 20 percent above your desirable weight, gradually lose weight prior to conception. If you are more than 10 percent below your desirable weight, gradually gain weight before conception.
3. Take a multiple vitamin and mineral that contains 100 to 150 percent of the Reference Daily Intakes (RDIs) for all vitamins and minerals, plus at least 400 mcg of folic acid and 18 mg of iron each day.
4. Stop drinking alcohol, using tobacco, or taking any medications or drugs not approved by your physician as safe during pregnancy.
5. If you are not already exercising regularly, begin a low-impact sport such as walking, bicycling, or swimming at least three days a week.

Gearing Up for Pregnancy

The first "big day" may be when your pregnancy test comes back positive, but in reality you may have been pregnant for weeks prior to this day, and in fact, your baby is well on his or her way to being a person. Before you even know you are pregnant, your baby's rapid growth is demanding a constant and hefty supply of all the essential nutrients, many of which will come from both your current dietary intake and the nutrient stores you accumulated prior to conception.

Most scientists and health experts agree that optimal nutrition before conception is critical to the prevention of many birth defects. In fact, the *preconception* visit may be the single most important health-care visit when viewed in the context of its effect on pregnancy. Gearing up for pregnancy should start long before you are actually pregnant. Ideally, you should be preparing for pregnancy at least one year before conception, or one year and four to six weeks before that pregnancy test. In short, it is not just a pregnant woman's nutritional status that is important; it is the nutritional status of any woman who *might become* pregnant.

Even for women who pay close attention to their diets, there is room for improvement as they prepare for pregnancy. In a recent survey of women's eating habits during pregnancy and breast-feeding, researchers at the U.S. Department of Agriculture's Human Nutrition Information Service found that women's diets fall far short of optimal. Although they use milk products (high-calcium foods) more than at any other time in life, pregnant women still don't consume enough to optimally nourish their babies and maintain their own bones. Likewise, they consume too few vitamin-rich fruits and vegetables; only two thirds of their needs for folic acid, the B vitamin essential in the prevention of birth defects; and less than half their requirements for iron.

In another study, conducted at the University of Maine, middle-income women in their first trimester met as little as 33 percent of their folic acid and iron needs and frequently consumed as little as half the recommended amounts of other nutrients, including zinc and vitamins A, B6, and C—nutrients essential for building a healthy baby. One in every three women smokes cigarettes during the childbearing years, a habit linked to birth defects, low birth weight, and low blood levels of many nutrients, including folic acid, vitamin C, and beta carotene.

A nutritionally well-stocked woman is better prepared for the first few weeks of her baby's life, when cell division and growth are so rapid that all of the vital organs have been formed before a woman even knows she is pregnant. She is also prepared for the nutritionally intense nine-month process of making a baby. Eating right also helps a mother recover quickly after the baby is born. The sooner you start, the better; however, it is never too late to begin. (Take Quiz 1.1 to get an objective view of your present diet.)

Quiz 1.1   My Diet: What Needs Improvement?

Thinking about getting pregnant or already there? Here's a quick assessment of how you are doing. Any questions answered no indicate areas that need improvement.

_____ **1.** I am within 10 percent of my desirable body weight.

_____ **2.** I consume at least 2,000 calories a day of nutritious foods and take a moderate-dose vitamin and mineral supplement that includes at least 400 mcg of folic acid and at least 18 mg of iron.

_____ **3.** I consume at least eight servings each day of fresh fruits and vegetables. At least two servings are vitamin C–rich selections, such as citrus fruit, and two servings are dark green leafy vegetables.

_____ **4.** I consume at least six servings each day of 100 percent whole-grain breads and cereals.

_____ **5.** I consume two servings each day of extra-lean meat (i.e., 9 percent fat or less by weight), poultry without the skin, seafood, or cooked dried beans and peas. At least one serving is beans or seafood. (If you are a vegetarian, you should consume daily at least four servings of cooked dried beans and peas.)

_____ **6.** I consume two or more servings each day of calcium-rich foods, such as low-fat or nonfat milk and milk products, dark green leafy vegetables (kale, chard, spinach, or romaine lettuce), or other alternative sources of calcium.

_____ **7.** I am fat-conscious and almost always bake, steam, broil, poach, or grill food rather than fry, sauté, or use sauces and gravies that contain fat; I avoid ordering fatty foods in restaurants and purchase mostly low-fat foods.

_____ **8.** I include one to two tablespoons daily of safflower oil in my diet.

_____ **9.** I drink at least five glasses of water and other nutritious fluids each day.

_____ **10.** I limit my intake of salty foods and avoid using salt in food preparation or at the table.

_____ **11.** I limit my intake of sweets.

_____ **12.** I avoid all alcoholic beverages and do not use alcohol in cooking.

_____ **13.** I limit coffee, caffeinated soft drinks, and other caffeine-containing beverages to one serving or less a day, and I do not take caffeine-containing medications.

_____ **14.** I feel, look, act, and function at my best.

Iron Blues

Iron is of particular concern for all women, but especially for a woman planning for pregnancy. Iron deficiency is common during the childbearing years and is a problem for up to 80 percent of active women. The developing baby and expanding blood volume will take a toll on a mother's iron reserves. If you enter pregnancy with these reserves already drained, it will be even more difficult to maintain optimal iron status. Hence you are likely to suffer more complications during your pregnancy, including fatigue, vaginal bleeding, an increased risk for delivering a low-birth-weight baby, and prolonged fatigue after the baby is born.

Routine blood tests, such as hemoglobin and hematocrit, reflect only final iron-deficiency anemia, so ask for more sensitive tests such as serum ferritin or total iron binding capacity (TIBC), which reflect tissue iron stores. Be your own health advocate and ask for a copy of the lab report; don't settle for an "everything is normal" verbal report from your health-care provider. Serum ferritin levels of less than 20 mcg/l or a TIBC of greater than 450 mcg/l is a sign your tissue iron levels are depleted.

If a blood test verifies that you are iron deficient, an aggressive supplement program should be undertaken several months prior to conception, since it takes three months or more to build iron reserves. Usually, physicians prescribe 60 to 120 mg of iron daily until blood values return to normal and 30 to 60 mg daily thereafter. Women who take therapeutic doses of iron also should increase their intakes of zinc (to at least 15 mg daily) and copper (to at least 2 mg daily) because high doses of iron can cause digestive-tract upsets such as constipation and can interfere with the absorption and use of these minerals. If these minerals are obtained from supplements, try to take them at opposite times of the day from your iron supplement (see Table 1.1). (There's more on dietary iron in chapters 3 and 5.)

Nutrition and Preventing Birth Defects: Folic Acid and Other Vitamins

Neural tube defects (NTD) are the second leading cause of death among infants who die from birth defects in this country (Down syndrome is the leading cause). Roughly one in every 1,000 babies born in the United States has an NTD. These defects occur within the first few weeks after conception, when the tube that

Table 1.1   Iron Up

You should consume at least 18 mg of iron each day prior to pregnancy. If a blood test shows you are iron deficient, your iron needs are even higher.

FOOD	AMOUNT	IRON (MG)
BEANS		
Tofu, firm	1 cup	26.4
Soybeans, cooked	1 cup	8.8
Baked beans	1 cup	5.0
Refried beans, fat-free	1 cup	4.5
Black beans, cooked	1 cup	3.6
Kidney beans, cooked	1 cup	3.1
DAIRY PRODUCTS		
Yogurt	1 cup	.2
Cheese	1 ounce	.1
Milk, whole or nonfat	1 cup	.1
FRUITS AND FRUIT JUICES		
Mango, fresh	1 cup sliced	2.1
Avocado	1 whole	2.0
Raisins	$^1/_2$ cup	1.5
Blackberries, fresh	1 cup	.8
Apricots, fresh	3	.6
Strawberries, fresh	1 cup	.6
Peach nectar	1 cup	.5
GRAINS AND BAKED GOODS		
Wheat germ	$^1/_2$ cup	3.3
Noodles, enriched egg, cooked	1 cup	2.5
Whole wheat bread	2 slices	2.4
Rice, white enriched, cooked	1 cup	2.3
Bagel	1	2.1
English muffin	1	1.7
Oatmeal, cooked	1 cup	1.6
White bread	2 slices	1.6

(continued)

Table 1.1   Iron Up (continued)

FOOD	AMOUNT	IRON (MG)
Rice, brown, cooked	1 cup	.8
Corn tortilla	1 6-inch	.6
MEAT, FISH, AND SHELLFISH		
Oysters, raw	1 cup	16.6
Liver, beef	3 ounces	5.8
Beef, extra-lean, cooked	3 ounces	2.0
Chicken, dark meat, cooked	3 ounces	1.3
Chicken, light meat, cooked	3 ounces	.9
Halibut, baked	3.5 ounces	.9
Pork, lean only, cooked	3 ounces	.9
Salmon, baked	3 ounces	.5
NUTS AND SEEDS		
Sunflower seed kernels	1/4 cup	2.4
Cashews, dry-roasted	1/4 cup	2.0
Almonds	1/4 cup	1.3
Peanut butter	2 tablespoons	.6
VEGETABLES		
Chard, cooked	1 cup	4.0
Spinach, cooked	1 cup	3.0
Beet greens, cooked	1 cup	2.7
Peas, green, cooked	1 cup	2.5
Spinach, raw	1 cup chopped	1.5
Beets, boiled	1 cup	1.1
Corn, cooked	1 cup	1.0
Broccoli, raw	1 cup chopped	.8
Lettuce, romaine	1 cup chopped	.6
Lettuce, iceberg	1 cup chopped	.3

should eventually become the baby's spinal cord and brain does not close properly, leaving an open seam. If the opening occurs in the spine, the baby is born with a portion of the spinal cord exposed or, less commonly, covered only with skin. This neural tube defect is called spina bifida. Two thirds of these babies survive into childhood and suffer from lack of bladder or bowel control, paralysis below the waist, and/or fluid accumulation in the brain leading to mental retardation. If the open seam occurs at the top of the neural tube, as is the case with anencephalic babies, the brain never develops and the baby dies within a few hours of birth.

There is something you can do to reduce your risk of giving birth to a baby with NTD: consume ample amounts of folic acid, a B vitamin, before and during your pregnancy. The vitamin study of the Medical Research Council (MRC) at the Medical College of St. Bartholomew's Hospital in London provided landmark evidence of a direct link between folic acid and NTD. This MRC study found that folic acid supplementation in high-risk women (women who already had given birth to a baby with NTD) around the time of conception and during pregnancy reduced the risk of both spina bifida and anencephaly.

Andrew Czeizel, M.D., director of the Department of Human Genetics and Teratology at the National Institute of Hygiene in Budapest, conducted a study that went one step further than the MRC study by investigating whether the occurrence of NTD could be reduced in low-risk women with no previous history of NTD. This study was of particular interest because 95 percent of women who have a fetus or infant with NTD have not previously had offspring with this defect. The women took multiple-vitamin preparations that contained 800 mcg of folic acid for one month prior to and for at least two months following conception. The results showed that while six cases of NTD were reported in the control group who took only trace-element supplements, there were no cases of NTD in the vitamin-supplemented group. In addition, the supplemented group experienced less morning sickness, had a 5 percent higher rate of conceptions, a nearly 50 percent higher rate of multiple births, and a significant decrease in the rate of major congenital abnormalities other than NTD, including limb defects, urinary defects, and cardiovascular malformations. Dr. Czeizel concluded that "a woman should supplement a folic acid–rich diet with a 400 mcg supplement of folic acid or, in the event her diet is low in folic acid, supplement with at least 800 mcg of folic acid prior to, and during, her pregnancy."

Preventing birth defects goes beyond including folic acid–rich fruits and vegetables in your diet. Dr. Czeizel emphasizes that other nutrients affect NTD occurrence, including vitamin B12, vitamin C, and possibly zinc. In many of the studies that showed a link between folic acid and reduced NTD incidence, the women were given multiple-vitamin supplements with added folic acid, not just folic acid alone. Other studies report similar results: women who take multiple-vitamin supplements prior to and during pregnancy are significantly less likely to give birth to babies with NTD as compared to women who do not supplement. The benefits are greatest when women take multiples for at least three months prior to conception and during the first trimester of pregnancy, but benefits are less pronounced if supplementation begins in the second trimester, and if started in the third trimester, it has little effect on preventing NTD.

Although the evidence is contradictory, there is reason to believe that some vitamins and minerals might help prevent other types of birth defects in addition to NTDs, including cleft palate and cleft lip. These forms of birth defects produce marked disfiguration of the mouth and might impair speech development. In one study, women who had previously given birth to babies with cleft lips or palates were given prenatal multivitamins at the first suspicion of and through the fourth month of pregnancy. At the end of the study, three cases of cleft palate and/or cleft lip were reported in the group who supplemented, while twenty-two cases were reported in the group who did not supplement. In another study, the incidence of these birth defects was greatly reduced in women who supplemented their diets prior to conception and through the first trimester compared to women who did not. However, the link between diet and cleft palate or cleft lip remains controversial, since other studies have shown little or no reduction in risks with supplementation.

Prepregnancy Reasons to Supplement

Should all women consider taking supplements prior to conception to prevent birth defects? Yes. Approximately one in every five women has low blood levels of folic acid even though she shows no signs of folic acid deficiency. Folic acid supplementation prior to conception can reduce the risk of recurrent NTDs by 71 percent. In addition, no toxicity symptoms from intakes greater than the RDA have been reported. While large doses of supplemental folic acid can mask a vitamin B12 deficiency, this is rare and is a possibility only when folic acid is consumed in amounts far in excess of 800 mcg. Therefore, because so many women consume too few folic acid–rich foods and because there is no health risk associated with supplementing with 400 mcg, all women of childbearing age should consume at least two servings daily of folic acid–rich spinach, chard, or other dark green leafy vegetables (a serving is one cup cooked) and/or take a moderate-dose multiple vitamin and mineral supplement that contains at least 400 mcg of folic acid. The Centers for Disease Control recommends that women who have given birth to babies with NTD should supplement with 4 mg of folic acid daily for at least four weeks prior to conception through the first three months of pregnancy (see Table 1.2).

Janet King, Ph.D., R.D., professor in the Department of Nutritional Sciences at University of California, Berkeley, supports the use of supplements for pregnancy, but cautions that "women who assume that supplements will meet all their needs and forget to also pay attention to their diets could be doing themselves more harm than good." While most women who take vitamin and mineral supplements do so responsibly, a few women believe that if some is good, more must be better—an assumption that could lead to tragic results. Vitamins A and D, for example, are potent teratogens (substances that can cause birth defects) when consumed in excessive amounts during pregnancy. There also is concern that the vitamin A derivative, tretinoin, which is used as a topical treatment for acne, might cause birth defects; however, this theory remains controversial.

To maximize the benefits and avoid the risks, consider taking a multiple-vitamin supplement that provides no more than 100 to 150 percent of the Reference Daily Intake (RDI) for all vitamins and minerals, with at least 400 mcg of folic acid. (See chapter 5 for guidelines on supplementation.)

Dispelling Myths and Debunking Misconceptions

People have been giving dietary advice to pregnant women since the dawn of civilization. Most of this advice about how food affects pregnancy is more fiction than fact.

The first and foremost myth regarding diet and pregnancy is that you can rely on your physician for all your nutritional needs. Although your ob-gyn is your ally and the expert in all medical-related issues regarding your pregnancy, most physicians spend little time talking about diet. Many pregnant women at best

Table 1.2   Fortifying Your Diet with Folic Acid

During childbearing years, women should consume at least 400 mcg of folic acid. While dark green leafy vegetables are excellent sources of this B vitamin, other foods also can be worthwhile sources.

FOOD	AMOUNT	FOLIC ACID (MCG)
Banana	1 medium	33
Brewer's yeast	1 tablespoon	313
Chick-peas (garbanzo beans), cooked	1 cup	160
Lentils, cooked	1 cup	358
Lima beans, dried, cooked	1 cup	156
Liver, chicken, cooked	3 ounces	655
Orange juice, frozen	1 cup	109
Pinto beans, cooked	1 cup	294
Red kidney beans, cooked	1 cup	229
Split peas, cooked	1 cup	123
Wheat germ, toasted	½ cup	199

receive booklets on the four food groups. Few are asked if they drink milk, take supplements, smoke or drink alcohol, or eat dark green, leafy vegetables daily. According to a survey conducted by New York Hospital and Cornell University Medical Center, more than half of the ob-gyns interviewed admitted they rarely questioned their patients about their diets. Thus, gearing up for pregnancy means doing your own nutrition homework.

Old Wives' Tales

Prior to this century, the links between diet and pregnancy were based on observation. Since science has developed methods for assessing a food's nutritional content only recently, beliefs about foods often were colored by the emotional and mystical aura surrounding the pregnant state. Salty and bitter foods were discouraged for fear the baby would be born with a "sour" disposition. A woman was told not to eat eggs because of their similarity to her own fertilized egg, or ovum. On the other hand, broth, warm milk, and ripe fruits were thought to soothe the fetus, prepare the uterus for delivery, and ease the birth process. Even the archaic and dangerous recommendations to limit weight gain that flourished in the 1800s and early 1900s were based on poorly understood beliefs about nutrient deficiencies, as well as on difficulties in delivering normal-weight infants from women with protracted pelvises caused by long-term vitamin D deficiencies (see pages 2–3). These recommendations agreed with the notion that a baby's weight was not influenced by how much weight the mother gained during pregnancy. This and other serious misconceptions about nutrition during pregnancy persisted into the 1970s and still flourish in isolated pockets of society.

THE LIVER SCARE: Some pregnant women have been advised to avoid eating liver, since large doses of vitamin A can cause birth defects. However, there is no evidence that eating up to 3 ounces of liver each week, which contains approximately 36,105 IU of vitamin A, is harmful; in fact, this amount provides a wealth of other nutrients, including the B vitamins such as folic acid, iron, zinc, copper, and other trace minerals. (The only time liver might pose a problem is when infants and children are fed liver daily, which could amount to potentially toxic levels of vitamin A.) To avoid the potential toxins that are assumed to accumulate in the liver, a pregnant woman might want to select calves' liver, which is high in the nutrients but is less likely to be a source of unwanted chemicals.

GERMS AND PREGNANCY: Listeriosis, a condition caused by the bacterium *Listeria monocytogenes*, can produce complications during pregnancy, including fever and heartbeat irregularities. A woman considering pregnancy or already pregnant should avoid food sources of this bacteria, including cooked and chilled foods that are inadequately reheated, prepacked salads and coleslaw, uncooked or undercooked meat and poultry, pâté, and unpasteurized milk.

Toxoplasma gondii bacteria are excreted in cat feces and, if ingested, can result in severe problems for the developing baby, including blindness and mental retardation. Treatment of the pregnant mother with antibiotics helps reduce transmission of the infection to the developing baby. However, prevention is the best treatment: a pregnant woman should avoid contact with anything that might be contaminated with toxoplasmosis, including uncooked or undercooked meat, unwashed fruits and vegetables, and cat feces. (Avoid the cat box, keep cats off kitchen and dining surfaces, and wear gloves when gardening.)

COMPUTERS AND PREGNANCY: Controversy persists over whether video display terminals (VDTs) increase the possibility of spontaneous miscarriages. The electromagnetic waves possibly emitted from VDTs are thought to be the potential cause of the problem. While there is no solid evidence to substantiate this claim, the National Association of Working Women recommends "prudent avoidance" of VDTs. A pregnant woman can switch to a laptop computer or a model with a liquid crystal display. Or she can turn off her machine when not using it, limit work in front of the VDT to no more than four hours a day (twenty hours a week total), or sit at arm's length from the computer screen and at least four feet from the sides and back of a VDT.

UNUSUAL DIETS: Suggestions to follow any restrictive or unusual diet should be considered suspect. Dietary imbalances that result from avoiding a wide variety of foods or from overemphasis on certain foods could have far-reaching yet poorly understood effects on the developing baby, especially in the first few weeks or months following conception. For example, researchers at the Beilinson Medical Center in Israel report that after giving birth to three healthy girls, a woman who wanted to bear a son followed her doctor's dietary advice to take a potassium-containing preparation, eat lots of salty beans, limit her intake of fruits and vegetables, and avoid all milk products. While following this diet over the course of several years, she conceived seven times and every fetus either spontaneously aborted or, as in the case of the last baby, was born malformed. This one case does not a conclusion make; however, at a time when you need to eat the very best diet possible, why play Russian roulette with experimental diets?

Thin Is Beautiful?

Although a relatively low percentage of women report that they are dieting to lose weight prior to pregnancy, many are consuming suboptimal amounts of calories, which implies that semifasting has become normal to many women. In fact, the average daily intake for women in the United States is approximately 1,600 calories. The "thin is beautiful" mystique that plagues American women prior to pregnancy could have lifelong damaging and irreversible effects on their developing babies and the outcomes of their pregnancies. Studies show that many women enter pregnancy concerned about weight gain and are plotting the return to their prepregnancy figures before their tummies even begin to bulge.

Pregnancy is not the time to worry about your hips and thighs. Most weight-loss diets are nutritional nightmares, lacking even marginal amounts of many vitamins and minerals, including iron and folic acid. While gearing up for pregnancy, focus on stockpiling the nutrient stores in your tissues and attaining or maintaining a desirable, healthy weight. Eating disorders, including anorexia, bulimia, and compulsive eating, can have serious and irreversible effects on an unborn child, so resolve these problems prior to considering pregnancy.

A woman who is below 10 percent of her desirable body weight prior to conception is at higher risk for complications during pregnancy that may affect the developing baby. Underweight women tend to have premature or low-birth-weight infants who have difficulty "catching up" in terms of growth and who show delayed neurological development and reduced IQ later in life. Underweight women also are more likely to develop anemia and premature rupture of the amniotic membranes during their pregnancies than are normal-weight women.

Overweight women—that is, 20 percent or more above desirable weight—should not attempt to use pregnancy as a way to use up extra body fat, since stored body fat is not the stuff from which babies are made. The obese woman entering pregnancy is more likely to develop complications, such as hypertension and diabetes, and to have more trouble during labor and delivery. Ideally, an overweight woman should lose excess body fat prior to the month or two before conception so that she enters pregnancy with well-stocked nutrient stores in her tissues and is within 10 to 20 percent of her desirable weight.

It is not only weight loss, however, but the *method* of weight loss that is important. According to Ralph LaForge, M.S., director of health promotion at the San Diego Cardiac Center and Medical Group, "It's an obsession with body shape that places a woman in the high-risk category for health problems." To attain unrealistic weights and shapes, women eat poorly, become overly stressed, or practice other unhealthy habits. Consequently, they regain the weight, possibly at a very high cost to their health, their baby's development, and the course of their pregnancies.

"It's a losing battle to attempt to lose weight if your lifestyle won't support it. People must deemphasize weight loss and emphasize healthy behaviors. Anyone can lose weight doing a variety of tricks, many of which, such as smoking cigarettes, are not healthful. For the vast majority of people it's exercise and a healthful diet that will keep the weight off," recommends David Williamson, Ph.D., at the Division of Nutrition at the Centers for Disease Control in Atlanta.

Ironically, a side effect of adopting a healthy lifestyle and following the Baby-wise Diet is that a woman usually loses weight. "Once people adopt lifelong healthful behaviors, the weight takes care of itself," says Dr. Williamson.

Women who lose weight by increasing their physical activity are more likely to keep the weight off and live longer, healthier lives than are people who lose weight without exercising. In addition, exercise must be combined with a low-fat diet that places the body in a fat deficit. Exercise without a low-fat diet doesn't work. And the combination must be a lifelong commitment. "Even if people lose weight, they must continue to eat low-fat foods and exercise daily, or it's a sure thing they'll regain the weight and place themselves in a higher disease-risk category," says Steven Blair, P.E.D., director of epidemiology at the Cooper Institute for Aerobics Research in Dallas. In short, if you are 120 percent or more of your desirable weight, begin losing weight slowly prior to pregnancy so you have attained a more healthful weight by the time of conception. (See Worksheet 1.1 for developing a good weight-loss program.)

Fertility Foods

While infertility (that is, the inability to conceive after twelve months or more of unprotected intercourse) occurs in only 1 percent of teenagers, the rate increases as people age, with up to 25 percent of couples in their mid to late thirties and as many as 50 percent of couples in their forties experiencing infertility problems. While what you eat may play a part in fertility, it is important to sift the few facts from the wealth of fiction when it comes to how much food can do for your conception rate.

Fertile Fiction

Since the beginning of civilization, people have turned to food to enhance fertility and sexual prowess. In fact, eating and loving are so closely entwined that we often speak of "eating our hearts out," "feasting our eyes," or having "lusty appetites." Before the turn of the century, people had little understanding of the chemical and nutritional contents of foods, so many of the fertility-food links were based on hundreds of years of symbolism. An age-old belief in the doctrine of signatures underlies many of these ancient beliefs about food. According to

Worksheet 1.1   Gearing Up for Pregnancy: A Sensible Weight-Loss Plan

Unless advised and monitored by a physician, you should lose no more than two pounds a week, with a long-term goal of achieving between 90 and 120 percent of your desirable weight prior to conception. To determine how long it will take you to reach this goal:

1. Identify your target weight and subtract that weight from your current weight to achieve the total pounds to be lost.
2. Divide this figure by 2 pounds per week.
3. Starting with this week, count off on the calendar the number of weeks it will take to reach your goal.
4. Use the following worksheet to track your success.

Current weight: _____   Target weight: _____
Pounds to lose: _____   Weeks needed (@ 2 pounds/week): _____

Once a week, fill in your weight in the lefthand column of the chart, beginning with your starting weight. Mark the appropriate box to the right and connect the marks to create a graph. (Each square represents two pounds.) See the filled-in chart on the next page for an example.

WEIGHT	PRE-PROGRAM	WEEK 1	WEEK 2	WEEK 3	WEEK 4	WEEK 5	WEEK 6	WEEK 7	WEEK 8	WEEK 9	WEEK 10	WEEK 11	WEEK 12
STARTING WEIGHT													

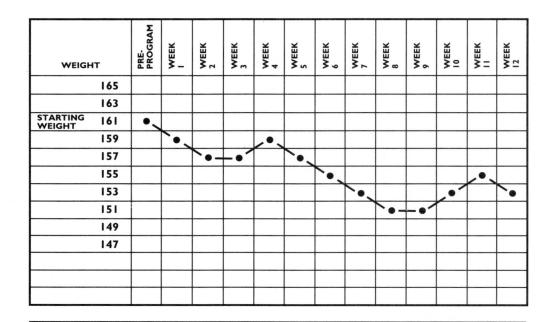

WEIGHT		PRE-PROGRAM	WEEK 1	WEEK 2	WEEK 3	WEEK 4	WEEK 5	WEEK 6	WEEK 7	WEEK 8	WEEK 9	WEEK 10	WEEK 11	WEEK 12
	165													
	163													
STARTING WEIGHT	161	●												
	159		●			●								
	157			●	●		●							
	155							●					●	
	153								●			●		●
	151									●	●			
	149													
	147													

this belief, nature provides clues to a plant's usefulness through its shape or appearance. Plants shaped like human sexual organs, such as onions, which resemble testicles, would enhance sexual potency. Oysters and figs resemble the female anatomy and were thought to increase sexual desire and fertility. The sexual organs of animals, eggs, and meat from animals known to reproduce easily—that is, rabbits as well as fish, clams, sea slugs, lobsters, goose, eels, snails, and snakes—have at one time or another been used to enhance fertility. Ripe fruit such as bananas, cherries, dates, peaches, and pomegranates and vegetables such as cucumbers, peppers, ginseng, and tomatoes were also believed to increase sexual desire. All of these beliefs are based on fiction, not fact.

The rise in blood pressure or pulse rate sometimes experienced after eating spicy foods such as those made with curry or chili peppers was mistaken for a sign of increased sexual potency. Rare or exotic foods also were thought to supply a fertility or potency factor; these included hippopotamus snout, hyena eyes, pine nuts, dried liver, camel's hump, shark's fin, and chocolate or cocoa. During Elizabethan times, prunes were considered such a powerful aphrodisiac that they were served in brothels. Again, not a word of this advice was true.

Some beliefs have survived into modern times. The ancient Greeks spread an offering of barley around the temple of Demeter to assure fertility. The custom was passed down to subsequent generations and is perpetuated today when we throw rice at the bride and groom at a wedding. It's a nice custom, but it doesn't do a thing for fertility.

Fertile Facts

While history is filled with food myths, are there any foods that increase a couple's chances of conceiving? Yes, no, and maybe. Though there is little research on how specific foods affect fertility, there is strong evidence that reversing the effects of general malnutrition will improve conception rates. For example, famines imposed by wars have resulted in dramatic drops in the birth rate, with as many as 50 percent or more of women experiencing cessation of menstruation during wartime. Menses returned to normal within six months after food intake was returned to pre-famine levels for women who were well nourished prior to the war; normal fertility took longer for women who were poorly nourished prior to the war.

The link between nutrition and fertility is not restricted to wartime. Any time a woman follows a strict diet that severely limits calories or any time she experiences severe weight loss (below 10 percent of desirable body weight) she is likely also to experience a disruption in ovulation. Men undergoing strict dieting also are likely to show reduced sperm formation. Usually, restoring healthful eating patterns helps normalize reproductive function. This is especially true for people with serious eating disorders (such as bulimia and anorexia), those who engage in frequent strenuous exercise, which often results in amenorrhea (cessation of the menstrual cycle), or even in women eating nutritionally unbalanced vegetarian diets. On the other hand, overnutrition in the form of obesity also affects the menstrual cycle and can interfere with ovulation and fertility, while gradual weight loss improves a woman's chances of conception. In short, too little or too much of either calories or body fat interferes with a woman's ability to conceive.

The belief that oysters increase fertility might have some scientific basis. Oysters are the richest dietary source of zinc, supplying as much as 13 mg of zinc per oyster. (The Recommended Dietary Allowance for adults is 12 to 15 mg.) Several studies have shown that even short-term inadequate intake of this trace mineral reduces fertility in men, including reduced semen volume, blood testosterone (the male sex hormone) levels, and zinc concentrations in semen. Zinc also plays a role in ovulation and fertilization in women. However, this research should be viewed in perspective. While attaining and maintaining normal zinc status by consuming 15 mg of zinc each day will help sustain a person's normal sexual function, consuming larger doses will not produce superhuman fertility rates or turn a jalopy-style reproductive system into a hot rod (see Table 1.3).

Other dietary and lifestyle habits have been linked to fertility. Researchers at the University of Wisconsin at Madison investigated the effectiveness of vitamin D supplements on reversing male infertility caused by poor diet, and they found that the combined effect of increasing vitamin D and calcium intake (to 400 IU and 1,000 mg, respectively) might improve fertility rates. Both excessive and inadequate intakes of selenium are linked to reduced fertility rates, while consuming selenium-rich foods such as seafood, whole grains, and extra-lean meats enhances conception.

Even carrots are under suspicion when it comes to fertility. One study published in 1983 reported that ten women who had consumed excessive amounts of beta carotene–rich foods—that is, one pound of carrots or 129,000 IU of beta carotene daily (the RDA is 4,000 IU)—showed elevated blood carotene levels and irregular or no menstruation. Cutting back on carrot intake helped these women normalize menstrual function. The link between carotene and menstruation remains speculative, however, since this nutrient is considered relatively nontoxic even in large doses and the results of this study have not been tested by other researchers.

Men who smoke benefit from increasing their intakes of vitamin C–rich foods such as orange juice, strawberries, and broccoli. Increasing vitamin C intake to at least 200 mg in smokers has helped reduce nicotine toxicity and improve all measures of sperm quality. However, since both smoking and exposure to other people's smoke can decrease fertilization rates, your best bet is to stop smoking and avoid passive smoke before, during, and after pregnancy.

Anyone wishing to get pregnant should eliminate coffee, tea, caffeinated soft drinks, chocolate, and other caffeinated substances. Allen Wilcox at the National Institute of Environmental Health Sciences reports that, according to his study, "women exposed to more than a cup-of-coffee's-worth of caffeine a day were about half as likely to become pregnant than women who drank less." Dr. Wilcox monitored approximately 100 women who were planning to get pregnant. After three months and again at six months, the women who limited or avoided caffeine were four times more likely to get pregnant than the caffeine guzzlers. In another study conducted at Yale University School of Medicine, researchers found that

Table 1.3 Galvanizing Your Reproductive System

A person should consume approximately 15 mg of zinc each day. Here are a few ways to increase your zinc intake.

FOOD	AMOUNT	ZINC (MG)
Amaranth grain	1 cup	6.20
Avocado	1	1.28
Baked beans, vegetarian	1 cup	3.55
Bean burrito	1	2.37
Cashews	½ cup	3.09
Cheese	1 ounce	.70–1.10
Chicken, dark meat	3 ounces	2.38
Chicken, light meat	3 ounces	1.05
Clams, canned	½ cup	2.18
Ground beef, extra-lean	3 ounces	4.44
Lentils, cooked	1 cup	2.50
Milk, nonfat	1 cup	.92
Oatmeal, cooked	1 cup	1.15
Oysters, raw	6 medium	76.70
Rice, wild, cooked	1 cup	2.20
Spinach, cooked	1 cup	1.37
Tofu, firm	½ cup	1.98
Wheat germ	½ cup	6.15
Yogurt, low-fat	1 cup	2.02

even one cup of coffee, or the equivalent of 150 mg of caffeine from any source including colas or tea, delayed conception by more than 10 percent; women who consumed 300 mg or more of caffeine (the amount obtained from more than three cups of coffee) daily had a 27 percent lower chance of conceiving compared to women who avoided caffeinated beverages.

In summary, to maximize your chances of conceiving, consume a nutrient-packed, low-fat diet that supplies all the vitamins and minerals in optimal amounts, as outlined in the Baby-wise Diet in chapter 2. Take a moderate-dose multiple vitamin and mineral supplement and maintain a desirable weight. If you are too thin, gradually increase your weight to above 90 percent of desirable levels. If you are too heavy, slowly reduce your weight to less than 120 percent of your desirable weight. These dietary habits combined with moderate exercise; daily relaxation (chronic stress also interferes with ovulation and fertility); avoidance of caffeine, alcohol, and tobacco; and medications limited to those prescribed by a physician may not be as enticing as rhino horn, ginseng, or fish eggs, but they will go much further in helping you optimize your chances of conceiving a healthy baby.

Just Say No to Caffeine, Tobacco, Alcohol, and Drugs

Gearing up for pregnancy is a great opportunity to clean up your act when it comes to health-damaging habits. Many medications, all street drugs, and even everyday substances such as the caffeine in cola or coffee, tobacco, and alcohol could have far-reaching effects on your unborn baby.

Coffee, Tea, or Baby?

On average, American women each guzzle 28 gallons of caffeinated beverages each year. While caffeine is found in tea, many soft drinks, cocoa, chocolate, some prescription and over-the-counter (OTC) drugs, and diuretics, the most concentrated source of caffeine is coffee.

Starting in the late 1970s, people became concerned about the safety of drinking coffee during pregnancy. Numerous studies on animals showed that even moderate amounts of caffeine caused birth defects, reduced fertility, increased the risk for low-birth-weight offspring, and caused other reproductive problems. In 1980, the U.S. Food and Drug Administration (FDA) warned pregnant women to restrict caffeine consumption. Despite the level of consumption and risk identified in animals, the research on caffeine during pregnancy in humans has remained contradictory (see Table 1.4).

Some studies have reported that caffeine might delay conception or increase the risk for a spontaneous abortion; others have shown no effect. Recent evidence, however, has tilted in favor of avoiding caffeine prior to and during pregnancy. In a study from the University of Montreal and McGill University in Montreal, the caffeine intakes of 331 women prior to and during pregnancy were compared to

Table 1.4   Caffeine Counts

To be safe, you should avoid caffeine prior to and during the first trimester of pregnancy. Although no limit has been set, it is best to limit caffeine in the last six months of pregnancy to no more than 200 mg a day, from all sources.

ITEM	CAFFEINE (MG)
Coffee (5-ounce cup)*	
Brewed, drip method	60–180
Instant	30–120
Instant with chicory, 6 ounces	38
Decaffeinated	1–5
Irish cream instant, 6 ounces	53
Orange cappuccino instant, 6 ounces	73
Suisse Mocha instant, 6 ounces	41
Vienna instant, 6 ounces	56
Tea (5-ounce cup steeped 4 minutes)*	
Darjeeling	65
English Breakfast	52–77
Red Rose	46
Lipton	38
Tetley	25
Instant	25–50
Iced (12-ounce glass)	67–76
Hot chocolate made with cocoa	
(5-ounce cup)	2–20
Chocolate milk (8 ounces)	2–7
Baker's chocolate (1 ounce)	25
Dark chocolate candy, semisweet	
(1 ounce)	5–35
Milk chocolate candy (1 ounce)	6
Chocolate-flavored syrup (1 ounce)	4
Chocolate desserts	
Instant pudding, 1/2 cup	5

*Caffeine content will vary depending on the strength of the brew.

(continued)

Table 1.4 Caffeine Counts *(continued)*

ITEM	CAFFEINE (MG)
Pudding pops, 1 pop	2
Mousse pie, ⅛ pie	6
Soft drinks, colas (12-ounce serving)	
Canada Dry Diet Cola	1
Coca-Cola/Diet Coke	46
Diet Pepsi/Pepsi Light	36
Diet-Rite	36
Dr Pepper/Sugar-Free Dr Pepper	40
Mountain Dew	54
Pepsi-Cola	38
RC Cola	36
Shasta Cherry Cola	44
Sugar-Free Mr. PIBB	59
TAB	47
Nonprescription drugs	
Anacin, Midol, Vanquish	33
Aqua-Ban diuretic	100
Dexatrim/Dex-a-Diet II/Dietac	200
Dristan	30
Excedrin	65
NoDoz/Appendrine	100
Prolamine	140
Vivarin	200
Prescription drugs	
Cafergot (migraine headaches)	100
Darvon compound (pain relief)	32
Fiorinal (tension headache)	40
Norgesic Forte (muscle relaxant)	60
Soma compound (pain relief)	32
Synalgos-DC (pain relief)	30

pregnancy outcome. The researchers found that women who consumed three cups or more of coffee daily during the months prior to conception had nearly twice as great a risk of losing their babies as women who drank less than half a cup a day. During pregnancy, as little as a cup of coffee daily (or five cups of tea or four cans of cola) doubled the risk of having a miscarriage. In fact, the effect was dose-dependent—that is, for every 100 mg of caffeine, a woman's risk increased by 22 percent.

Caffeine consumption produces birth defects in rats, but whether or not human infants are affected is unclear. It does seem likely, however, that caffeine interferes with normal growth of the developing baby. Researchers at the University of California at Berkeley reported that women who consumed more than 300 mg of caffeine each day doubled their risks of having low-birth-weight infants compared to women who avoided caffeinated beverages prior to and during pregnancy. A study at the Department of Medicine at the University of Laval in Quebec also concluded that caffeine consumption—from coffee, cola, tea, or chocolate—increased the risk of intrauterine growth retardation by up to 50 percent. Other studies have reported similar findings and have noted a reduction in head circumferences in infants born from mothers consuming approximately three 5-ounce cups of coffee or more each day.

Brenda Eskenazi, Ph.D., associate professor of maternal and child health in the School of Public Health at the University of California, Berkeley, says, "The most consistent findings, if any, are with fetal growth retardation and low birth weight. Women who consume 300 mg or more of caffeine daily are at highest risk." That's the equivalent of three 5-ounce cups of coffee. It also appears that pregnant women who smoke and drink coffee have even greater risks for giving birth to babies with stunted growth; however, the smoking is by far the greater sin.

No one is sure how caffeine exerts its effects prior to pregnancy. Although coffee and tea consumption is suspected to increase the loss of some minerals essential for health and fertility, such as calcium, iron, and magnesium, the evidence is inconclusive that this effect is substantial.

During pregnancy, researchers speculate that caffeine can decrease blood flow through the placenta (the nutritional superhighway between the mother and baby) and, thus, restrict nourishment to the developing baby. Another theory links caffeine to zinc. Animals that consume caffeinated diets develop congenital malformations, show decreased brain weight, and have low zinc concentrations in the brain. Because zinc plays an essential role in growth and development (see chapter 3), the significant decrease in brain zinc levels that results from caffeine intake could affect the developing brain, which in turn might lead to an increased risk for miscarriage, retarded growth, or other problems. Studies conducted at Louisiana State University Medical Center in New Orleans show that increasing the zinc intake in these animals helps offset the harmful effects of caffeine, including greater brain and total body weights. However, zinc supplementation did not return brain zinc levels to normal as long as the animals continued to consume caffeine.

If caffeine intake contributes to miscarriage, complications, and birth defects, it could affect your baby before you know you are pregnant. "Most women do not recognize they are pregnant until the middle or the end of the first trimester and do not receive prenatal care until the 10th week of gestation when [development of most organs in the unborn baby] is almost complete and most spontaneous abortions have occurred," says Dr. Eskenazi.

Another concern is that although women avoid coffee while they are nauseated in their first trimester, they often turn to diet colas, which also are a source of caffeine, or return to coffee in the last trimester when infant growth is at its peak, says Dr. Eskenazi. Caffeine consumption (in amounts greater than 200 mg per day) in the later stages of pregnancy affects the unborn directly, including a disruption in normal sleep and activity patterns. Although a safe dose of caffeine has not been established, your best bet is to avoid all caffeinated beverages prior to and during the first trimester of pregnancy; then, if you do drink caffeinated beverages in the second and third trimesters, do so in moderation.

Smoking and Pregnancy

Tobacco smoke contains thousands of chemicals, many of which are toxic, including nicotine, cadmium, carbon dioxide, aromatic hydrocarbons, and vinyl chloride. Many of these pollutants found in cigarette smoke migrate into seminal fluids, are carried by the sperm cells when they fertilize the ovum, and continue to bombard the developing baby when the mother smokes or is exposed to tobacco smoke. The carbon monoxide in tobacco smoke constricts the blood vessels to the placenta and interferes with the oxygenation of the blood. Since the baby depends on the placenta for a constant supply of oxygen and nutrients, every time a woman puffs on a cigarette or inhales other people's smoke she is suffocating her baby.

Women who smoke have smaller babies who are more likely to die soon after birth than do women who avoid tobacco. Prepregnancy smoking doubles the risk of having a growth-retarded infant or of having an ectopic pregnancy, in which the fertilized egg implants somewhere other than the uterus. In addition, women who smoke are more likely than nonsmokers to experience complications such as pre-eclampsia during pregnancy, preterm labor, premature rupture of membranes, and premature delivery. Even exposure to other people's smoke, called passive smoking, can increase a mother's risk for having a low-birth-weight baby. Men who smoke have considerably higher risks of having children with birth defects and childhood cancer, possibly as a result of smoking's effect on lowering vitamin C levels in seminal fluids and sperm.

The harmful effects of prenatal exposure to tobacco smoke persist into childhood, with children born to mothers or fathers who smoked during the pregnancy having significant increased risks for developing cancer. In addition, children whose mothers smoked ten or more cigarettes daily during pregnancy score lower on intelligence tests later in life compared to children born in smoke-free environments, suggesting that smoking impairs nerve development in the unborn baby.

Smoking goes hand-in-hand with poor eating habits. Smokers' consumption of essential nutrients for the baby's growth, such as zinc, iron, and the B vitamins, is often suboptimal, which only increases their risks for complications during pregnancy and health problems in the newborn. For example, smokers have low blood levels of vitamin B12, a nutrient essential in the formation and maintenance of red blood cells and in protein metabolism.

Smoking also depletes the tissues of many essential nutrients. Each cigarette smoked depletes the mother's body of 25 mg of vitamin C, the amount found in a cup of pineapple or half a cup of strawberries. The vitamin C level in the amniotic fluid and in the unborn baby's blood also is lower in women who smoke as compared to women who avoid tobacco. This vitamin is essential for tissue formation and iron absorption. Smoking also escalates calcium loss from the bones, which might interfere with skeletal development in the baby.

Finally, women who smoke are twelve times more likely to die prematurely from lung cancer and three times more likely to die from strokes than are nonsmokers. Therefore, they are much less likely to live to see their children grow up or be there when their grandchildren are born.

The bottom line obviously is to not smoke if you are trying to conceive and to avoid all tobacco smoke prior to, during, and following pregnancy. For the future health of your child, keep your home smoke-free. If you can't quit smoking, at least cut back to fewer than ten cigarettes a day, smoke outdoors where the air will help dilute the sidestream smoke, don't expose your children to smoke, and limit the time you spend with other smokers.

What About Alcohol?

Alcohol and pregnancy don't mix. Alcohol freely crosses the placenta, directly exposing the developing baby to its toxic effects. In fact, the alcohol travels in the baby's bloodstream in the same concentration as that of the mother. So if you drink enough to feel "tipsy," your baby is tipsy, too. However, the baby's immature nervous system, liver, and kidneys are not prepared to detoxify alcohol as quickly or as efficiently as an adult's body. Consequently, alcohol lingers in the unborn's body much longer than in the mother's body.

Alcohol can have a devastating and irreversible effect on your baby. Many babies born to women who drank alcohol during their pregnancies have a condition called fetal alcohol syndrome, or FAS. They are shorter and lighter in weight than other babies, and they don't catch up, even with special postnatal care. They have abnormally small heads, facial irregularities, joint and limb abnormalities, heart defects, and poor coordination. Many are mentally retarded and may develop behavior problems as they grow up, including hyperactivity, extreme nervousness, and poor attention spans. Some babies develop all of these physical and emotional problems; others develop varying degrees of some of these problems; still others show no signs until irreversible behavioral and learning disabilities surface when the child enters school. Alcohol consumption also increases the risk for miscarriage, stillbirth, and death in early infancy; heavy drinkers are two to four times more likely to have miscarriages between the fourth and sixth month of pregnancy than are women who don't drink.

The strongest relationship between the mother's alcohol consumption and FAS seems to exist between the month prior to conception and the first missed menstrual period or the pregnancy test, although alcohol can exert its effects anytime during pregnancy. The risk of birth defects increases with even two ounces of alcohol, or the equivalent of two drinks. You also can't "save up" by abstaining all week then downing six drinks on Saturday night; even a single high dose during one night or weekend of heavy drinking could be all it takes to change the course of your baby's life.

There are several other links between alcohol and nutrition. Alcohol often replaces more nutritious foods, reduces the absorption of some nutrients, and increases the need for, and the urinary loss of, other nutrients. Consequently, nutritional needs go up as the supply goes down. These alcohol-induced nutrient deficiencies further aggravate the effects of alcohol or produce secondary problems. For example, inadequate intake or absorption of vitamin B1 results in further nerve damage, while alcohol's toxic effects on the developing baby are amplified in the presence of a folic acid deficiency. Alcohol increases magnesium losses, resulting in insufficient magnesium for optimal growth. Bone density is reduced in the mother because the alcohol-damaged liver no longer can convert vitamin D to its active form, thus also jeopardizing infant growth. Liver and blood levels of zinc decrease, which might impair the transport of nutrients through the placenta to the baby, reduce oxygen supply to the baby, alter DNA production that interferes with normal cell growth and differentiation, and increase damage to the developing tissues. In fact, numerous marginal nutrient deficiencies that result from alcohol intake also can cause birth defects, including deficiencies in vitamin A, the B vitamins, vitamin C, vitamin D, vitamin E, calcium, magnesium, copper, iodine, manganese, and zinc.

Since alcohol causes permanent physical and mental birth defects and no safe amount has been found, you should avoid all alcoholic beverages prior to and during pregnancy. Heavy drinkers should avoid pregnancy until they are certain they can abstain from alcohol for the entire time—from preconception through birth (and after the baby is born if you plan to breastfeed). Be aware of the alcohol content of foods and drugs you might not suspect; for example, Irish coffee, wine coolers, rum and fruit cakes, liquor-laced desserts, and cough medicines contain alcohol. Also limit cooking with alcohol, since as much as 50 percent of the alcohol remains intact even after prolonged heating.

Drugs: Illicit, Prescription, and Over-the-Counter

In the past, doctors believed the placenta formed an impenetrable barrier that protected the developing baby from any harmful substances. Today, we know this is not true. Although the placenta is amazing, it is not flawless. Most drugs, chemicals, and other substances can cross it so that the baby is an unprotected recipient. While most people are well aware of the harm "hard" drugs such as heroin can have on maternal and infant health, some people are more lax when it comes to other street drugs, such as marijuana or cocaine, or commonly used over-the-counter or prescription medications. Approximately one in every ten babies born in the United States has been exposed to one or more illicit drugs.

Even moderate use of street drugs can affect fertility and could have lifelong and serious consequences on the developing infant. For example, marijuana can lower sperm count in men and might affect menstrual cycles and ovulation in women, which are reversed when the drug is discontinued. Sudden infant death syndrome (SIDS) is the third leading cause of infant mortality, with a sixfold increased risk for SIDS when the mother uses opiates such as heroin and a threefold increased risk with cocaine use. A woman who uses cocaine is also five times more likely to deliver prematurely and to give birth to a baby with a small head circumference, decreased birth weight, and reduced mental and motor development. Combine cocaine use with other drugs and the effects on the baby can be even more serious. On the other hand, children who were born to mothers who used marijuana during pregnancy show learning deficits and short attention spans later in life.

While optimal nutrition might help buffer some of these effects, it cannot compensate totally for the devastating effects of drugs. More likely, drug use goes hand-in-hand with poor eating habits; consequently, nutrient deficiencies take an even greater toll on the baby's chances of developing normally. The recommendation for taking any type of street drug prior to and during pregnancy is as simple as "Don't, not even a little."

Fortunately, most women have a healthy skepticism about taking over-the-counter (OTC) or prescription medications. On the other hand, people are accustomed to popping a pill at the first sign of an ache, pain, cold, or cough under the assumption that if it is readily available without a prescription, it must be safe to take during pregnancy. While some of these medications are safe, others are not; almost all medication—OTC or prescription—come with risks as well as benefits. Even more important is that many of the potential physical defects to the unborn child caused by drugs occur within the first few weeks before you know you are pregnant.

For example, the female hormones estrogen and progestin taken during the first few weeks of pregnancy can increase the risks for birth defects, including limb and heart defects, and increase the likelihood that a baby girl will develop cervical cancer later in life. For this reason, women who discontinue taking the birth control pill, which contains these hormones, should wait at least three months before attempting to conceive and should use another form of birth control in the meantime.

Antibiotics and tranquilizers are other examples of where the risks sometimes outweigh the benefits. Tetracyclinelike antibiotics taken during pregnancy cause permanent discoloration of the child's teeth, while erythromycin might cause liver damage and streptomycin can cause nerve deafness. The tranquilizers—Librium, Miltown, and Valium—taken by the mother during pregnancy might increase the risk that her baby will be born with a cleft lip or palate. Even aspirin should be taken only with physician approval. Aspirin and many other pain relievers contain a compound called salicylate that might prolong pregnancy and labor and may cause excessive bleeding before and after delivery.

A general rule of thumb is to never self-medicate when you are planning to get pregnant or during your pregnancy. Medications that are safe when you are not pregnant can be toxic to your developing baby. On the other hand, many prescription and OTC medications are safe before, during, and following pregnancy. So always confer with your physician before taking any medication, even if it is something as simple as cough syrup or a painkiller.

Genetics, Drugs, and Russian Roulette

With any drug, including tobacco, alcohol, and caffeine, most people know someone who used it before and/or during her pregnancy with no apparent harm. It's true: every woman who smokes will not give birth to a low-birth-weight infant, just as every woman who drinks coffee will not miscarry. The research is based on averages and trends; that is, women who drink coffee, take cocaine, or drink alcohol are more likely to have problems and place their babies at risk than are women who avoid these substances.

No one knows exactly why there is such a wide variation, but genetics is probably a factor as well as other contributing lifestyle patterns. So what is lethal or harmful to one baby may have little effect on another. Of course, the combination of two or more harmful drugs, such as smoking cigarettes and drinking coffee or alcohol, ups the ante for health risks to you and your baby. Since the primary cause of hospitalizations in babies can be traced back to the mother (and to a lesser extent the father) not taking care of herself during pregnancy, why take the chance?

Get Moving: Exercise and Your Prepregnancy Plan

In the past, pregnancy was the time when a woman was told to slow down and "take it easy." Not anymore, at least when it comes to moderate activity. The key is to start before you are pregnant so that you are physically fit and in shape ahead of time. Pregnancy is not the time to begin a rigorous exercise program, but most physicians agree that a pregnant woman can continue an exercise program started prior to pregnancy, usually with some modification during the second and third trimesters.

Why is exercise important during pregnancy? Physical activity improves your sense of well-being. You are also likely to have fewer pregnancy complications, a more timely onset of labor, a shorter labor, less difficulty with labor pain, and fewer obstetric interventions. In addition, babies born to moms who burned 1,000 calories a week through exercise weigh 5 percent more than infants born to inactive women; moms who burn 2,000 calories a week have children who are 10 percent heavier than the norm. This increase in weight shouldn't be taken lightly, since researchers say that heavier babies are healthier and better able to fight infection than are smaller babies. Exercise also helps prevent abnormalities in blood-sugar regulation that are more frequent during pregnancy, helps you sleep better at night, and assists in controlling excessive weight gain. (The more active you are the more calories you can eat without gaining too much weight.)

In general, the 1985 guidelines of the American College of Obstetricians and Gynecologists recommend against vigorous exercise during pregnancy for previously sedentary women or for women with prior adverse outcomes or symptoms in the current pregnancy, such as premature labor, a history of miscarriages, bleeding, or ruptured membranes. For women who started exercising prior to conception, the guidelines suggest limiting exercise in terms of activity type, intensity (less than or equal to 140 heartbeats per minute), and duration. In addition, a woman should exercise no fewer than three days a week, rather than sporadic or intermittent activity, and she always should warm up and cool down before and after exercise.

These recommendations are conservative and were developed to serve a diverse population, so they might not apply to a physically fit woman who is used to daily intense exercise. (See chapter 6 for a detailed description of exercise guidelines during pregnancy.) Most important, you should monitor your body-temperature response to exercise during early pregnancy (that is, from conception through the first trimester), since limited evidence suggests that an increased body-core temperature could adversely affect the developing baby. As part of this temperature regulation, remember to drink ample amounts of fluids prior to and following exercise. In all cases, consult with your physician, preferably several months before you conceive, to develop a physical activity plan that is safe and will fit into your daily schedule.

The Prepregnancy Diet

Starting now and continuing through your pregnancy and up until your baby's first birthday, you should follow the guidelines outlined in the Baby-wise Diet in chapter 2. The guidelines differ from prepregnancy through the trimesters of pregnancy and during the recuperation year following pregnancy only in the minimum number of servings recommended from each of the six food groupings:

1. Calcium-rich foods
2. Vegetables
3. Fruits
4. Extra-lean meats and legumes
5. Grains
6. Quenchers

Of course, the maximum number of calories, and therefore the amount of food, you consume is based on your height and desirable body weight, your activity level, and your individual metabolism. In all cases, when you must cut back on servings to maintain your weight, cut fat and sugar before you reduce the number of servings of the more nutritious foods recommended. In general, to ensure well-stocked nutrient stores, you should consume (ideally for one year, but at least for three months prior to conception) at least:

2 servings from the Calcium-Rich Group
5 servings from the Vegetable Group (at least 2 of
these should be from the selections marked with
an asterisk in the "Fantastic Vegetables" list on
page 51; these are folic acid–rich selections)

3 servings from the Fruit Group (2 of these should be from the selections marked with an asterisk in the "Fabulous Fruits" list on page 51; these are vitamin C–rich selections)

6 servings from the Grains Group (at least 4 of these should be from the selections marked with an asterisk in the "Great Grains" list on page 52; these are trace mineral–rich selections)

2 servings from the Extra-Lean Meats and Legumes Group, with at least 1 serving of fish or legumes (see page 52)

5 servings from the Quenchers (beverages) Group (see page 53)

To make your own diet checklist, see Worksheet 1.2, below.

Worksheet 1.2   My Prepregnancy Daily Checklist

Copy this master sheet to complete daily.

FOOD GROUPS	MINIMUM SERVINGS	ACTUAL INTAKE
Calcium-rich foods	2	_____
Vegetables (at least 2 folic acid–rich choices)	5	_____
Fruits (at least 2 vitamin C–rich choices)	3	_____
Grains (at least 4 whole-grain choices).	6	_____
Extra-lean meats and legumes	2	_____
Quenchers	5	_____

Did I reach my goals? _____

What needs improvement? _____

What will I do differently next week? _____

Prepregnancy Meals and Snacks

The following seven days of menus are examples of how to apply the guidelines of the Baby-wise Diet when gearing up for pregnancy. You should tailor the daily calorie count to meet your individual needs and maintain a desirable weight. Keep in mind that the Recommended Dietary Allowances (RDAs) for iron and zinc are difficult to meet when dietary intake falls below 2,500 calories, while vitamin D needs are guaranteed only when at least three cups of vitamin D–fortified milk are consumed each day.

Day 1

BREAKFAST

¹/₂ grapefruit
1 cup Shredded Wheat cereal with:
    1 cup 2% low-fat milk

SNACK

10 low-fat whole wheat crackers
1¹/₂ ounces part-skim mozzarella cheese
1 medium orange
1 cup sparkling water

LUNCH

Turkey sandwich:
    2 slices whole-grain bread
    3 ounces sliced turkey breast
    2 tablespoons low-calorie
        mayonnaise
1 raw carrot, cut into sticks
¹/₂ cup raw cauliflower florets
1 cup lemon-flavored sparkling water

SNACK

1 plain bagel topped with:
    2 tablespoons fat-free cream
        cheese
1 cup fresh strawberries
2 cups water

DINNER

3 ounces cod fillet, broiled
1 medium sweet potato, baked
1 cup broccoli florets, steamed
1 dinner roll with:
    2 tablespoons light margarine
1 cup herbal tea

SNACK

3 fig bar cookies

Daily totals: 1,983 calories; fat 23%; protein 21%; carbohydrate 56%; fiber 37 grams; salt (sodium) 2.5 grams*

*Sodium will be higher if salt is added to foods.

Day 2

BREAKFAST

1 cup cooked oatmeal with:
   2 teaspoons brown sugar
   2 tablespoons toasted wheat germ
   1 tablespoon raisins
   $\frac{1}{2}$ cup 2% low-fat milk
1 cup grapefruit juice

SNACK

1 cup low-fat plain yogurt with:
   $\frac{1}{2}$ cup fresh fruit
1 cup sparkling water

LUNCH

Peanut butter and jam sandwich:
   2 slices whole-grain bread
   2 tablespoons peanut butter
   1 tablespoon all-fruit jam
1 cup sliced raw vegetables
1 cup 2% low-fat milk

SNACK

1 tangerine
1 soft pretzel
2 cups water

DINNER

3 ounces roasted pork loin
1 baked potato with:
   1 teaspoon light margarine

2 tablespoons nonfat sour cream
1 cup spinach salad with 2 teaspoons
   low-fat dressing

SNACK

1 medium orange, sliced
1 cup air-popped popcorn
1 cup decaffeinated tea

Daily totals: 1,976 calories; fat 27%;
protein 18%; carbohydrate 56%; fiber
30 grams; salt (sodium) 2 grams*

Day 3

BREAKFAST

1 cinnamon-raisin bagel, toasted,
   with:
   2 tablespoons fat-free cream cheese
1 cup low-fat plain yogurt with:
   1 tangerine, sectioned
   $\frac{1}{4}$ cup cubed pineapple
1 cup decaffeinated tea with lemon

SNACK

1 cup 1% low-fat cottage cheese
1 cup sliced melon
1 cup sparkling water

LUNCH

2 cups minestrone soup
2 whole wheat rolls with:
   2 teaspoons light margarine

*Sodium will be higher if salt is added to foods.

1 orange
1 cup iced tea with lemon

SNACK

Trail mix:
   $\frac{1}{2}$ ounce almonds
   2 tablespoons golden raisins
   3 tablespoons semisweet chocolate
      chips
2 cups water

DINNER

3 ounces salmon fillet, broiled
1 cup cooked linguini
1 cup steamed fresh spinach
1 cup steamed cauliflower florets
1 tablespoon light margarine

SNACK

1 carrot, sliced into sticks, with:
   3 tablespoons sour cream dip
$\frac{1}{2}$ cup 2% low-fat milk

Daily totals: 2,012 calories; fat 27%;
protein 23%; carbohydrate 50%; fiber
34 grams; salt (sodium) 4.5 grams*

Day 4

BREAKFAST

1 ounce Grape-Nuts cereal with:
   1 banana, sliced
   $\frac{1}{2}$ cup 2% low-fat milk

1 slice whole wheat toast with:
   1 teaspoon light margarine
1 cup herbal tea

SNACK

5 mini rice cakes
1 cup low-fat plain yogurt with:
   1 cup fresh blueberries
1 cup sparkling water flavored with lime

LUNCH

2 slices vegetarian pizza with extra
   vegetables
Tossed salad:
   1 cup romaine lettuce
   $\frac{1}{4}$ cup sliced fresh mushrooms
   2 teaspoons low-calorie dressing
1 cup iced herbal tea

SNACK

1 cup orange juice
3 graham crackers
1 cup baby carrots

DINNER

3 ounces roasted turkey breast
1 cup zucchini, steamed
$\frac{1}{2}$ cup mashed potatoes with:
   1 teaspoon butter
$\frac{1}{2}$ cup three-bean salad
1 cup decaffeinated tea

*Sodium will be higher if salt is added to foods.

SNACK

1 slice raisin toast topped with:
    1 tablespoon fat-free cream cheese
    $1/3$ cup fresh raspberries

Daily totals: 2,015 calories; fat 19%; protein 20%; carbohydrate 62%; fiber 34 grams; salt (sodium) 3.5 grams*

Day 5

BREAKFAST

2 slices whole wheat toast with:
    2 teaspoons peanut butter
    2 teaspoons jam
$1/4$ cup stewed prunes
$1/2$ cup 2% low-fat milk

SNACK

1 medium orange
$1/2$ pita bread with:
    2 tablespoons fat-free cream cheese
    5 cucumber slices
1 glass iced tea with lemon

LUNCH

Roast beef sandwich:
    2 slices whole-grain bread
    2 ounces extra-lean roast beef
    1 teaspoon mustard
    2 lettuce leaves
    2 tomato slices

1 cup tossed salad with:
    $1/4$ cup kidney beans
    1 tablespoon low-fat dressing
1 medium apple
1 glass sparkling water

SNACK

10 low-fat whole-grain crackers
$1 1/2$ ounces part-skim mozzarella
    cheese
1 cup broccoli florets
2 glasses water

DINNER

1 cup spaghetti, cooked
$1/2$ cup marinara sauce
1 ounce Parmesan cheese, grated
1 cup steamed green beans
Spinach salad:
    1 cup raw spinach
    1 tablespoon diced red onion
    2 tablespoons sliced mushrooms
    2 tablespoons chopped tomato
    1 tablespoon light Russian
        dressing
1 cup decaffeinated tea

SNACK

5 vanilla wafers

Daily totals: 2,071 calories; fat 27%; protein 18%; carbohydrate 55%; fiber 41 grams; salt (sodium) 3.8 grams*

*Sodium will be higher if salt is added to foods.

Day 6

BREAKFAST

1 poached egg
1 English muffin, toasted, with:
   2 teaspoons light margarine
1 cup orange juice
1 cup herbal tea

SNACK

1 whole wheat bagel with:
   1 tablespoon fat-free cream cheese
2 kiwis
1 glass water

LUNCH

1½ cups split pea soup
1 whole-grain dinner roll with:
   1 teaspoon light margarine
1 carrot, cut into sticks
1 cup 2% low-fat milk

SNACK

1 cup grapes
1 cup 2% low-fat milk
1 glass water

DINNER

4 ounces baked red snapper fillet
1 cup cooked wild rice
1 cup steamed broccoli

Tossed salad:
   1 cup chopped romaine lettuce
   ¼ cup sliced mushrooms
   ¼ cup alfalfa sprouts
   2 tablespoons sliced radishes
   1 tablespoon low-fat dressing
1 cup decaffeinated tea

SNACK

1 slice angel food cake topped with:
   1 cup fresh blueberries
1 glass water

Daily totals: 1,944 calories; fat 16%; protein 20%; carbohydrate 64%; fiber 36 grams; salt (sodium) 3 grams*

Day 7

BREAKFAST

2 toasted frozen whole wheat waffles with:
   3 tablespoons berry syrup
   ½ cup fresh berries
1 banana
2 cups herbal tea

SNACK

2 cups 1% cottage cheese
1 cup sliced melon
1 glass orange-flavored sparkling water

*Sodium will be higher if salt is added to foods.

LUNCH

Chicken salad:
    2 cups mixed salad greens
    3 ounces cubed chicken
    1/4 cup chopped celery
    2 teaspoons light mayonnaise
    1/4 cup chopped tomato
    2 tablespoons chopped red onion
    1/4 cup grated carrots
    1 teaspoon roasted sunflower seeds
    1 ounce mozzarella cheese, grated
    3 tablespoons light Italian dressing
1/2 fresh papaya
1 glass water

SNACK

1 cup mixed raw vegetables
1 glass sparkling water flavored with
    lemon

DINNER

3 ounces salmon fillet, baked
1/2 cup cooked pasta
8 asparagus spears, steamed
1 tomato, broiled
1 slice 7-grain bread
1 cup decaffeinated tea

SNACK

10 mini rice cakes dipped in:
    6 ounces apple-cinnamon yogurt

Daily totals: 2,054 calories; fat 21%;
protein 28%; carbohydrate 51%; fiber
25 grams; salt (sodium) 3 grams*

* Sodium will be higher if salt is added to foods.

CHAPTER TWO

The Baby-wise Diet

While the rest of the chapters in this book provide a detailed and extensive review of the what, why, and when of nutrition for pregnancy, this chapter spells out exactly how you should be eating before, during, and following pregnancy. If you do nothing else but follow the guidelines for the Baby-wise Diet, you will be well on your way to giving your baby the best start toward a happy and healthy life.

The guidelines are simple and easy to follow. This is not a time to "diet." It is a time for planning your meals and snacks around fresh fruits and vegetables, grains, and legumes, with ample amounts of calcium-rich and protein-rich foods. The Baby-wise Diet is based on six food groupings:

1. Calcium-rich foods
2. Vegetables
3. Fruits
4. Extra-lean meats and legumes
5. Grains
6. Quenchers

These food groups are outlined in Table 2.1 and the lists on pages 51–53. On page 53 you'll find additional high-value foods that can be consumed in moderation, and page 55 lists foods to be avoided.

The number of servings from each of the six food groups varies somewhat depending on your stage of pregnancy, from preparing for pregnancy, through the three trimesters, to restocking your body's nutrient stores after the baby is born. Later chapters in this book provide specific guidelines on how to apply the Baby-wise Diet to each of these specific stages of pregnancy.

You still can eat your favorite foods, enjoy your favorite recipes, and go to your favorite restaurants; just make sure you eat the number of nutritious foods in the Baby-wise Diet. When, where, and how much you eat is flexible and often is governed by necessity. You might choose a snack for breakfast and a large evening meal during the first trimester if you suffer from morning sickness, but select a larger breakfast and a light evening meal in the last trimester when heartburn is more of a problem.

Table 2.1   Calcium-Rich Goodies

A cup of milk provides approximately 300 mg of calcium. The following foods supply a similar amount of calcium. Gearing up for pregnancy, you should consume 800 mg to 1,000 mg of calcium (at least two servings of the following calcium-rich foods, plus calcium from other sources). During pregnancy, you should consume at least 1,000 mg (or three servings); during breast-feeding, this amount should increase to 1,200 mg (or four servings).

FOOD	AMOUNT
Milk, nonfat or 1% fat	1 cup
Milk, evaporated skim	½ cup
Black-eyed peas, cooked	1½ cups
Bok choy, cooked	2 cups
Broccoli, cooked	3 cups
Cheese	1½ to 2 ounces
Collard greens, cooked	2 cups
Cottage cheese, low-fat	2 cups
Dandelion greens, cooked	2 cups
Kefir beverage	1 cup
Mustard greens, cooked	1½ cups
Spinach, cooked	1¼ cups
Tofu, firm	¾ cup
Turnip greens, cooked	1½ cups
Yogurt, low-fat	¾ cup

Fantastic Vegetables

In general, one portion is equal to one cup raw, one whole piece (such as one carrot), or ½ cup cooked. Vegetables marked with an asterisk are high in folic acid. Gearing up for pregnancy and in your first trimester, you should include at least five portions daily of these foods. During the second two trimesters of pregnancy and during breast-feeding, consume at least six servings daily.

Asparagus*
Bean sprouts
Beans, green
Beets
Broccoli*
Brussels sprouts
Cabbage
Carrots
Cauliflower

Chard*
Collards*
Dandelion greens*
Eggplant
Kale*
Mustard greens*
Okra
Pea pods
Peas, green*

Romaine lettuce*
Spinach*
Squash, winter
Succotash
Sweet potato
Tomato
Turnip greens*
Zucchini

Fabulous Fruits

In general, one portion is equal to one piece, 1½ cups cubed or sauced (including whole grapes), or 1 cup whole (for strawberries or cherries). The fruits marked with an asterisk are especially high in vitamin C. Gearing up for pregnancy and during the first trimester, you should include at least three portions daily of these foods. During the second two trimesters of pregnancy and during breast-feeding, consume at least four servings daily.

Apple
Applesauce
Apricots
Banana
Berries:
   Blackberries
   Blueberries
   Strawberries*
Cantaloupe*

Casaba melon
Cherries
Fruit cocktail
Grapefruit*
Grapes
Kiwi*
Honeydew melon*
Mandarin oranges*
Nectarine

Orange*
Papaya*
Peach
Pear
Pineapple
Plum
Prunes
Tangerine*
Watermelon

Great Grains

In general, one portion is equal to one slice of bread; 1/2 bagel, English muffin, or pita pocket; 1/2 cup cooked pasta, rice, or cereal; or 1 ounce of ready-to-eat cereal. Foods marked with an asterisk are especially high in trace minerals. Gearing up for pregnancy and during the first trimester, you should include at least six portions daily of these foods. During the second two trimesters of pregnancy and during breast-feeding, consume at least seven servings daily.

Bagel, whole wheat*
Bagel, egg, raisin, or plain
Bread, whole wheat*
Bread, white, French, or sourdough
Cereal, cooked—oatmeal, barley, farina*
Cornbread
Crackers, low-fat
English muffin
Hamburger bun
Hot dog bun
Noodles or pasta, whole wheat*

Noodles or pasta, enriched or egg
Pancake
Pita bread, whole wheat*
Popcorn, plain, air-popped
Pretzels
Rice, brown*
Rice, white
Rice cakes
Tortilla
Waffle
Wheat germ*

Extra-Lean Meats and Legumes

In general, a portion is 3 ounces of cooked extra-lean meat, skinless poultry, or fish or 3/4 cup cooked dried beans and peas.

Cooked dried beans and peas, such as kidney, black, garbanzo (chick-peas), great northern, or lima beans; lentils; split peas; or soybeans
Beef, such as chipped beef, flank steak, London broil, round steak, stew meat, or ground round marked as 9% fat by weight
Pork, such as boiled ham, lean pork roast, and tenderloin
Poultry
Seafood
Veal, such as chop, steak, or roast
Luncheon meat (95% fat-free)
Egg (limit to no more than three per week)
Egg substitute

Quenchers

In general, a portion is one 8-ounce glass. Drinks marked with an asterisk are especially high in vitamin C; drinks marked with a pound sign (#) are especially high in beta carotene. Gearing up for pregnancy and during your first trimester, include at least five glasses daily of these fluids, more if you exercise. During the second two trimesters of pregnancy, you should drink at least six glasses, and during breast-feeding, drink no fewer than eight glasses of fluid daily.

Water
Sparkling water
Juices:
    Apple
    Apple cider
    Apricot nectar#
    Carrot#
    Grapefruit*
    Grape

Orange*
Papaya nectar
Passion fruit#
Peach nectar
Pear nectar
Pineapple
Prune
Tomato
V-8

Nutritious Additions

The following foods are high in fat or sugar, but also supply a hefty dose of vitamins and minerals. They can be included in the diet in moderation.

Avocado
Cake, angel food
Cookies—vanilla wafers or animal crackers
Dried fruit—dates, figs, and raisins
Ice cream, preferably low-fat or fat-free varieties
Nuts—almonds, cashews, peanuts, pecans, pistachios, or walnuts
Peanut butter
Pudding
Seeds—pumpkin, sesame, or sunflower

How Often Should I Eat?

How you mix and match these selections is up to you. Keep in mind that vitamins and minerals are best absorbed and a desirable body weight is best maintained when food is divided into small meals and snacks evenly distributed (for example, every four hours during waking hours) throughout the day. Ideally, you should aim for an eating plan that includes three meals and two to three snacks, each snack including at least one fruit or vegetable and one serving from the other food groups, such as grains or calcium-rich foods. The menus at the end of chapters 1, 5, 6, 7, and 9 are based on this eating style.

However, you are most likely to stick with an eating plan if it fits into your schedule. So if "three square meals" is your eating style, then plan your meals accordingly. As your pregnancy progresses, everything from morning sickness in the first trimester to a bulging tummy in the third trimester might dictate when and how much you eat at any one sitting.

Start the Day Off Right

One rule in the Baby-wise Diet is that you must eat breakfast. At no other time in life is breakfast more important than during pregnancy. Breakfast will help you maintain a more desirable weight and will help prevent fatigue. Women who skip breakfast in an effort to cut calories often do more snacking later in the day and overeat at evening meals. In addition, a woman who skips breakfast may initially feel energized in the morning, but waning blood sugar levels eventually lead to fatigue. In fact, even if you try to catch up by eating a well-balanced lunch, you'll never regain the energy you would have had if you had taken ten minutes to eat a nutritious breakfast. Finally, allowing too much time to lapse between meals can be stressful to your baby during pregnancy, since a constant supply of nutrients and calories is needed for the minute-by-minute growth that is taking place.

So even if you are not particularly hungry, eat at least a small snack in the morning, preferably one that includes some protein and some carbohydrate. Even a toasted English muffin with a slice of cheese or a small bowl of ready-to-eat cereal with milk will suffice.

What About Foods Not On the Lists?

The basic foods in the Baby-wise Diet are low in fat, salt, and sugar. In fact, if you follow this meal plan, you will automatically consume about 2,000 calories with 25 to 30 percent of those calories coming from fat and very little or none coming from refined sugars. This meal plan also provides about 25 to 35 grams of fiber. If you exercise daily and/or can maintain a desirable weight on more calories, then feel free to include other foods, such as ones listed as "Nutritious Additions" on page 53.

The No-No List for Pregnancy

The following foods supply few nutrients; are very high in fat, sugar, or salt; or contain harmful substances. They should be avoided or consumed in very small amounts.

Alcohol, including hard liquor, wine, and beer
Caffeinated beverages, such as coffee, colas, or tea
Candy
Candied fruit, including maraschino cherries
Cereals sweetened with sugar
Cookies, cakes, pies, brownies, or commercial sweetened pie fillings
Doughnuts
Fruit drinks made with sugar, concentrated pear, or high-fructose corn syrup (HFCS)
Luncheon meats that are less than 95% fat-free
Nondairy creamers
Olives
Potato chips, corn chips, and other commercial snack foods high in fat and salt
Relishes and pickles
Soda pop
Soups, commercial dry or canned varieties that are not "low sodium"
Sour cream (unless it is fat-free)
Sugar, corn syrup, honey, or fructose
Sundae toppings
Whipping cream or commercial whipped toppings

Vegetable oils used in food preparation or in salad dressings, convenience snack foods such as chips and granola bars, and desserts also can be included in your meal plan, but ideally only after you have met the recommended number of servings from each of the six food groups in the Baby-wise Diet. "The general public has been educated on the need to cut the fat and increase high-quality complex carbohydrates [whole grains, legumes, fruits, and vegetables], but the same guidelines are not being emphasized for pregnant women, even though they are just as important," says Janet King, Ph.D., R.D., professor in the Department of Nutritional Sciences at University of California, Berkeley. "Those simple guidelines alone would improve the mother's overall health during pregnancy and could increase the nutrient supply to the developing baby."

Basically, there is nothing wrong with a few high-fat or high-sugar foods as long as they don't replace more nutritious foods. Problems arise when potato chips, greasy fast foods, fried foods, cookies, salad dressings, cake, pies, and other sweet-and-creamy foods are chosen instead of fruits, vegetables, and whole grains. Salt is discussed in more detail in chapter 6.

Now I Can Eat All I Want, Right?

Not quite. Your daily energy needs increase by only 300 calories (100 calories is equivalent to a slice of bread and a small piece of fruit) during the second and third trimesters, with an average of 2,000 to 2,200 calories during the prepregnancy period and the first trimester and 2,300 to 2,500 calories for the remaining two trimesters. (Small or sedentary women will need to be on the lower end of this calorie range, while tall or active women might need as much as 3,000 calories or more.) On the other hand, vitamin and mineral needs are high from conception to delivery; consequently, a woman must consume more nutrients for the same—or only slightly more—calories.

Your best bet is to consume foods that are as close to their natural, wholesome forms as possible. That is, choose minimally processed whole grains, such as whole wheat or brown rice, more often than highly refined grains, such as white bread or white rice. Opt for low-fat milk instead of ice cream and fresh fruit instead of fruits canned in heavy syrup. Just as you wouldn't dream of feeding your newborn a diet of hot dogs, cola, and French fries, remember to give your unborn the same consideration.

But that does not mean you can't enjoy your favorite foods. Just make sure nutritious foods far outnumber fatty, sugary, or salty items. You still can eat pizza on occasion; just say no to the fatty salami and sausage and complement the pizza with a large salad and a glass of nonfat milk. (For a list of foods to avoid, see "The No-No List for Pregnancy" on page 55.)

Unplanned eating is likely to get you into trouble. You find yourself nibbling from the refrigerator when you return home from work, grab a candy bar at a vending machine or a cinnamon roll while shopping, or order your turkey sandwich without specifying you want it on whole wheat bread. While these eating habits have only minor effects on your overall health at other times of life, they are indiscretions you can't afford to tolerate before, during, and following pregnancy. So think before you eat and make every bite count. Plan ahead so you won't be caught hungry with only the vending machine to curb your appetite.

On the other hand, think before you don't eat. Your nutritional needs are at an all-time high for pregnancy and your baby will need a constant supply of calories, fluids, and nutrients. You can't afford to skip meals now, but must adapt to eating regularly, or approximately every four hours.

Protein, Carbs, and Fat

The pregnant woman needs more protein than at any other time in her life, but the extra servings of nonfat or low-fat milk and extra-lean protein-rich foods recommended in the Baby-wise Diet will more than accommodate any increases in protein needs. There is no reason to use protein powders or tablets. A woman following a strict vegetarian diet that does not include any foods of animal origin must be particularly careful to include ample amounts of protein-rich legumes, nuts, and soy products.

Starches and other complex carbohydrates remain the mainstay of the diet, just as they did prior to pregnancy. However, now they may serve an added bonus by helping fend off morning sickness. In addition, researchers at St. Louis University Medical School speculate that carbohydrate loading—the same dietary practice used by athletes prior to a marathon—might increase tissue glycogen stores and help supply extra energy for labor and delivery.

Fat adds calories without much nutritional clout, and should be limited to no more than 25 to 30 percent of total calories. At least some of this fat should come from safflower oil, a vegetable oil rich in the essential fatty acid linoleic acid, and oils from fish. So if you use oil in cooking or in salad dressing, choose linoleic-rich safflower oil, preferably the cold-pressed versions, which contain more vitamin E than the bleached and more highly processed oils. And include at least two to three servings of fish during the week. (See chapter 3 for more information on fish oils.)

Vitamins and Minerals: How Much of What and Why?

All nutrition experts agree that the best place for a mother-to-be to get her vitamins and minerals is from food. However, the trick is getting enough of these essential nutrients.

The fruits and vegetables in the Baby-wise Diet supply beta carotene, vitamin C, and folic acid. All of these nutrients are essential for your baby, although folic acid has received particular attention because of its ability to help prevent birth defects. (See chapters 1 and 3.)

The whole-grain breads and cereals in the Baby-wise Diet contribute B vitamins and trace minerals such as chromium, iron, and selenium. They also provide fiber to help prevent constipation, hemorrhoids, and other inconveniences of pregnancy. The nonfat and low-fat dairy products, especially milk, supply calcium, vitamin D, vitamin B12, vitamin B2, and magnesium—nutrients essential for normal bone, muscle, and nerve development and function. The two to three servings of extra-lean meat and legumes provide iron, magnesium, zinc, vitamin B6, vitamin B12, and other B vitamins.

Avoiding any of these foods can result in nutrient deficiencies that could have far-reaching effects on the developing infant and your pregnancy. For example, low calcium intake increases the risk for elevated blood pressure in both the mother and the newborn, while calcium intakes of 1,000 mg or more each day lower blood pressure and reduce the risk of eclampsia in pregnant women. A vitamin B6 deficiency is linked to reduced Apgar scores, increased irritability (and resistance to soothing in the infant), and reduced mother-infant bonding. (The Apgar score reflects a baby's condition sixty minutes after delivery, based on heart rate, respiratory effort, muscle tone, reflexes, and color.) Marginal zinc intake increases the risk for pregnancy complications and premature delivery.

Since marginal vitamin and mineral intakes are common in women and can have far-reaching effects on the health of the baby even before a woman knows she is pregnant, it is wise to consider taking a moderate-dose vitamin and mineral supplement that contains at least 400 mcg of folic acid and 18 mg of iron. (See chapters 3 and 5 for more on vitamin and mineral supplements.)

How Do I Change My Eating Habits?

We have a love-hate relationship with food. While we know fat, sugar, and salt are at the root of everything from heart disease and hypertension to tooth decay and obesity, at the same time even Herculean efforts to cut these foods from the diet result in paltry drops in our food cravings. We can't live with desserts, commercial snack foods, and fast foods, but why can't we live without them?

The problem might not be what, but how, we attempt to change our eating habits. For example, recent research shows that fat intake is regulated not only by willpower but also by a stewpot of brain chemicals that rebel against drastic changes in food intake. Elliott Blass, Ph.D., at Cornell University speculates that when people attempt restrictive diets or reduce fat intake too quickly they may set up a rebound effect in these brain chemicals, which inevitably swings their appetite pendulums from abstinence to binge eating. A similar response also may hold true for salt and sugar.

Sarah Leibowitz, Ph.D., a professor of neurobiology at Rockefeller University in New York, who has pioneered research on the control center for food intake, agrees: "Quick weight loss diets cause [brain chemicals] to go berserk." Dr. Leibowitz recommends that gradually making changes in the diet is the most effective way to work with the appetite-control chemicals and avoid the rebound effect.

The good news is you can reprogram your taste buds to enjoy healthful fare. Researchers at the Cancer Research Center in Seattle surveyed 448 women who had participated in nutrition classes to lower their fat intakes. More than half of the participants reported that their love for fatty foods changed to a growing dislike for the creamy, greasy taste the longer they remained on low-fat diets. More than 60 percent said they actually felt physical discomfort after eating high-fat foods.

By slowly making changes in your diet during the months prior to conception, you will take much of the stress out of habit change and will increase your chances of eating well throughout your pregnancy. Make the Baby-wise Diet your goal and slowly work toward that goal. Become a fat, sugar, and salt sleuth by learning what foods are high in these substances. Then slowly reduce them in your diet while emphasizing vegetables, fruits, and grains.

In most cases, only minor changes in fat, sugar, or salt intake make dramatic differences in the nutritional quality of a day's menu. For example, reducing butter from 1 tablespoon to 2 teaspoons (a difference of only 1 teaspoon) might drop the fat calories from 39 to 31 percent for one day's breakfast. Sprinkling a quarter, rather than a half, teaspoon of salt on a meal can cut the day's sodium intake by 25 percent or more. Switching from fruited yogurt to plain yogurt with fresh fruit can reduce your sugar intake by several teaspoons.

While fat, salt, and sugar should be reduced, they shouldn't be eliminated. Fat is needed to help absorb the fat-soluble vitamins (A, D, E, and K), supply the essential fat called linoleic acid, and add variety to the diet. Your body needs some sodium during pregnancy to regulate muscle and nerve function and maintain natural fluid balance. Sugar adds taste and pleasure to a meal or snack. So set your sights on reducing, but not eliminating, this trio.

One benefit of reducing your fat intake is that the quantity (and quality) of the diet increases to make up for the lost calories. You can actually eat more food for fewer calories! In addition, it is the entire day's fat, sugar, and salt intake that is important. Consequently, don't worry if some meals are higher in fat, sugar, or salt as long as the overall intake is low.

Finally: don't sweat the small stuff. Minor fluctuations in fat, salt, or sugar have little or no impact on the total day's food intake. Sodium might fluctuate 100 mg or more; fat intake may vary a few percentage points; a teaspoon of sugar one way or the other is not important. Your goal is not a food-by-food or even a meal-by-meal inventory but, rather, an overall daily and weekly reduction in fat, sugar, and salt.

The Vegetarian Diet and Pregnancy

Avoiding meat is no longer fringy business. With meat linked to everything from heart disease to cancer, many women have taken the plunge and gone vegetarian. But are vegetarian diets the best, or even safe, during pregnancy and nursing? Can you meet all of your increased nutrient needs without a meat-and-potatoes diet? Must you resort to bizarre foods and eating habits to ensure optimal nutrition for you and your baby? You might be surprised at the answers to those and other important questions.

Several studies show that meat consumption, with its high amount of saturated fat and cholesterol, is positively correlated with heart disease in both men and women. Women who daily eat meat have a 50 percent higher risk of developing heart disease compared to vegetarian women. In fact, disease risk increases as both the length of time and frequency of meat consumption increases. Consequently, people who adopt a vegetarian diet early in life have a lower risk of disease than do people who wait until after age 50 to switch from meat to beans.

In all fairness to meat, it may not be the harmful effects of a T-bone steak per se, but the protective effects of other foods in the vegetarian diet that is the real issue, according to Paul Mills, Ph.D., research epidemiologist at the National Institute for Occupational Safety and Health in Cincinnati. Dr. Mills spent ten years studying the link between vegetarian diets and cancer in a group of 35,000 Seventh-Day Adventists, a group with a high percentage of vegetarians and a lower cancer rate than that found in the general public. "We were surprised to find that meat was not a significant factor in the development of certain types of cancer," says Dr. Mills. "However, we did find that people who ate lots of fruits, legumes, and vegetables were at much lower risk for certain cancers, probably because they simply didn't have as much room in their diets for other fattier foods."

Whether it's an issue of a lower meat intake, a higher intake of fruits, vegetables, and legumes, or both, vegetarian diets can be a safe and healthful alternative to typical Western diets when you're pregnant. "The vegetarian diet is a good thing [for your health]," recommends Bonnie Worthington-Roberts, Ph.D., professor of nutritional sciences at the University of Washington in Seattle. "But, even with a good thing, you must do it right." With careful planning, both a lacto vegetarian (who eats milk products) and a lacto-ovo vegetarian (who eats milk products and eggs) diet can supply all the necessary vitamins, minerals, protein, and other nutrients essential to health.

"The research on Seventh-Day Adventists shows there are good reproductive outcomes with vegetarian diets," says Johanna Dwyer, D.Sc., R.D., professor at Tufts University School of Medicine and the Director of the Nutrition Center at the New England Medical Center in Boston. In fact, most women who eliminate meat from their diets actually consume a more nutrient-rich diet than meat eaters, probably because they include more fruits and vegetables and fewer fatty animal products.

Women on lacto- or lacto-ovo vegetarian diets should consume basically the same diet plans when gearing up for pregnancy, minus the meat and with extra servings of cooked dried beans and peas. Moderate-dose vitamin and mineral supplements that include iron, zinc, and folic acid should fill in the gaps and help vegetarian women gear up for pregnancy.

Women on strict vegetarian diets (who consume only whole grains, fruits, vegetables, cooked dried beans and peas, and nuts and seeds) have greater nutritional challenges. These women must consume adequate calories to ensure optimal weight and to spare protein from being used for energy. As mentioned above, they also must choose several servings of high-quality protein by combining grains and legumes.

Without milk, these women must look for other sources of vitamin D, vitamin B2, vitamin B12, and calcium. Increased amounts of iron, zinc, and other trace minerals must be consumed to compensate for the lack of meat and the added phytates (in unleavened whole grains), oxalates (in spinach and other dark green vegetables), and fiber in these diets, which interfere with mineral absorption.

The strict vegetarian diet should include at least:

- 7 servings of vegetables
- 3 servings of fruits
- 6 to 11 servings of whole grains
- 4 servings of cooked dried beans and peas, nuts, and seeds
- 4 servings of calcium-rich foods
- A source of vitamin B12

Fermented soy products such as miso and tempeh, brewer's yeast, wheat germ, and vitamin and mineral supplements also are nutrient-rich sources in the strict vegetarian's diet. In general, most strict vegetarians gearing up for pregnancy would benefit from multiple vitamin and mineral supplements that contain 2 mcg of vitamin B12 and 400 IU of vitamin D.

The Bottom Line

Eating well is essential for the health of your baby—from conception throughout life. It does not mean resorting to odd eating habits or having to eat bizarre foods. Eating well does mean planning your meals and snacks around foods of plant origin plus two to three servings daily of both protein-rich and calcium-rich foods. Three rules of thumb are:

1. Two thirds to three quarters of your plate should be heaped with a variety of grains, vegetables, fruits, and legumes, with the rest coming from extra-lean protein-rich and low-fat calcium-rich items. Another way to say this is that for every one protein-rich or calcium-rich food you consume, choose at least three servings of fruits, vegetables, grains, and legumes.
2. Include at least one grain and one fruit or vegetable at every snack and vary your choices.
3. Before you eat something, always ask yourself, "Is this good for me and my baby?" If you answer yes, then go ahead and eat it. If you answer no, try to find something that will satisfy the same taste and hunger needs, but will be a healthier choice.

Finally, this eating plan is a family affair that includes you, your unborn baby, and dad. The father-to-be will need his stamina just as much as mom. He also plays an important role in supporting her nourishing efforts during pregnancy and will be a major role model for the child in the coming years. So choose foods that look good, taste good, and are good for you and your family.

Stocking the Kitchen

Eating well begins with taking stock of your kitchen and learning a few shopping tips to survive the supermarket experience. Take a quick trip through your cupboards and refrigerator. What takes up the most room? Are your shelves jammed with canned beans, fruit canned in their own juices, and bags of whole wheat noodles? Or do you see dried soup mixes, bags of potato chips, and gravy mixes? Is your freezer filled with frozen plain vegetables and concentrated orange juice, or ice cream and bags of frozen French fries? Is your refrigerator bulging with nonfat milk, yogurt, and fresh fruits and vegetables, or with bottles of soda pop, luncheon meats, and margarine? Is what you see what you want to feed your baby?

Not-so-nutritious foods can be tempting. So your first step is to discard anything in the kitchen that will interfere with your eating plans. Basically, you want to keep the wholesome foods and limit the highly processed ones. Granted, the old standby "Out of sight, out of mind" isn't foolproof, but it will help you stay on track. Remember, the father-to-be is part of this team effort. One way he can help is by not bringing home foods that will tempt you to revert to less nutritious eating patterns.

Your next step is to assemble a list of healthful foods that you enjoy and that complement your favorite recipes. The "Sample Shopping List" on page 65 provides a workable model that you can revise to fit your needs. Remember, to avoid impulse buying, always shop from a list and never shop when hungry. In addition, planning the week's menus in advance allows you to shop only once a week, which can save precious time.

At the Store

Selecting nutritious foods is as easy as one, two, three.

ONE: Read the food label, not the claims. Learn to identify which foods contain fat. A rule of thumb is to select foods that contain no more than 3 grams of fat for every 100 calories. (That is, if a food supplies 300 calories per serving, it should contain no more than 9 grams of fat per serving.) Ignore the "Calories from Fat" and the "% Daily Value" on the label; these numbers provide little practical information for planning menus.

Unfortunately, food labels lump together all sugars, both natural and refined. Consequently, a food low in refined sugar, such as plain yogurt or fruit canned in its own juice, may appear high in sugar only because the food contains natural sugars, such as lactose or fructose. The only way to identify sugar-laden foods is to eyeball the ingredients list. If sugar, sucrose, corn syrup, high fructose corn syrup, or other added sugars appears in the first three items, it is a good bet the food is high in refined sugar.

A Sample Shopping List

The following shopping list is a sample of the types of foods recommended in the Baby-wise Diet.

WHAT	HOW MUCH
AT THE PRODUCE DEPARTMENT	
Fresh fruits and vegetables	Purchase enough for 8–10 servings daily
AT THE BAKERY	
Bread, bagels, bread sticks, tortillas, muffins	Purchase enough for 6–8 servings daily
AT THE DAIRY CASE	
Nonfat or low-fat milk or yogurt, low-fat cheeses, eggs or egg substitutes	Purchase enough for 2–4 servings daily; limit eggs to no more than 3 per week
AT THE MEAT DEPARTMENT	
Extra-lean cuts of beef, chicken, pork, turkey, or veal	Purchase enough for 1–2 3-ounce servings daily
AT THE SEAFOOD COUNTER	
Fresh fish and shellfish	Purchase enough for at least 1–2 3-ounce servings weekly
ALONG THE CANNED AND DRY GOODS AISLES	
Dried beans and peas, pasta, rice, flour, and other grains; canned fruit; nonfat evaporated milk, low-fat soups, fat-free tomato sauce	Purchase enough for at least 1 serving daily; keep the kitchen shelves well stocked, preferably with whole-grain varieties; select fruit canned in its own juice; keep 1–2 cans each of soups and sauces in the cupboard

(continued)

A Sample Shopping List (continued)

WHAT	HOW MUCH
ALONG THE CEREAL AISLE	
Cooked cereals—oatmeal, barley, farina; ready-to-eat low-fat, whole-grain cereals, such as Grape-Nuts, Shredded Wheat, Nutri-Grain; wheat germ	Keep a supply on hand
AT THE FROZEN FOODS DEPARTMENT	
Concentrated fruit juice, low-fat frozen entrees, whole wheat waffles	Keep a supply on hand
NUTRITIOUS ADDITIONS	
Dried fruit, nuts and seeds; popcorn, low-salt pretzels, oven-baked chips; angel food cake, vanilla wafers	As needed
HERBS, OILS, AND CONDIMENTS	
All-fruit jam, herbs and spices, ketchup, lemon juice, mustard, nonfat salad dressings, safflower oil, salsa, vanilla	As needed

---

TWO: The more refined and processed a food, the higher the fat, sugar, salt, and calorie content is likely to be and the lower the vitamin, mineral, and fiber content. For example, a potato is a fat-free source of vitamins, minerals, and fiber. In contrast, a package of frozen scalloped potatoes contains 1 teaspoon of fat per serving and a bag of potato chips contains several teaspoons of fat, while the vitamin, mineral, and fiber content is dramatically reduced.

THREE: Be wary of label claims and promises. The new food labels require a greater degree of truth in advertising; however, terminology still may imply something that the product is not. For example, although foods labeled "low-

---

Table 2.2   Fat Gram Quota: Deciphering the 30 Percent Rule

The Baby-wise Diet supplies no more than 30 percent of calories as fat, but what does this mean? To translate 30 percent fat calories to just plain calories or grams of fat, locate your daily calorie allotment below. The "Fat Calories" column represents how many calories as fat you can eat daily to remain at 30 percent. The corresponding grams of fat are given, too. You can use this guideline when reading labels or designing menus.

DAILY CALORIES	FAT CALORIES	GRAMS OF FAT
1,800	540	60
2,100	630	70
2,400	720	80
2,700	810	90
3,000	900	100

---

calorie" must contain no more than 40 calories per serving, check the serving size to make sure it is not unrealistically small! Low-fat milk contains 2 percent fat *by weight*, but 35 percent of the calories come from fat! When in doubt, return to the rule of 3 grams of fat per 100 calories and read the ingredients list for sources of sugar and fat.

Finally, shop primarily around the periphery of the grocery store. Choose a wide variety of fresh fruits and vegetables from the produce department; a mix of whole grains from the bakery section; nonfat or low-fat milk products from the dairy case; and extra-lean meats, poultry, and fish from the meat department. Venture into the middle aisles to purchase low-fat cereals and crackers, dried beans and peas, and low-fat convenience foods (see Table 2.2).

Health Food Store Survival

You don't have to frequent a health food store to buy healthy foods. In addition, just because a food is in a health food store does not mean it is healthful. The same implied health claims, label misinformation, and "labelese" are used for health foods as are used for flavored sugar beverages, puffed and sugary cereals, and other highly processed items in a regular grocery store.

On the other hand, there are some worthy choices that grace the shelves of most health food stores. For example, you are more likely to find a wider assortment of grains, from amaranth to triticale, than are stocked at most grocery stores. Grains, dried fruits, and other foods in bulk are also usually less expensive here. However, always check the freshness of these items, since contamination and rancidity are more likely when bulk foods are exposed to air. Low-fat acidophilus milk, kefir, and soy milk are found in some supermarkets, but people who cannot find these nutritious beverages at their neighborhood store may want to try the local health food store.

Keep a wary eye on the desserts and the misuse of "natural" ingredients. Health food stores often stock desserts that contain honey, fructose, and date sugar, which are fancy names for sugar. Many items also contain coconut oil, which sounds natural but actually is almost as saturated as lard. In addition, "organic" eggs are just as cholesterol-dense as other eggs.

Is organic better? Recent legislation has placed some restrictions on and set new guidelines for what can be labeled as organic, which has added some credibility to the term. However, an "organic" label does not guarantee clean or nutritious food. Organic food can still be contaminated with pesticides from neighboring fields, irrigation water, or pesticide traces found in the soil from previous use. In essence, there is too much background chemical pollution on our farmlands to make a blanket guarantee of residue-free food. There also is no definite research to show that organic food is more nutritious than regular produce, grains, beans, and other items. However, since you don't have to peel organic produce to remove the wax and trapped pesticides often found in other produce, you will consume more fiber and nutrients that are concentrated in the skin of vegetables and fruits.

The bottom line is that fresh, certified organic foods probably contain fewer pesticides and residues than other foods and buying them supports environmentally sound alternatives to conventional farming practices. They are a worthwhile choice when available and affordable.

Menu Planning

When you sit down to plan your menus, plan for the whole week. This saves time, helps prevent last-minute food choices, and allows a more varied and appealing eating plan. A seven-day plan also makes it easier to do your grocery shopping; clean and store enough raw vegetables for several days; cook enough of some foods to use for more than one meal; and plan for social engagements. Of course, you probably will modify the plans throughout the week, but you are more likely to follow the dietary guidelines in the Baby-wise Diet when you have stocked your kitchen with the necessary supplies. If you can plan for only three or four days at a time, then schedule more planning time midweek. Remember, failure to plan is planning to fail.

Plan meals and snacks with vegetables, fruits, and grains in mind. Since nine out of every ten women do not consume even five servings daily of fresh fruits and vegetables, it probably will take an "attitude shift" to make sure you get enough of these nutrient-packed foods. In general, include vegetables in everything you prepare. Rather than 6 ounces of beef and an iceberg lettuce salad, be creative and add vegetables to the following:

- Spaghetti and pizza sauce: add grated carrots, mushrooms, green or red peppers, onions
- Lasagna: substitute a layer of broccoli or spinach in place of all or part of the meat and cheese
- Casseroles: stir in green peas, corn, green beans, carrots, celery, onion, green/red/yellow peppers, squashes, sweet potatoes
- Baked beans, chili, meatloaf: blend in grated carrots, extra tomato sauce, canned tomatoes, green beans
- Potato salad: add carrots, peas, peppers, red onions
- Canned soups: add extra vegetables such as potatoes, corn, beans, peas, carrots, squash
- Baked potatoes: stuff with spinach and low-fat yogurt; broccoli, mushrooms, and part-skim ricotta cheese; or nonfat cottage cheese and salsa
- Cornbread and muffins: stir in grated carrots, zucchini, corn, green chilies
- Shish kabob: use at least twice as many vegetables, including mushrooms, carrots, eggplant, cherry tomatoes, zucchini, onion, or potato, as extra-lean meat, chicken, or shellfish
- Tortillas: fill with ricotta or cottage cheese and spinach with a sprinkle of nutmeg; black beans, plain nonfat yogurt, and salsa; grated carrot and zucchini, low-fat cheese, and green chili peppers; nonfat refried beans, cilantro, tomato, and grated carrot

Cooking to Keep Nutrients, or Don't Throw the Baby Away with the Bathwater

The folic acid content of foods can be reduced to a fraction of the original content if foods are handled poorly or overcooked. To retain nutrients during cooking, prepare fresh foods using the shortest cooking time and the least amount of water. In addition:

• Wrap foods well and promptly refrigerate.
• Wash produce quickly; do not soak.
• Cook produce only until tender-crisp in a steamer or microwave.
• Roast meats at moderate temperatures of 325° F to 375° F.
• Do not use baking soda when cooking vegetables because it destroys nutrients.
• Use the liquid from cooking vegetables and meats (defatted) for soups and sauces.
• Reheat only the portion of leftovers or prepared-ahead foods that will be eaten.

• Salads: vary with carrots and raisins; Waldorf (apples, celery, green pepper, nuts); spinach and orange slices; or marinated vegetables such as carrots, celery, tomatoes, broccoli, cauliflower, beans, yellow squash, mushrooms combined with a low-fat or nonfat vinaigrette dressing (see "Cooking to Keep Nutrients," above)

Recipe Makeover

Gradually converting your eating style to one that will nourish your growing baby does not mean you must throw out all your favorite recipes. Most recipes just need a low-fat facelift. Those that include a mixture of ingredients, such as most soups, stir-fries, bean dishes, or tomato sauces, will adapt well, as will recipes that feature vegetables, grains, and small amounts of extra-lean meat and milk products. Quick breads, muffins, and other desserts also can be easily revised. Try reducing the fat and sugar by half in a recipe and continue to cut back as you reeducate your palate. Even packaged grain dishes, such as rice or noodle side dishes, can be fat-modified by eliminating the suggested added fats and using nonfat or 1 percent low-fat milk instead of whole milk or cream. Eating aspartame-sweetened desserts and reducing the serving size of packaged desserts are two ways to cut back on sugar. Many of the commercial nonfat desserts, such as cakes and cookies, have increased the sugar content to make up for the lack of fat, so never assume that a low-fat food is a low-calorie food— always read the label.

The Working Mother: Quick Meals and Snacks on the Job

Pregnant women get hungry at the oddest times. At the library, on the bus, at the makeup counter of a department store, at the playground, or while waiting in rush-hour traffic. More likely than not, you'll be hungry some place other than in your kitchen, so you had best plan ahead. Stock your purse, briefcase, glove compartment, and/or office desk drawer with healthful snacks such as fat-free whole-grain crackers, bread sticks, fresh fruit, crunchy vegetables, or dried fruit. Take a thermos of nonfat milk, fruit juice, or vegetable juice or a small brown-bag lunch wherever you go.

Brown-bag lunches and snacks are a must for any expectant mother. First, invest in an insulated lunchbox with a dry-ice unit that can be refrozen at night. Second, pack your lunch the night before to save time in the morning. Here are a few ideas for carry-along lunches:

- Include leftovers from the previous night's dinner, such as soup, pizza, spaghetti, or chicken breast and rice casserole. (You can pack your lunch as you clean up after dinner.)
- Pack sandwich fillings and bread separately to avoid soggy sandwiches.
- Prepare an assortment of raw vegetables, whole-grain crackers, and a filling dip made from well-seasoned thick bean soup.
- Stuff whole wheat pita bread with meatloaf (made from extra-lean meat) and salad greens or chicken salad and sprouts.
- Make a rolled sandwich from a warmed whole wheat tortilla, mashed beans, and crumbled feta cheese. Pack a cup of salsa in which to dip the rolled sandwich.
- Pack a tortilla, a container of leftover vegetables, and some grated cheese. Combine the ingredients just before warming.

- Stuff a baked potato with part-skim ricotta cheese and steamed vegetables.
- Bring hot soup in a thermos and a fruit salad.
- Pack two muffins with two slices of low-fat cheese, an orange, and a bag of baby carrots.
- Top a portion of fat-free cottage cheese or low-fat yogurt with a mixture of cut-up fresh fruit and a topping of low-fat granola or wheat nugget cereal.
- If you have a microwave at work, pack a frozen entree (purchased or prepared at home) and cook it at lunchtime.
- Always pack cut-up vegetables to eat with lunch or as emergency snacks.

The vending machine might be your only option at work if you forget to bring a snack or lunch. For the most part, office vending machines should be viewed as reminders of the importance of planning ahead. They typically are filled with high-sugar, high-fat items that feed your fatigue and mood swings. If you are in need of a snack with only a vending machine as a cure, quickly scan for the best options, including fruit, fruit juice, whole-grain crackers, fig bar cookies, or low-fat or nonfat milk. If all else fails, choose starch over candy, preferably pretzels, but potato chips or corn chips are last-resort options. The latter are high in fat but have less sugar than candy.

The Five-Minute Meal

If you have time to pull in to a drive-up window at a fast-food restaurant or grab a box of buttered popcorn at the movies, then you also have time to eat right in order to feel your best. The tricks to preparing quick, low-calorie meals and snacks are advanced planning, a basic inventory of ingredients, and the right time-saving equipment.

A well-stocked pantry and freezer will provide your basic ingredients. Time-saving cooking equipment includes a microwave oven for reheating foods and cooking vegetables and fish, and a slow-cooker for meals that can be started in the morning and are ready when you get home in the evening. (You also can slow-cook brown rice on high for two to three hours in a slow-cooker.) A wok or a large nonstick skillet is handy for stir-frying vegetables. A blender is great for whipping up a fruit-and-milk smoothie at breakfast.

Some foods are quicker to prepare than others. For example, fish is the fastest-cooking animal protein. A fresh fish fillet or fish steak can be cooked in the microwave in less than 10 minutes. A frozen fish fillet can be oven-baked in less than 30 minutes. Soup and salad are a fast and satisfying quick fix for lunch or dinner. You can start with a low-fat, low-sodium canned soup from your pantry and tailor it to your taste by adding fresh or frozen vegetables, canned kidney beans, or extra noodles. Or you can reheat a homemade soup from a previous meal and add fresh vegetables, herbs, or a fast-cooking grain like quick-cooking rice or bulgur wheat. Another five-minute meal is to toss a salad from your already-prepared stash of vegetables and toast a piece of whole-grain bread while the soup is heating.

Another way to save meal preparation time is not to cook at all. Serve raw vegetables and fruits or foods that come straight from the refrigerator and cupboard. For example, serve cold chicken or tofu salads on a bed of fresh greens, surrounded by marinated vegetables and whole-grain crackers. Even a few slices of low-fat turkey, a hunk of low-fat cheese, a handful of whole wheat crackers, and a bag of baby carrots can be a nutritious quick meal. Or you can choose from the wide variety of frozen entrees that are low in fat and sugar, and supplement them with a salad, frozen vegetables, orange juice, and/or milk. Other ideas include:

- *Breakfast foods for dinner:* Scramble low-fat egg substitute with a small amount of low-fat bacon and serve with whole-grain toast and fresh fruits. Or make pancakes and serve with pureed fruit toppings and nonfat yogurt.
- *Chef's salad:* Layer salad greens, chopped vegetables, beans, sliced chicken or turkey, grated low-fat cheese, sweet potato strips, and/or pretzel bits. Serve with a nonfat dressing, whole-grain roll, and fresh fruit.
- *Baked sweet potatoes:* Top with fat-free sour cream, yogurt, or cottage cheese. Serve with steamed broccoli sprinkled with nutmeg and cinnamon.
- *Grilled sandwiches:* Use whole-grain bread, low-fat cheese, deli-sliced lean meat, grated carrots, and a nonstick pan. Serve with fat-free baked tortilla chips and fruit slices.

There is no excuse for not eating a nutritious breakfast. To speed the process on hectic mornings and reduce your chances of skipping the day's most important meal, try the following:

1. Set out bowls, plates, silverware, and cups the night before.
2. Assemble dry ingredients for hot cereal in a bowl the night before. In the morning, add the liquid and microwave the cereal.
3. For a breakfast burrito, chop an onion and low-fat turkey bacon and store in the refrigerator the night before. In the morning, sauté the onion and bacon until tender in a nonstick skillet coated with vegetable spray. Add prepared fat-free egg substitute and scramble until done. Roll up in a whole-wheat tortilla.
4. Split a whole-grain bagel and sprinkle low-fat or fat-free grated cheese on each half. Wrap in plastic and store in refrigerator. In the morning, add slices of fresh tomato or apple and microwave.
5. Peel, wrap, and freeze chunks of bananas or other fruits in advance. In the morning, toss frozen fruit chunks in the blender with nonfat yogurt and orange juice. Toast a bagel while your shake blends until smooth.

Snack Right

Does snacking elicit thoughts of sneaking cookies from the cookie jar? Perhaps it means tiptoeing to the vending machine to grab a candy bar at your afternoon break. Feeling a bit naughty because you stash chips in your desk drawer for a quick energy fix? Put aside the guilt. With two thirds of Americans doing it, snacking has come out of the closet and into the nutritional limelight. Besides—snacking is good for you!

Snacks play an important role in the Baby-wise Diet. They provide up to 25 percent of a woman's calorie intake and, if properly selected, can be prime sources of nutrients. As a further benefit, women who eat more frequently throughout the day have an easier time maintaining desirable weight gain during pregnancy than women who stick to "three square meals."

But before you race to the vending machine with a license to snack, keep in mind that nibbling can make or break the nutritional quality of your diet, your stamina, and your baby's development. It all depends on what you choose.

The number one rule for healthy snacking is to keep it simple. A nutritious snack must be convenient—that is, it must be readily available, take little time to prepare, and taste great.

Second, consider snacks as part of your total diet. Snacks are a perfect way to meet your daily quota for nutrient-packed, low-fat, and low-sugar foods. Include at least two of the following groups at any one snack and make one choice either fruits and vegetables or whole grains.

1. Fresh fruits and vegetables
2. Whole-grain breads and cereals
3. Nuts and seeds
4. Nonfat or low-fat milk products, such as yogurt or cheese
5. Cooked dried beans and peas
6. Extra-lean meats

Third, minimally processed foods should outnumber highly processed snack items. Most commercial cookies, chips, flavored popcorn, and candy are high in fat, salt, or sugar. Choose fruit, unsalted pretzels, apple-cinnamon rice cakes, bagels, crunchy carrots, and other nutritious snacks instead.

Finally, listen to your body and your mood, and snack only when you're hungry. In addition, consider these snack ideas:

• Fruit slices dipped in nonfat yogurt with cinnamon
• Raw vegetables with a garbanzo or black bean dip and salsa
• A slice of whole wheat toast or a bagel with fruit topping
• A handful of mini rice cakes topped with low-sugar applesauce
• Pretzels with chilled vegetable juice
• A cup of fresh strawberries with nonfat whipped topping
• Bite-size wheat biscuit cereal with nonfat milk or yogurt

Very cold or very hot foods that are crunchy or chewy also are satisfying. Consider these hot or cold examples:

- A bowl of hot soup with crisp-tender vegetables
- A cup of sugar-free, nonfat cocoa topped with nonfat whipped topping
- A nonfat milkshake made from frozen berries and/or banana chunks and nonfat milk
- Frozen peas

Healthy snacking takes some, but not much, planning. It means getting rid of the tempting "bad" snacks in the cupboards and freezer and replacing them with convenient "good" snacks. Include healthy snacks on your shopping list. Prepare vegetables and fruits before you refrigerate them, so they are ready to go when you are in a hurry. Take nutritious snacks everywhere with you—on planes and to office meetings, the gym, the movies, or the ballgame. That way you're always prepared to fuel your body and soothe a craving.

Eating Out and Other Social Graces

Even the most conscientious person can find eating away from home a challenge. Social and situational pressure and the disruption of daily habits can undermine the best intentions. Sometimes the stress of travel can foster emotional eating, sleep disturbances, or other moods that, in turn, cause you to throw dietary caution to the wind.

Occasional social events or restaurant meals probably will have little impact on your overall plan, even if you "just wing it"—that is, as long as you don't allow a minor slip to progress to a major relapse. However, unless you exercise regularly, you probably are on a tight nutritional budget during pregnancy and need to make every bite count. The good news is that most restaurants are willing to accommodate special requests, especially for a pregnant woman!

In general, the same rules apply to eating out as they do for eating at home: choose low-fat fare, fill your plate with vegetables and grains, and complement the meal with moderate amounts of low-fat, protein-rich, and calcium-rich foods. Never assume anything; always ask how a food is prepared ("grilled" may mean grilled in butter) and request lower-fat preparations where needed.

Parties and social engagements at other people's homes are another chance to test your assertiveness skills. If you know the person well, you can discuss your food preferences openly and can offer to bring something to add to the meal. For example, you may want to bring sparkling water if only alcoholic beverages or soda pop will be served. If you do not know your hosts well, you must decide whether you want to risk eating a high-fat and/or high-sugar meal, avoid the high-fat or high-sugar foods that are served and risk having less to eat, or discuss your eating plan with the hosts and offer to bring something to add to the meal. In all cases, making specific plans ahead of time will help you avoid spur-of-the-moment decision making.

Take Charge

Now is the best time to make changes in what and how you eat. You probably want the very best for your baby, so you'll be more motivated to spend the extra time it takes to develop new eating habits. Once established, these habits will be yours and your baby's for life. Getting by is no longer good enough. Now you should be striving for the optimal. So take charge of your *kitchen* (by stocking only nutritious foods), *shopping* (by reading labels and by not being swayed by advertising gimmicks), and *meal preparation* (by revising recipes and always carrying nutritious snacks wherever you go).

CHAPTER THREE

The Nutrition Primer for Pregnancy

Eating well prior to, during, and following pregnancy is one of the most important ways you can contribute to both your baby's lifelong health and your own well-being. Unfortunately, people do not instinctively choose a good diet. If they did, sales of soda pop would not have skyrocketed in the past two decades, while consumption of dark green leafy vegetables went from too little to even less. The first step in guaranteeing an optimal intake of all the nutrients essential for you and your baby is to understand what you need, why you need it, and what foods are the best sources. Here is a quick course on the nutrients most important as you gear up for and then carry through on your pregnancy.

The Calorie-Containing Nutrients

Protein, carbohydrate, and fat are the calorie-containing nutrients. They supply the energy you and your baby will need to produce the miracle of life. Protein and carbohydrate (including both sugar and starch) supply 4 calories per gram, while fat supplies 9 calories. Except for sugar (which is pure carbohydrate) and oils, butter, and other fats (which are pure fat), most foods are a combination of two or more of these nutrients. For example, a bowl of oatmeal is primarily carbohydrate, but it supplies a little protein and a trace of fat. A protein-rich chicken breast also contains some fat, while peanut butter is high in fat, but contains protein and carbohydrate.

Protein

Your protein needs prior to and during the first trimester of pregnancy are the same as during any other time in your adult life. However, during the second and third trimesters of pregnancy you will need more protein. The extra servings of nonfat milk and low-fat protein-rich foods, such as cooked dried beans and peas, chicken without the skin, fish, and milk, recommended in the Baby-wise Diet will more than accommodate this increased requirement. In fact, protein is the least likely nutrient to be low in the diet, since most Americans consume more than twice their protein need.

For most women, there is no need to take extra protein in the form of powders or tablets. In fact, eating too much protein might impair normal growth and could be harmful to your developing baby. Women following a strict vegetarian diet, however, must be very careful to plan adequate amounts of protein into the daily menu, since poor protein intake can reduce placental growth and function, limit the growth of the baby, impair normal brain development, and jeopardize survival rates. Several servings daily of cooked dried beans and peas combined with whole grains and pasta, as well as tofu, soymilk, and nuts, will help ensure adequate protein intake for strict vegetarians.

Carbohydrate

Starches and other complex carbohydrates remain the mainstay of the diet. Carbohydrate comes in two packages: the complex starches in breads, pasta, rice, grains, potatoes, legumes, and vegetables; and the simple sugars naturally found in milk (lactose) and fruit (fructose) or the refined or concentrated sugars in table sugar, honey, brown sugar, corn syrup, and "raw" sugar.

The starches and naturally occurring sugars come packaged with vitamins, minerals, fiber, fluid, and other essential nutrients. Wholesome, minimally processed, low-fat versions of these foods are essential to building a healthy baby and are the mainstay of the Baby-wise Diet. On the other hand, prior to and during pregnancy you should minimize or eliminate the foods high in refined sugars, including desserts, sweet snack foods, sweetened fruit drinks, and convenience foods with added sugar, since there is little room in your diet for these nutrient-poor selections. Inevitably, they either replace more nutritious foods and jeopardize your health and your baby's welfare or are eaten in addition to all the other nutritious foods you need, thus contributing to excessive weight gain.

Fat

Fat adds calories without much nutritional clout and should be limited to 25 to 30 percent of total calories. Few studies support the safety to the developing baby or a benefit to the mother of cutting fat below 25 percent during pregnancy, unless there are other health risks, such as diabetes or heart disease. In those cases where pregnancy raises blood cholesterol levels as much as 40 percent, reducing fat intake to less than 25 percent of total calories might be warranted but should be recommended and monitored by a physician and dietitian. (See chapter 6 for more on diabetes during pregnancy.)

In addition, not all fats are created equal. Some, in fact, are essential to your baby's growth and development. Linoleic acid, a polyunsaturated fat found in vegetable oils such as safflower oil, is essential for you and your baby. This fat is a type of fatty acid (a component of triglycerides, the saturated and unsaturated fats in foods) that cannot be made from the breakdown of other substances and so must be provided in the diet. Developing infants especially need linoleic acid, so it is no coincidence that breast milk is high in this fatty acid. For example, young infants fed diets low in linoleic acid develop thickening and dryness of the skin and skin eruptions in the diaper area. Dry, itchy, flaky skin sometimes is a sign of linoleic acid deficiency in adults. One to two tablespoons daily of safflower oil, such as in salad dressing, baked goods, or cooking, is all you need to ensure adequate intake of linoleic acid.

Another type of polyunsaturated fat, called the omega-3 fatty acids, including docosahexanenoic acid (DHA), is found in fish and also is critical to normal eye and vision development. These fatty acids normally account for greater than one third of the total fatty acids in the brain and the retina of the eye. In studies on animals, offspring born to mothers who had DHA-deficient diets have behavioral problems and abnormal visual acuity, and their eyes do not respond correctly to changes in light. The risk for nerve and visual damage is highest in premature infants and is potentially irreversible. Although most of the accumulation of DHA and possibly other omega-3 fatty acids in the brains and eyes of human infants occurs in the last trimester, consuming these fats prior to and throughout pregnancy is important. Fish oils also are beneficial in preventing or helping to treat some pregnancy-related disorders such as pre-eclampsia and high blood pressure. (See chapter 6 for more information on fish oils and pregnancy-related disorders and chapter 9 for more information on fish oils and infant formulas.)

On the other hand, some altered fats in processed foods might be harmful during pregnancy. Hydrogenated fats are liquid vegetable oils made creamy when manufacturers convert some of the unsaturated fats into saturated ones through a process called hydrogenation. This process also rearranges some of the remaining unsaturated fats so their natural shape, called the "cis" formation, is transformed into an abnormal "trans" shape. These fats are known as trans fatty acids, or TFAs.

While TFAs are found naturally only in minute amounts, they constitute up to 60 percent of the fat in processed foods that contain hydrogenated fats, such as cookies, potato chips, and other snack foods. Studies show that TFAs, in amounts typically consumed by people in developed countries, raise LDL levels and increase the heart disease risk by as much as 27 percent. In short, these unsaturated fats act like saturated fats. In addition, they might accumulate in the baby's tissues and have been associated with lower birth weights. Researchers at the University of Munich in Germany who studied the effects of TFAs during pregnancy caution that their findings shed doubt on the safety of these processed fats during pregnancy and the perinatal period (the months preceding and following birth). (See "Reading Between the Lines," below.)

Reading Between the Lines: Trans Sleuthing

The new food labels do not require that the trans fatty acid (TFA) content be listed directly on the label. However, they also do not allow any unsaturated fat that has been converted to a trans fatty acid to appear as part of the total fat content. So when it comes to TFAs, what you don't see is what you get. For example, a label on a bag of corn chips might read:

Total fat: 15 grams
    Polyunsaturated fat: 5 grams
    Saturated fat: 2 grams
    Monounsaturated fat: 1 gram

The remaining 7 grams of fat (15 grams − 8 grams = 7 grams) probably are trans fatty acids.

You can't eat butter because its high saturated fat content increases the risk for heart disease, and now margarine is a no-no. Is this a nutritional catch-22? No. The bottom line is eat less fat. Limit your intake of any processed product that contains hydrogenated vegetable oil in the ingredient list. Use diet or whipped margarine in moderate amounts, since both contain fewer TFAs than tub or stick margarine, or make your own spread by whipping a stick of butter with half a cup of canola oil. This blend is lower in saturated fat than butter and is trans-free.

Vitamins and Minerals: What You Do and Don't Need

All nutrition experts agree that the best place for a mother-to-be to obtain all the essential vitamins and minerals is from her diet. However, the trick is getting enough. As long as you follow the Baby-wise Diet, your food will supply ample amounts of all the vitamins, minerals, and other health-enhancing substances. A moderate-dose multiple-vitamin supplement that contains extra iron and folic acid will fill in any nutritional gaps (see Table 3.1).

The following has been organized by food groups that, in general, are the best sources of the listed vitamins and minerals. Keep in mind, however, that all wholesome, minimally processed foods supply varied combinations of nutrients, so that while vegetables are generally a good source of vitamin C, beta carotene, and/or folic acid, some vegetables also are excellent sources of vitamin B2 and calcium (nutrients typically high in milk products), while other vegetables are better sources of vitamin E or copper. Low-fat milk products are excellent sources of calcium, vitamin B12, and vitamin B2, but some also supply ample amounts of zinc.

Fruits and Vegetables: Vitamin C, Beta Carotene, and Folic Acid

The fruits and vegetables in the Baby-wise Diet supply beta carotene, vitamin C, and folic acid. All of these nutrients are essential for your baby. For example, folic acid is essential in the prevention of neural tube defects (see chapter 1) and also is associated with a lower risk of growth retardation and an increased birth weight.

Beta carotene is converted to vitamin A in the body, a fat-soluble vitamin

Table 3.1   The Recommended Dietary Allowances (RDAs) vs. Optimal Daily Intakes (ODIs) During Pregnancy

NUTRIENT	RDA	ODI
Vitamin A	4,000 IU	4,000 IU
Beta carotene	NA	10 mg
Vitamin D	400 IU	400 IU
Vitamin E	10 mg	20 mg
Vitamin B1	1.5 mg	2.0 mg
Vitamin B2	1.6 mg	2.0 mg
Niacin	17 mg	20 mg
Vitamin B6	2.2 mg	3.0 mg
Folic acid*	800 mcg	800 mcg
Vitamin B12	2.2 mcg	3 mcg
Vitamin C	70 mg	150 mg
Calcium	1,200 mg	1,200 mg
Copper	1.5–3.0 mg	3.0 mg
Iodine	175 mcg	175 mcg
Iron*	48–78 mg	30–78 mg
Magnesium	320 mg	400 mg
Zinc	15 mg	20 mg

*The current RDAs (1989) have substantially reduced levels for these nutrients and have been met with considerable controversy. Previous RDA levels (1980) are used here.

essential in reproduction, the immune system, vision, and cellular differentiation. The latter function is particularly critical during periods of rapid growth and tissue development, as in pregnancy, infancy, and early childhood. During pregnancy, and especially during the first trimester, the supply must be closely regulated to ensure that the developing baby is exposed to neither too little nor too much vitamin A, since both conditions can cause birth defects. Fruits and vegetables are the best place to get your vitamin A, since it is virtually impossible to consume a toxic dose of beta carotene from dietary sources.

Vitamin C is essential in the formation and maintenance of collagen, a protein that forms the basis for the most abundant tissue in the body, connective tissue. The shape and function of all tissues depend on collagen, which acts as a cementing substance between cells. Collagen is found in the bones and teeth, tendons, skin, the cornea of the eye, and blood vessel walls. It maintains the shape of the discs of the backbone, allows the joints to move, and binds muscles together. In addition to its role in collagen formation, vitamin C helps maintain the immune system by strengthening resistance to infection and disease, promotes the healing of tissues, and helps prevent the development of numerous diseases from cancer to heart disease.

Beta carotene, vitamin C, and folic acid are packaged in foods that taste good—juicy, sweet fruits and crunchy raw vegetables. These foods supply a wealth of other nutrients, fiber, and health-enhancing nonnutritive substances called phytochemicals. It is no wonder that women who include plenty of fruits and vegetables in their diets during pregnancy are most likely to give birth to healthy babies. In fact, one study from the University of Pennsylvania School of Medicine reported that women who consumed the most fruits and vegetables during pregnancy also were the most likely to have babies at low risk for developing tumors later in life.

Whole Grains: Trace Minerals, B Vitamins, and Fiber

The whole-grain breads and cereals in the Baby-wise Diet contribute trace minerals, such as chromium, iron (see chapters 1 and 6), and selenium, and some of the B vitamins. They also provide fiber to help prevent constipation, hemorrhoids, and other inconveniences during pregnancy. Chromium is essential for the normal regulation of blood sugar and, in concert with insulin (the hormone secreted from the pancreas that regulates blood sugar levels), stimulates the synthesis of protein in the unborn's developing tissues. Consequently, poor chromium intake is associated with pregnancy-induced diabetes, also called gestational diabetes (see chapter 6), and possibly poor fetal development.

Limited evidence shows that pregnancy might be associated with chromium depletion because of either poor dietary intake or increased requirements. This is not surprising, since nine out of ten adults consume suboptimal amounts of this mineral. It is essential that several servings daily of chromium-rich foods, including whole grains, wheat germ, and orange juice, be included in the diet. (Refined and "enriched" breads, rice, and noodles are poor sources of this essential nutrient.)

Selenium is an antioxidant mineral that is important for your body's defense against disease. As a component of the antioxidant enzyme called glutathione peroxidase, selenium protects red blood cells and cell membranes from damage by highly reactive oxygen fragments called free radicals. Selenium also is important for maintaining strong immune systems in both the mother and her baby. Studies on animals show that a deficiency during pregnancy can have irreversible effects on the baby's development and growth, and can have detrimental effects on the formation of the immune system.

While no studies have been conducted on people, there is evidence that blood selenium and glutathione peroxidase levels decrease during pregnancy, suggesting that unless you take nutrition seriously, your typical diet might not be adequate to maintain normal body stores. Whole grains are excellent sources of selenium, supplying approximately 12 mcg per serving; six servings daily will supply 72 mcg or 110 percent of the Recommended Dietary Allowance for pregnant women. Optimal intake of these and other trace minerals improves your chance of having a healthy, full-term baby.

Whole grains also are excellent sources of several of the B vitamins, including vitamin B1, vitamin B2, niacin, and pantothenic acid. Because these B vitamins function primarily in the release of energy from the calorie-containing nutrients—fat, carbohydrate, and protein—their need increases in proportion to the increase in calories during the second and third trimesters. Optimal intake ensures a readily available supply of energy to fuel the processes of developing a baby and building the support tissues of pregnancy, such as the placenta.

The Baby-wise Diet emphasizes whole grains. Don't waste your carbohydrate quota on too many "enriched" processed grain products, such as white bread, white rice, or egg noodles. While vitamin B1, vitamin B2, and niacin have been added back to these refined grains, they are poor nutritional alternatives when it comes to other B vitamins such as folic acid, vitamin B6, and pantothenic acid. They also contain as little as 4 percent of the original amount of vitamin E, fiber, magnesium, zinc, chromium, copper, and manganese. In addition, whole grains, vegetables, and fruits, as well as legumes and nuts, are good dietary sources of fiber, including the soluble fiber that lowers your risk for developing heart disease and diabetes and the insoluble fiber that protects against cancer and constipation.

Iodine and Fluoride: Minerals Without a Home

Iodine and fluoride are two minerals essential to your baby's health that do not have a reliable dietary source, so they must be added to the diet through fortified salt (in the case of iodine) or water (in the case of fluoride). Iodine is a component of the hormone thyroxine, which regulates the body's metabolism, including when, where, and how much energy is used for any given task. Inadequate intake of iodine causes thyroxine levels to drop. The thyroid gland tries to compensate by working harder and a condition called goiter results. During pregnancy, an iodine deficiency can cause permanent malformations and mental retardation, a condition called cretinism, primarily because the nervous system requires adequate thyroid hormone exposure for normal development. Until iodine was added to salt in the 1920s, goiter and cretinism were common in the United States; now these conditions are rare. Using iodized salt sparingly during pregnancy plus consuming other sources of iodine, such as milk, brewer's yeast, and eggs, will help you meet your needs for this mineral.

Fluoridation of water (at a level of one part per million, the equivalent of a few drops in a swimming pool) is the most efficient and economical way to reduce tooth decay. Fluoride helps bond calcium and phosphorus in bones and teeth, making them strong and resistant to decay. Your baby's teeth begin to form about the tenth week of pregnancy; permanent molars and incisors begin developing in the second and third trimesters. Although the evidence is not conclusive, preliminary studies show that fluoride even in these early stages may help prevent tooth decay later in life.

Low-Fat Milk Products: Calcium, Magnesium, and Vitamin D

Low-fat milk products, including nonfat and low-fat milk, yogurt, and cheese, supply calcium, vitamin B12, vitamin B2, and magnesium—nutrients essential for normal bone, muscle, and nerve development and function. Fortified milk is the only reliable dietary source of vitamin D; all other milk products, from yogurt to cottage cheese, contain little or no vitamin D.

CALCIUM: Approximately 200 mg of calcium per day is deposited into the baby's skeleton during the last trimester of pregnancy. A similar amount is secreted daily in breast milk, although this varies depending on how much breast milk is produced, with some women secreting more than 300 mg daily. The total calcium cost of pregnancy for a woman who has had two babies and has breast-fed them both for three months is approximately 100 grams or 100,000 mg!

The bones are the storage area for 99 percent of the body's calcium. If you do not consume enough of this essential mineral to ensure optimal growth of the baby's skeleton, either the baby's growth is affected or calcium is drained from your bones. Marginal calcium deficiency also might be associated with reduced bone mineral content in the developing baby, while optimal calcium intake has been linked to a decreased risk for pregnancy-induced high blood pressure in the mother, lowered blood pressure in the infant (see chapter 6), and reduced lead toxicity in both the mother and developing baby. Granted, even when dietary intake is low, the body has backup systems to help ensure adequate availability of calcium during pregnancy, such as increased intestinal absorption of calcium. However, making sure you consume enough every day is still important.

Claims that milk can cause a number of health problems have been made, but most of these are unsubstantiated. However, concerns over the link between milk and heart disease are legitimate—although the main issue here is really the fat found in milk products. Milk fat is a blood vessel's worst nightmare. A cup of whole milk supplies 8 grams of fat—the equivalent of almost 2 teaspoons of grease; 1 teaspoon of that is the type of saturated fat that heads for your arteries. But with an abundance of low-fat and nonfat milk and yogurt products and literally hundreds of new low-fat cheeses on the market, there is no reason for anyone more than two years old to drink whole milk.

People who switch from whole to nonfat milk might even lower their risks for heart disease. At the University of Minnesota in Minneapolis, healthy young men consumed low-fat diets with the only difference being that one group drank whole milk and the other group drank nonfat milk. After six weeks, the men drinking nonfat milk had blood cholesterol levels 7 percent lower than the whole-milk group, a drop that equates to a 14 to 21 percent reduction in heart disease risk. Even their LDLs (the "bad" cholesterol) decreased by 11 percent.

The outcry that milk causes diabetes is another case where a little information was taken too far. A few preliminary studies have found a link between a series of amino acids in cow's milk, called ABBOS, and juvenile-onset diabetes in young children with a genetic predisposition to the disease. When these children ingest ABBOS, it triggers an immune response that not only attacks milk protein but also attacks the insulin-producing cells in the pancreas. Over time, the cells are destroyed and the child becomes diabetic.

Juvenile-onset diabetes is a very serious condition. In addition to requiring daily insulin shots, this form of diabetes can lead to blindness, kidney problems, foot amputations, and heart disease. However, the evidence linking milk to diabetes is inconclusive. In fact, the only proven fact is that breast-feeding is protective against the development of diabetes, not that cow's milk or formulas made with cow's milk are necessarily harmful. If there is a link between cow's milk and diabetes it is most likely only in babies less than one year old whose digestive tracts are still permeable, allowing large chunks of protein like ABBOS to enter the blood and start a reaction. The American Academy of Pediatrics for two decades has warned against feeding cow's milk to infants because milk is a poor source of iron and can cause bleeding in the digestive tract, leading to anemia. There is no solid evidence yet that anyone other than the under-one set, even children and adults genetically at risk for diabetes, is harmed by drinking milk— that is, unless they are milk intolerant.

While milk allergy receives a lot of attention, in reality few people are truly allergic to milk. The 1 to 2 percent of young children who develop allergic symptoms—bronchitis, eczema, and asthma—usually outgrow the problem by the time they are two years old; milk allergy is rarely diagnosed in adults.

On the other hand, lactose intolerance, caused by insufficient amounts of the digestive enzyme lactase, is relatively common; the incidence ranges from as low as one in every ten people of northern European descent to as high as 90 percent of African Americans, Asians, Jews, Native Americans, and Arabs in some areas.

The prevalence of lactose intolerance has been greatly exaggerated primarily because of studies in the 1960s that showed many people developed severe symptoms when they consumed 50 to 100 grams of lactose on an empty stomach. The assumption was that if lactose could do this to you, so would milk. In the mid-1970s, this assumption was proved wrong. Research at Cornell University showed that most lactose-intolerant adults could consume at least 15 grams of lactose—the amount found in $1\frac{1}{4}$ cups of milk—on an empty stomach without symptoms. Other studies confirmed that while many people were lactose intolerant, few were milk intolerant, especially if they drank small amounts of milk with meals, switched to yogurt (the ones made with the bacteria called *Lactobacillus bulgarius* or possibly *Lactobacillus acidophilus* are the best) or hard cheeses that have a lower lactose content, or drank milk treated with lactase, such as Lactaid. Unfortunately, frozen yogurts are a poor alternative, since freezing kills the beneficial bacteria.

Is milk for everybody? While the evidence is straightforward that children should drink milk each day, that these guidelines hold true for adults is controversial. "Early in life children need ample amounts of calcium to build strong bones," says Walter Willett, M.D., Dr.P.H., chairman of the Nutrition Department at Harvard School of Public Health. "Later in life the importance of milk is not so clear-cut."

Granted, no one needs to drink milk, but people in Western countries are hard-pressed to meet their nutrient needs without it. For example, milk supplies up to 75 percent of an adult's calcium intake. "It is very difficult to get enough calcium from diets that exclude milk because there are so few foods as rich in calcium that people are willing to eat frequently," states Bess Dawson-Hughes, chief of the Calcium and Bone Metabolism Laboratory at USDA Human Nutrition Research Center at Tufts University in Boston. Janet King, Ph.D., R.D., a professor in the Department of Nutritional Sciences at University of California, Berkeley, agrees and adds, "A woman must keep in mind that milk also supplies other essential nutrients, such as vitamin D and vitamin B2, that are difficult to get anywhere else." Since few pregnant women consume even one serving daily of dark green leafies, how realistic is it to expect them to eat the eight cups of cooked collard greens it would take to meet daily recommendations for calcium?

A long-held belief is that the protein in milk interferes with calcium metabolism. "Parts of the world where milk consumption is highest also have the highest incidence of hip fractures," says Dr. Willett. "Although it's clear we need to conduct more studies, it could be that the type of protein in milk increases urinary calcium loss."

"This statement is partially true and mostly wrong," says Robert Heaney, M.D., a calcium expert at Creighton University in Omaha. A high-protein diet does increase urinary excretion of calcium. "Sulfur-containing amino acids in all dietary protein act much like acid rain on limestone in flushing some calcium out of the body," says Dr. Heaney. However, these amino acids are found in all protein foods, from milk and meat to beans and grains. According to Dr. Heaney, it is the ratio of calcium to protein that is important, and it is here that milk comes out a winner. A cup of milk supplies 300 mg of calcium for only 8 grams of protein (a ratio of 37 to 1), while a 3½-ounce hamburger supplies up to 32 grams of protein but only 5 mg of calcium (a negative ratio of 1 to 6.4); even a cup of black beans contains twice the protein but only one sixth the calcium of milk (a ratio of 3 to 1).

In short, the protein issue is more theory than fact. "Protein's effect on calcium metabolism is primarily theoretical; no one has proved that the amounts typically consumed in this country are harmful," says Dr. Dawson-Hughes. If protein is a factor in osteoporosis, it is more likely that our high meat intake is to blame, not milk.

The majority of women consume less than the Recommended Dietary Allowance of 800 mg for calcium. Many researchers suspect this 800 mg limit might not be high enough to prevent age-related bone loss and osteoporosis, and that 1,200 to 1,500 mg might be a better goal. Some researchers recommend up to 2,000 mg for women preparing for and during pregnancy. "Women's calcium needs are greater than we previously thought and might be as much as four to five times higher than they are getting from their diets," says Dr. Heaney. An overwhelming amount of research shows that a high calcium intake protects against age-related bone loss and prevents fractures. "The effect is most strongly associated with calcium," says Heaney, "however, since milk is the best dietary source of calcium, the weight of the evidence comes down on the side of including milk in the diet."

Of course, you can take several calcium pills each day instead of drinking milk, but this goes against all dietary recommendations to turn first to food and then to supplements only as a last resort. "There is no evidence that calcium supplements are superior to milk [in preventing osteoporosis] and food always should be a person's first choice when it comes to obtaining optimal nutrition," says Dr. Dawson-Hughes.

There are several reasons to take this advice seriously. First, milk contains other factors that enhance calcium absorption and help prevent osteoporosis. The most important of these is vitamin D, a deficiency of which results in poor calcium absorption and rapid bone loss. In fact, Dr. Dawson-Hughes's research shows that increasing vitamin D intake, even without extra calcium, can help reduce bone fractures and slow the progression of osteoporosis.

However, for those women who cannot meet the goal of two to three servings of low-fat milk and other calcium-rich foods daily, then supplements are a must. "It's prudent to take a 1,000 mg supplement of calcium, since most women average only 500 mg of calcium from their diets," says Dr. Heaney. In addition, avoid the "natural source" calcium pills such as oyster shell and bone meal, since they might contain the toxic metal lead.

The hullabaloo over milk is more smoke than fire, since milk is a lot closer to the perfect food than to poison. Except for infants or people who are intolerant to even small dollops of yogurt, most women considering pregnancy would improve their diets by consuming more, not less, milk. So for those women who aren't willing to triple their current intake of green leafies, won't realistically drink calcium-fortified soymilk on a regular basis, and don't have enough mouth-watering recipes for canned salmon, the best bet is to follow mother's advice and drink milk—but make it low-fat or nonfat.

Dental caries are common in pregnant women, which has fueled the myth that the calcium drain of pregnancy causes a woman to lose a tooth for every baby. Several studies that have analyzed the chemical composition of teeth in both animals and people have not shown a link between pregnancy and calcium loss from the teeth. In one study, in which a dog was fed a calcium-deficient diet, the bones became so porous from loss of calcium that they hardly were detectable on X-ray film; however, the teeth showed no change. Changes in the pH of the mouth are more likely the cause of dental decay during pregnancy, and can be prevented with good dental hygiene and avoidance of sugary foods.

MAGNESIUM: Calcium is well publicized as the anti-osteoporosis mineral. Iron is famous for its role in red blood cells and the prevention of anemia. Chromium receives acclaim as the blood sugar regulator. Even fluoride is noteworthy for its role in the prevention of tooth decay. But seldom do you read about magnesium. Despite the lack of press, magnesium actually may be one of the most important nutrients during pregnancy and for the prevention of numerous health problems, from heart disease and high blood pressure to diabetes.

Magnesium functions in more than 300 processes essential to the development of a healthy baby, including the metabolism of carbohydrate, protein, and fat. It is one of the most abundant minerals in muscle, liver, heart, and other soft tissues, and is essential in the regulation of insulin and blood sugar levels, nerve transmission, the manufacture of proteins that synthesize the cells' genetic material, and in the removal of toxic waste products from the body. Magnesium also aids in muscle (including the uterus) contraction and relaxation. In fact, optimal blood levels of magnesium during pregnancy might help maintain uterine relaxation up until the thirty-fifth week, while dropping levels thereafter might favor the onset of labor.

Accumulating evidence also shows a direct link between magnesium intake and heart disease, with low dietary intake increasing a person's risk for arrhythmias, heart attack, and high blood pressure. Magnesium metabolism is altered in diabetics and might contribute to the development and progression of pregnancy-induced diabetes. (See chapter 6.)

Magnesium and calcium work as a team. For example, excess intake of magnesium inhibits bone formation, while consuming too much calcium interferes with magnesium metabolism. The balance between these two minerals is reflected in their roles in muscle contraction: calcium stimulates muscles to contract while magnesium relaxes muscles. Milk is one food that supplies both calcium and magnesium.

When it comes to magnesium, Americans don't get enough. The Recommended Dietary Allowance (RDA) is 320 mg for a pregnant woman, but a typical diet in the United States provides 120 mg of magnesium for every 1,000 calories; consequently, a woman consuming less than 2,000 calories will consume suboptimal amounts of magnesium. In addition, many researchers suspect the RDAs are inadequate to help prevent heart disease, high blood pressure, and diabetes. The RDAs for magnesium are based on 2.1 to 2.3 mg for every pound of body weight. However, studies show some people require up to 2.7 mg or more per pound of body weight, the equivalent of 368 mg for a 135-pound woman.

You will obtain optimal amounts of magnesium if you follow the Baby-wise Diet, which contains ample supplies of magnesium-rich foods, including milk, nuts, cooked dried beans and peas, whole-grain breads and cereals, soybeans, and seafood. Exceptions to this rule are women who have lost extra magnesium because of chronic diarrhea or repeated vomiting. In these cases, additional magnesium-rich foods should be consumed or a moderate-dose supplement that contains approximately 400 mg per day should be considered (see Table 3.2).

VITAMIN D: As mentioned above, vitamin D is essential for the absorption and use of calcium in the body. Studies show that animals born of mothers who consumed vitamin D–rich diets have better bone and skeletal development compared to those born of deficient mothers. But this fat-soluble vitamin is scarce in the diet. Studies in Europe and other countries show that vitamin D deficiency during pregnancy adversely affects growth, bone mineralization, tooth enamel formation, and even normal calcium balance in the unborn child. More low-birth-weight infants are born to vitamin D–deficient women than are born to well-nourished women. Congenital rickets, a condition in the newborn characterized by malformed bones, knocked knees or bowlegs, skull malformations, and

Table 3.2   What Foods Supply Magnesium?

FOOD	QUANTITY	MG
Wheat germ	1/4 cup	112
Peanuts	1/4 cup	63
Banana	1 medium	58
Avocado	1/2	56
Cashews	9 medium	52
Milk, low-fat	1 cup	40
Brewer's yeast	2 tablespoons	36
Mustard greens	1 cup	31
Bread:		
whole wheat	1 slice	19
white	1 slice	5

deformed rib cage, is the most common result of a mother's poor dietary intake of vitamin D. When a woman is breast-feeding, low vitamin D intake results in reduced amounts of the vitamin in the milk, which can be compensated for only by the baby's exposure to sunlight.

Sunlight is a major vitamin D source, since ultraviolet light triggers the conversion of a cholesterol-like compound in the skin to vitamin D. People who live in Florida, southern California, Italy, and other sunny climates are at low risk for vitamin D deficiency, while people living in northern climates are at increased risk. The diet becomes even more important as a source of this essential nutrient when direct sun exposure is limited because of cloudy weather conditions; the use of sunscreens, hats, and clothing; or sunlight that is filtered through windows and screens.

The only naturally occurring sources of vitamin D include sardines, mackerel, herring, salmon, and other fatty seafood that most people consume sporadically. That is why vitamin D–fortified milk is the only reliable or realistic dietary source; however, a pregnant woman must drink four glasses—or one quart—of low-fat milk to reach her RDA of 400 IU (or 10 mcg) or she must make sure she is out in the sun on a regular basis.

While getting enough vitamin D is essential, getting too much can be dangerous. Vitamin D is a fat-soluble vitamin and can accumulate in the body to potentially toxic levels with excessive intake. So make sure your total day's intake from fortified foods, milk, and supplements does not exceed 100 to 200 percent of the RDA for vitamin D, or a total of 400 to 800 IU. Don't worry about sun exposure; your body will regulate how much vitamin D is made based on need, not exposure.

Extra-Lean Meats and Legumes: B Vitamins and Trace Minerals

Legumes supply iron, magnesium, zinc, vitamin B6, and other B vitamins. Beans, dried peas, and lentils also are excellent sources of fiber and, except for soybeans, are essentially fat-free. Extra-lean meat, chicken, and fish also supply vitamin B12.

VITAMIN B6: Vitamin B6 is essential in the buildup and breakdown of carbohydrates, proteins, and fats; however, its main function is in protein metabolism. That means vitamin B6 is essential in the formation of all tissues, from the brain and nervous system to the muscles. Hormones, enzymes, red blood cells, and neurotransmitters (the chemicals that relay messages from one nerve cell to the next) are all protein-derived substances dependent on vitamin B6. Consequently, it is not surprising that low dietary intake of this B vitamin could have far-reaching effects on the physical, mental, and emotional development of a baby.

Mothers who consume suboptimal amounts of vitamin B6 during pregnancy are more likely than other mothers to give birth to babies who are irritable and not easily soothed. A deficiency also is linked to reduced Apgar scores. Mothers and babies who have low blood vitamin B6 levels also have trouble bonding after delivery.

The RDAs suggest a daily intake of 2.2 mg of vitamin B6 during pregnancy—a 0.5 mg increase over the nonpregnancy allowance. Many women consume much less than this, averaging as little as 54 percent of the RDA. In one study, only 6 percent of 400 pregnant and breast-feeding women met or exceeded the RDA for vitamin B6. In addition, the adequacy of the RDA has been questioned. Blood vitamin B6 levels drop during pregnancy when women consume only RDA levels, but are maintained with intakes two or more times higher than this, thus raising suspicion that RDA levels might not be enough to maintain optimal nutritional status. On the other hand, a pregnant woman should not consume more than 20 mg of vitamin B6 without her physician's consent and monitoring, since this B vitamin can cause nerve damage at high doses.

VITAMIN B12: This vitamin differs from other B vitamins in that it is found only in foods of animal origin, such as meat, milk, and eggs. If a plant contains this B vitamin, it is because of bacterial contamination or fermentation, as is true in the case of fermented soybean products such as miso. Thus, strict vegetarians who avoid all foods of animal origin must be especially careful to consume either vitamin B12–fortified soymilk, supplements, or hefty amounts of other B12 sources, since there are reports of vitamin B12–deficient infants born to vegetarian mothers.

Vitamin B12 is important in the normal processing of energy from carbohydrates, protein, and fats; in the formation and maintenance of the nervous system; in the correct replication of the genetic code within each cell; and in the formation of all body tissues. Consequently, vitamin B12 has been related, along with folic acid, to the prevention of birth defects, such as neural tube defects.

The most common symptom of vitamin B12 deficiency is a special type of anemia called macrocytic anemia (or pernicious anemia when the deficiency is caused by a lack of a digestive factor necessary for normal absorption of vitamin B12). In addition, the nerves do not form or function correctly as a result of deficiency, causing disorientation, numbness and tingling in the extremities, moodiness, irritability and agitation, dimmed vision, and dizziness. Digestive-tract disorders develop as a result of poor cell formation in these tissues. Fatigue and memory loss occur from the breakdown of the nervous system. Increased susceptibility to colds and infections result from faulty formation of white blood cells and other immune-system cells and tissues. Poor cell production in the skin causes dermatitis and changes in the lips and tongue. While pregnancy does not dramatically increase vitamin B12 needs (from 2.0 to 2.2 mcg), consuming enough to ensure optimal health and development of the baby is essential.

IRON: A woman's biggest nutritional challenge is iron. As many as 80 percent of active women and 20 percent of women in general are iron deficient. Compared to men, women have almost twice the daily requirement for iron, but consume half as much food. Pregnancy more than doubles a woman's iron requirement, but has a minimal effect on her food allowance; consequently, the iron dilemma intensifies prior to, during, and following pregnancy.

According to Fergus Clydesdale, Ph.D., professor and head of the Department of Food Science at the University of Massachusetts in Amherst, a well-balanced diet supplies approximately 6 mg of iron for every 1,000 calories. Based on this ratio, women must consume at least 2,500 to 3,000 calories to meet their nonpregnancy RDA of 15 to 18 mg (prepregnancy iron requirements are even higher for women with heavy menstrual losses or who have used intrauterine devices for birth control). But women average well under 2,000 calories daily and consume as little as 8 mg of iron; consequently many women enter pregnancy already iron depleted.

Iron deficiency is a subtle menace, so a woman who feels sluggish may unknowingly reach for a cup of coffee, when her real problem could be iron. (See chapter 6 for more on iron and fatigue.) As a component of hemoglobin in the blood and myoglobin within the cells, iron is the key oxygen-carrier in the body. When iron levels decrease, the tissues become oxygen starved, resulting in fatigue, poor concentration, and reduced work performance. Iron-deficient exercisers also experience reduced muscle strength, tire easily, and recover slowly after exercise. Poor regulation of body temperature and suppressed immunity resulting from iron deficiency increases susceptibility to infections and disease. All of these symptoms worsen as iron deficiency progresses to anemia. Pregnancy is likely to be the final factor that tips the scale from marginal to overt deficiency unless you increase iron intake ahead of time.

Iron deficiency is common in pregnancy, but it should be differentiated from normal changes in blood iron levels. The expanding blood volume during pregnancy dilutes the concentration of iron-containing substances, such as the hemoglobin in red blood cells, that carry oxygen to the tissues. Consequently, it is normal for hemoglobin and hematocrit values (typical tests for iron status) to fall. However, these tests measure the final stages of iron deficiency, so a drop to a level well below normal, nonpregnant values indicates that a woman has been iron deficient for some time.

Serum ferritin, as discussed in chapter 1, is a much more sensitive indicator of tissue iron stores and the early stages of iron deficiency anemia. In one study, 112 out of 120 pregnant women (93 percent) had depleted their tissue iron stores to levels of less than 20 mcg/l, even though all of these women had hemoglobin and hematocrit values within the normal range and were not anemic. To determine your iron needs, see Quiz 3.1.

Iron deficiency during pregnancy can have serious consequences. Poor iron

Quiz 3.1   What Is Your Risk for Iron Deficiency?

Answer the following questions yes or no.

_____ **1.** When not pregnant, do you have heavy menstrual bleeding?
_____ **2.** Do you eat less than 3 ounces of red meat every day?
_____ **3.** Do you often avoid a vitamin C–rich fruit, such as an orange or strawberries, with your meals or as snacks?
_____ **4.** Do you consume fewer than 2,500 calories daily of wholesome, minimally processed foods?
_____ **5.** Do you exercise regularly?
_____ **6.** Do you regularly take aspirin?
_____ **7.** Have you donated blood in the past year?
_____ **8.** Are you currently pregnant?
_____ **9.** Have you been pregnant with another baby in the past two years?
_____ **10.** Do you take iron supplements sporadically or not at all?

Although there is no set number of yes answers that will guarantee you are iron deficient, the more times you answered yes to the above questions, the more likely you are to be only marginally nourished in this essential mineral. The best way to check is to request a serum ferritin test from your physician and ask to see the results. A score less than 20 mcg/l is a clear sign you are iron deficient.

intake means fewer red blood cells to carry oxygen to your tissues and your baby. Your heart must pump harder and faster to compensate for iron-poor blood, consequently you are likely to tire more easily. The developing baby also is starved for oxygen. Pregnancy outcome is jeopardized; an anemic mother is three times more likely to deliver a low-birth-weight infant and twice as likely to deliver a premature infant than is a nonanemic woman. Blood loss during delivery can stress an already depleted system; the blood loss from a cesarean birth further depletes iron levels. Recovery after the baby is born also takes longer, leaving you with less physical and emotional energy to adjust to your new baby.

The iron costs of pregnancy are high. More than 246 mg of iron is stockpiled in the baby's tissues prior to delivery, another 134 mg is taken up by the placenta, and about 290 mg is used to expand the volume of the mother's blood.

The Balancing Act

Iron intake is more a balance between iron promoters and iron inhibitors than it is just eating iron-rich foods. Here are a few ways to maximize your promoters to guarantee you get the most from your diet:

1. Always consume a vitamin C–rich food with every meal, such as orange juice, a tossed salad, broccoli, or most fruits. Vitamin C dramatically improves the absorption of non-heme iron and counteracts some of the inhibitors in foods, such as phytates in whole grains and tannins in tea and coffee.
2. Consuming small amounts of heme iron in red meat, such as extra-lean beef, with large amounts of nonheme iron, such as in beans, increases the absorption of nonheme iron. Pork in a vegetable stir-fry and spaghetti with meatballs are other examples.
3. Cook in a cast-iron skillet.
4. Select iron-fortified foods.
5. If you drink tea and coffee, do so between meals, since substances called tannins in these beverages can reduce iron absorption by 80 percent or more.
6. Take iron supplements on an empty stomach to improve absorption.

That equates to about 2.4 mg a day during pregnancy just to cover the iron costs of pregnancy. In addition, 1.0 mg or more is needed to maintain the mother's normal body processes. Since you absorb only about 10 percent of dietary intake (although iron absorption increases to as much as 50 percent during pregnancy in some women), you must consume from 30 to 60 mg or more of iron daily to ensure optimal iron status.

The Baby-wise Diet will provide about 18 mg of iron daily, so you will need to consider a supplement. Even with a good diet and supplementation, it may take up to two years to restock iron stores after pregnancy and return serum ferritin levels to optimal levels. (See chapter 1 for more information on iron and the prepregnancy diet and chapter 10 for more information on iron and preparing for the next pregnancy; see also "The Balancing Act," above.)

COPPER: This trace mineral is found in all tissues, but it is especially high in the brain, heart, kidney, and liver. It is essential for the development and maintenance of your baby's heart, arteries, and blood vessels; the skeletal system; and the nervous system. Copper also is important in the development and mainte-nance of red blood cells, normal hair, and skin color.

Studies on animals show that a copper deficiency during pregnancy can cause birth defects and spontaneous abortions, while increasing copper intake improves survival rates and reduces nerve damage and spontaneous abortions. The only reported risk for copper deficiency in humans is when pregnant women take the drug penicillamine, which depletes copper from the tissues. However, the diets of many pregnant women might be marginal, since blood levels often are low and optimal copper status often is achieved only when women take multiple vitamin and mineral supplements that contain copper. The Baby-wise Diet supplies at least the recommended intake of 1.5 to 3.0 mg, so a supplement should not be necessary if you are eating according to this plan.

On the other hand, beware of cooking acidic foods, such as spaghetti sauce, in copper cookware. Cooking in copper pots destroys vitamin C, vitamin E, and folic acid and can increase the copper content of food to potentially toxic levels. While copper-bottomed stainless-steel cookware is safe, avoid using copper pans that are not well lined.

ZINC: Zinc plays center stage from conception through delivery. This trace mineral is essential for the formation of the sperm and the ovum, ovulation, and fertilization. Even a marginal zinc deficiency can increase a woman's chance of having a spontaneous abortion and other complications, pregnancy-related tox-emia, an extended pregnancy or premature delivery, and prolonged labor.

The baby also suffers. In studies on animals, pups born to mothers who are marginally deficient in zinc have an increased likelihood of malformation includ-ing cleft palate and lip, brain and eye malformations, and numerous abnor-malities of the heart, lung, and urogenital system), retarded growth, poor bone development, reduced taste acuity, visual impairment, and low birth weight. Similar problems have been noted in humans. For example, malformations, pre-term deliveries, and spontaneous abortions are more common in women with low blood zinc levels than in women with optimal zinc status. In fact, zinc status is so important for pregnancy outcome that researchers at the University of Alabama recommend checking the mother's blood zinc concentration during early preg-nancy as a screening technique for preventing low-birth-weight infants.

Zinc also has lifelong effects on the well-being of your baby. Low zinc intake has been linked to the development of neural tube defects. Zinc-deficient babies

Table 3.3   Where to Get Vitamins and Minerals

NUTRIENT	SOURCES
Vitamin A	Liver, eggs
Beta carotene	Dark green or orange vegetables, cantaloupe, peaches
Vitamin D	Fortified milk, fatty fish, egg yolk
Vitamin E	Wheat germ, safflower oil, spinach
Vitamin K	Dark green leafy vegetables
Vitamin B1	Whole grains, wheat germ, brewer's yeast, peanuts, green peas, dark green leafy vegetables
Vitamin B2	Milk, avocado, dark green leafy vegetables, salmon, asparagus
Niacin	Chicken, fish, peanut butter, green peas, wheat germ, brewer's yeast
Vitamin B6	Chicken, fish, avocado, potatoes, bananas
Folic acid	Dark green leafy vegetables, orange juice, wheat germ
Vitamin B12	Meat, chicken, fish, eggs, milk
Biotin	Oatmeal, soybeans, peanut butter, fish, milk, brown rice
Pantothenic acid	Chicken, fish, eggs, milk, peanut butter, bananas, oranges, brown rice, wheat germ
Vitamin C	Citrus fruit, Brussels sprouts, strawberries, dark green leafy vegetables
Calcium	Low-fat milk products, sardines, canned salmon with bones, tofu, dark green leafy vegetables, dried beans and peas
Chromium	Whole grains, wheat germ, orange juice
Copper	Chicken, fish, meat, avocado, potato, soybeans, dark green leafy vegetables
Iron	Lean meat, dried apricots, dark green leafy vegetables, raisins, dried beans and peas, potatoes
Magnesium	Low-fat milk, peanuts, bananas, wheat germ, dark green leafy vegetables, oysters

NUTRIENT	SOURCES
Manganese	Raisins, spinach, carrots, broccoli, oranges, green peas
Molybdenum	Lean meat, whole grains, dried beans and peas, dark green leafy vegetables
Potassium	Fruits, vegetables, fish, peanuts, potatoes
Selenium	Whole grains, seafood, lean meat, low-fat milk products
Zinc	Lean meat, turkey, dried beans and peas, wheat germ

also are less likely to survive, have compromised immune systems and are more susceptible to infections, show developmental and behavioral problems, and have a delayed onset of puberty later in life.

Why is zinc so critical to growth, development, and pregnancy outcome? Zinc is needed every minute of pregnancy for all phases of growth and tissue maintenance. It stabilizes the genetic code in every cell and, therefore, maintains normal tissue growth and differentiation during pregnancy. Zinc also plays an active role as a component of insulin, the hormone that regulates blood sugar—the primary energy source that fuels the baby-making process. In addition, zinc helps maintain the normal acid-base balance in the body, helps produce hormonelike compounds called prostaglandins that regulate numerous body processes, and aids in the functioning of the oil glands of the skin.

Pregnant women's diets are often low in zinc. The RDA during pregnancy is 15 mg (reduced from 20 mg in the previous 1984 RDA, not because 15 mg was optimal but because few people were consuming 20 mg). Yet many women consume only 9 to 10 mg daily. Your zinc needs will be met if you follow the Babywise Diet; however, if you cannot always eat well, a moderate-dose multiple vitamin and mineral supplement that contains 15 to 20 mg of zinc provides safe nutritional insurance (see Table 3.3).

The Food or Supplement Dilemma

Eating well is a must during pregnancy. In every case, wholesome, minimally processed foods are your best sources of vitamins, minerals, fiber, other nutrients, and nonnutritive substances such as the phytochemicals. For one thing, food supplies these nutrients in the proper ratio and balance, so your chances of consuming too little or too much, or of creating a secondary deficiency by consuming excessive amounts of one at the expense of other nutrients, is not likely.

In addition, a nutrient never works alone; vitamins and minerals always act as a team in any and all body processes. Calcium builds strong bones, but only with the help of magnesium, vitamin D, zinc, and other nutrients. Iron builds oxygen-rich blood, but only if the diet also supplies ample amounts of vitamin B12, folic acid, vitamin C, vitamin B6, and other vitamins and minerals. Science understands only a small part of this teamwork; until more is known, it is safe to say Mother Nature probably knows best how to mix and match nutrients for your baby's well-being.

Finally, science knows even less about the nonnutrient, health-enhancing compounds in foods called phytochemicals. Although we know that chemicals called indoles in cabbage reduce your risk for cancer and saponins in beans might lower your cholesterol, how these—and other as yet unidentified—compounds work together or with other nutrients is still to be explored, so a good diet is essential, with supplements as a backup for nutritional insurance. (See chapter 4 for more on the phytochemicals.)

It's obvious that women must take nutrition more seriously, because adequate isn't good enough when it comes to building a better baby. You can't afford to take your diet for granted. Small changes are worthwhile, but don't stop there. You know how to push the limits when it comes to everything, from exercise to work deadlines. Now it's time to stretch a little to reach your nutritional potential for the health of your baby and the ease of your pregnancy. Making changes *is* time-consuming at first, but the extra time up front is worth it when those goals become habit and you know you have given your baby the best possible start in life.

II.

During Pregnancy

CHAPTER FOUR

Your Changing Body:
What to Expect

Whether you are in touch with your body or you race through life barely aware of its subtle ups and downs, your nine months of pregnancy (as well as the first few months after the baby is born) are likely to bring some surprises—physically, emotionally, and mentally.

Whereas a slight slump in your afternoon energy level prior to pregnancy was a minor inconvenience, it seldom interfered with your schedule; the same symptom during pregnancy may escalate rapidly to exhaustion with no warning. The shrimp salad that sounded so good when you ordered it might trigger an overwhelming surge of nausea when it is set in front of you. You may be in a great mood one minute and sobbing the next. Even women who pride themselves on their self-control say they often had no idea how they would be feeling from one minute to the next during their pregnancies. While the first pregnancy usually brings the most surprises, subsequent pregnancies are seldom carbon copies of the first and usually come packaged with their own set of experiences.

Pregnancy can be one of life's little lessons, reminding us that we are only partly in control. On the other hand, at no other time in life is a woman more aware of her connection to a greater purpose. Many of the ups and downs of pregnancy are natural rhythms resulting from dramatic physical changes that must take place to build a new person. You can't stop Mother Nature—she's doing what she does best—but you do have some say over how you react to these changes.

Learning about your body's changes during pregnancy can help you understand why you are exhausted one minute and elated the next, why you crave foods

Take Care of Yourself

Before and throughout your pregnancy be sure to:

1. Follow the Baby-wise Diet.

2. Exercise daily.

3. Refrain from smoking, drinking alcohol, or taking any drugs or medications (without physician approval).

4. Keep all of your physician appointments. If you miss one, call and reschedule rather than wait until the next month.

5. Wear your seat belt.

6. Brush and floss your teeth daily and see your dentist at least every six months. (Also, brush your teeth immediately after any bout of vomiting.)

7. Avoid hot tubs or saunas, especially during the first trimester when the risk for birth defects is highest.

8. Notify health-care providers that you are pregnant before having any X rays.

9. Read all labels for warnings and directions before you use cleaners, bug sprays, paint, and other chemicals.

you never would have eaten before pregnancy, or why at nine months it takes you longer to get off the couch than it used to take to run a mile! (One friend confessed she got stuck in an overstuffed chair in her ninth month and had to wait for her husband to come home to help her out!) Your body will be experiencing some very dramatic changes, and it knows how to do it all with no help from you. Knowing how you will be forming a new life can help you be patient with the process and develop a deep appreciation for the miracle that is happening inside you; this positive attitude will help foster an easier pregnancy and a healthy baby. (For some general tips on living with your pregnancy, see "Take Care of Yourself," above.)

Table 4.1   Hormones During Pregnancy, to Name a Few

HORMONE	PRIMARY SOURCE	FUNCTION
Estrogen	Placenta	Influences mood; alters thyroid function; controls growth and function of uterus; increases flexibility of connective tissues, which facilitates delivery; causes fluid retention and puffiness or swelling; alters taste and smell
Progesterone	Placenta	Slows stomach emptying; stimulates fat accumulation in mother; increases urinary loss of salt; influences mood; relaxes uterus to allow growth; relaxes other muscles in digestive tract, which allows increased nutrient absorption and constipation; increases respiration
Human placental lactogen (HPL)	Placenta	Increases availability of blood sugar
Human growth hormone (HGH)	Pituitary (brain)	Increases blood sugar, stimulates bone growth
Human chorionic thyrotropin (HCT)	Placenta	Stimulates thyroid function
Thyroxine	Thyroid gland	Regulates metabolism
Parathyroid hormone (PTH)	Parathyroid gland	Increases calcium absorption
Insulin	Pancreas	Reduces blood sugar levels; promotes energy production; aids in fat storage
Glucagon	Pancreas	Increases blood sugar
Calcitonin	Thyroid gland	Inhibits calcium loss from bone
Aldosterone	Adrenal glands	Maintains salt balance
Cortisone	Adrenal glands	Helps regulate glucose and protein metabolism
Renin-angiotensin	Kidneys	Salt and water retention; increases thirst

Your Pregnant Body, from Head to Toe

Every part of your body, from the top of your head to the tips of your toes, is affected by the baby-making process. Long before the tummy begins to protrude or the scale shows a gain in weight, you'll feel the changes.

Throughout pregnancy, the most obvious changes are in your uterus, blood, breasts, and fat stores. In addition, the pulse rate increases, skin temperature rises, appetite fluctuates from nil to famished, nutrient absorption increases in the intestines, and the ligaments soften. The pregnant woman secretes more than thirty different hormones, many of which are present only during pregnancy while others such as estrogen are normally present, but now their levels of secretion are altered by the pregnant state (see Table 4.1).

For example, the uterus, which is usually a solid, pear-shaped organ, will expand and increase hundreds of times in volume. The walls will thicken to protect the fragile developing baby, and later will thin to accommodate changes in your growing baby's size and position. The lower end of the uterus, called the cervix, softens during pregnancy and forms a mucous plug that protects the uterus from bacterial infection.

If you are healthy and eat well, your blood volume will increase by about 50 percent. This increase is an indicator of pregnancy outcome, since women who have small increases in blood volume compared to women with normal increases are more likely to have stillbirths, spontaneous abortions, and low-birth-weight infants. Another example is your skin. Both the "pregnancy glow" you have heard about and the dark blotches on the face, upper lip, cheeks, or forehead (a condition called chloasma or pregnancy mask) could result from changes in hormones.

Since the physical changes of pregnancy are too complicated to describe in detail, the following is a summary of how the changes in your body correspond to the growth of your baby.

The First Trimester (Weeks 1 through 13)

During the first three months of pregnancy, your body must adapt to very dramatic changes. The female hormones—estrogen and progesterone—are elevated, while another hormone called human chorionic gonadotropin (HCG) enters the bloodstream. (This is the hormone that eventually will give you a positive reading on your pregnancy test.)

SETTLING IN: The first signs of pregnancy are subtle: a missed period, tender breasts (probably as a result of increased estrogen levels), frequent urination (caused by the expanding uterus pushing against your bladder), or a sleepy haze that comes over you late in the afternoon (possibly caused by elevated progesterone levels). These are just the tip of the iceberg, however, in terms of what is going on inside.

The fertilized egg is dividing at a rapid rate as it moves down the fallopian tubes toward the uterus, which will be its home for the next nine months. By the time it implants in the uterus, about six to eleven days later, it is already a hollow ball made up of at least 100 individual cells. Some of these cells create a bubble that fills with fluid; this eventually will become the amniotic fluid where the baby develops, lives, and is cushioned and nourished. Out of this bundle of cells, which is increasing in number every hour, the inner cells differentiate and go about becoming a baby, while the outer cells will form the placenta and other membranes. (See "The Placenta: The Nutrient Highway," page 110.)

By the second week, some of the new cells form a type of barrier surrounding the embryo, which now contains three layers of immature tissues that will continue to differentiate into the entire body. The outer layer, or the ectoderm, will develop into the brain, nervous system, hair, and skin. This layer develops quite rapidly in the early days of pregnancy. The middle layer, or the mesoderm, develops into the muscles, bones, cardiovascular and excretory systems. The inner layer of cells, the endoderm, will develop into the digestive tract, lungs, and glands. This marks the end of the first phase of pregnancy, called the blastogenesis stage. At this point, if your menstrual periods are very regular, you will notice you have missed a period and might suspect that you are pregnant.

WEEKS 3 THROUGH 8: The second phase of pregnancy is called the embryonic stage, which begins about the third week and lasts through the second month. Your baby now is one tenth of an inch long and has developed a rudimentary brain with two lobes and the beginnings of a spinal column. On about the twenty-fifth day, the heart is beating, blood is flowing, and arm "buds" appear, followed two days later by leg "buds." By the fourth week, other organs, such as the liver, kidneys, and thyroid gland, are visible and the embryo is about the size of a grain of rice (10,000 times larger than the original fertilized egg!), has a primitive vascular system, but has no face.

The Placenta: The Nutrient Highway

The placenta is the nutritional highway between you and your baby. In addition to its role in producing several of the hormones responsible for the regulation of your growth and development, it is the vital pipeline for nutrients to and waste products from the baby, and it forms a somewhat permeable barrier against some harmful substances.

The placenta is a network of blood vessels and tissues attached to the uterine lining and to the baby via the umbilical cord. The umbilical cord contains one blood vessel that carries oxygen and nutrient-rich blood to the baby and two different blood vessels that return waste products and carbon dioxide to the placenta. These umbilical blood vessels branch out into the placenta in fingerlike projections called villi. Blood vessels from the mother also project into the placenta and blood pools around the fetal villi. It is here that nutrients, oxygen, and waste products are exchanged.

One of the unique capabilities of the placenta is that it contains two separate blood supplies—the mother's and the baby's—that communicate, but never touch. Consequently, when the mother eats and digests food, the nutrients enter her blood system and make their way to the blood vessels in the placenta. Here, the fetal blood vessels pick up the needed nutrients, fluids, oxygen, and other substances and release waste materials that are excreted by the mother via the kidneys.

The placenta is not a true barrier and cannot protect the baby from harmful substances. Size and chemical structure, not potential toxicity, determine what crosses from the mother's blood into the baby's environment. Consequently, many drugs, chemicals, and medications can pass into the baby's bloodstream and influence development. Other substances, such as alcohol or vitamins A and D, can accumulate to toxic levels in the developing baby if the mother's blood levels remain high.

The placenta forms in the first few weeks of development and continues to grow until the final month of pregnancy. (At birth, a well-developed placenta will weigh between 1 ½ and 2 pounds and is eight inches wide and an inch thick.)

A well-nourished woman builds a better placenta. Research shows that the growth of the placenta is directly related to the mother's food intake. Even a marginal nutrient deficiency can have significant effects on the size and functioning of the placenta, which in turn affects the nutrient supply to the developing baby.

Table 4.2   Red Flags of Concern

While most of the changes, discomforts, and symptoms a woman experiences during pregnancy are normal, there are a few warning signs that should be immediately checked by a physician.

SYMPTOM	CONCERN
Bleeding or cramping	Could be a sign of miscarriage (often accompanied by the absence of pregnancy symptoms; that is, you no longer feel tired or nauseous, or your breasts are no longer tender). An ectopic pregnancy (when the fertilized egg implants outside the uterus) also may cause bleeding and pain and is life-threatening to the mother. Bleeding late in pregnancy could indicate problems with the placenta.
Pain	Continuous pain could signal nonpregnancy problems such as appendicitis, or could be a sign that something unusual is happening with the pregnancy. Abruption—premature separation of the placenta from the uterine wall—also causes pain.
High blood pressure	Usually identified by your physician during your routine checkup. Also called pregnancy-induced hypertension or PIH, pre-eclampsia, and/or eclampsia, it will cause no symptoms, but often is accompanied by sudden weight gain of more than 2 pounds in a week and swelling of the face and hands. Headaches, pain, or blurred vision (seeing spots) also are late signs of PIH. Left untreated, PIH can progress and cause seizures in the mother and a stillborn baby.

It is about this time that you will experience more pronounced physical changes. Nausea, vomiting, food aversions, or food cravings might begin. You also may be overcome with fatigue as your body adapts to the radical changes. Changes in blood pressure might make you feel dizzy or faint when you stand up too quickly, so avoid sudden movements. The increased levels of estrogen and progesterone also might be the cause of bleeding, inflamed, or tender gums called pregnancy gingivitis (see Table 4.2 for symptoms that may be cause for concern).

Emotional changes crop up, probably a result of the hormone storms. You may feel more irritable, weepy, depressed, or anxious. On the other hand, you may experience a newfound joy, elation, and excitement about life, which may spill over into an increased sex drive. Many normal emotions are amplified during the first months of pregnancy. If this is an unwanted pregnancy, you may be angry or in denial; if it is a wanted pregnancy, you may be fearful of a miscarriage (in reality, about 10 percent of women experience an early miscarriage, while ectopic or tubal pregnancies affect only one in every 100 women).

By the fourth week, your baby's eyelids are beginning to appear and will be formed and closed around the developing eyes within another week. By the thirty-seventh day, the nose has formed, while the ears take shape around the fifth or sixth week and rudimentary hearing begins during the second month. During the second month, the kidneys begin to function, the stomach produces some digestive juices, and blood is forming in the liver. Muscles also are developing and lengthening.

Even though your baby is only slightly larger than a coffee bean by the sixth week, the skeleton has already formed. The early skeleton is composed of cartilage; cartilage makes way for calcium-containing bone around the forty-eighth day. The fingers you will eventually count and the toes you will kiss also have taken shape.

By the end of the second month, the embryo is now called a fetus and is about the size of your big toe, with arms and legs thinner than spaghetti noodles and skin as thin as waxed paper. You barely know you are pregnant, but your baby has weathered its most critical time. Developing properly during these first two months greatly increases the baby's chances for survival.

As early as the first month or two you will notice changes in your breasts. Your milk glands and ducts enlarge and fatty tissues form to prepare for breast-feeding. You may even experience tingling in your breast tissue during this time. Increased blood supply to the breast may cause blue veins to become temporarily noticeable, while the areola around the nipples may darken. Raised white areas, called Montgomery's glands, begin to secrete oil to keep the nipples lubricated.

THE THIRD MONTH: While your uterus grows to the size of a grapefruit and your waistline thickens, your baby is developing a rudimentary personality. The first ridges of the fingerprints appear, a lifelong mark of individuality. As internal organs and the nervous system mature enough to communicate back and forth, the brain can begin to send signals to the body. If you feel a fluttering (called quickening) in your abdomen as if you had swallowed a butterfly (or as if someone is blowing a fine stream of bubbles inside your belly), it could be your four-inch-long baby letting out a kick with its fragile legs and newly formed muscles. Most women feel these tumbles by weeks 16 to 20.

Babies at this stage also can bend their wrists and elbows or form a fist. Your baby's face looks much more human now and can make facial expressions, such as a frown or a squint. The vocal cords also begin to develop around the tenth week. The ribs and vertebrae have begun to calcify, bones are forming in the hands, the nail beds have started to form, and tooth formation has begun.

The two bony plates that make up the palate are combining at this stage. By the twelfth week, the baby is developing sexual organs. In fact, by the end of the first trimester, the baby has developed all of its major systems and is giving clues as to whether he or she will be rambunctious or quiet.

Your blood volume has increased 30 to 40 percent. You also may be thirsty or perspiring more as result of increased fluid requirements and metabolic rate.

Fortunately for many women, by the end of the first trimester much of the hormonal upheaval that caused the fatigue, nausea, mood swings, and other annoying symptoms has subsided and the body is in full pregnancy swing. Even though a frequent need to urinate may disrupt sleep patterns, many women report feeling better by the end of the first trimester, and some say the nausea and fatigue seem to vanish overnight, leaving them feeling calmer, more accepting, and more energetic. For other women, symptoms lessen, but they still set aside time for a quick nap in the afternoon or continue to experience nausea. A few women battle serious nausea, fatigue, or other discomforts well into the second trimester or even throughout their pregnancies.

The Second Trimester (Weeks 14 through 27)

Many women consider the second trimester the easy part. Most women no longer have the fatigue, nausea, and mood swings of the first trimester, while the awkwardness that comes in the final weeks of pregnancy is far away. The size of your baby rapidly increases in the second trimester. In the fourth month, your baby could fit into a teacup, by twenty weeks it is half the birth length, and by the end of the second trimester your baby will be 12 inches or longer and will weigh about $1\frac{1}{2}$ pounds.

The bones continue to develop, which causes the fetus to straighten from its curled position. The tiny heart is pumping quarts of blood through its body, the facial features are becoming more distinct, hair is beginning to grow, and the air passageways are developed even though the baby isn't able to breathe. The muscles are more developed, so the gentle flutters you felt before now turn to tumbles, rolling waves, kicks, pokes, and even hiccups as your small baby still has plenty of room inside the uterus to test his or her new abilities. Some women say that during the second trimester it feels as if the baby were playing Tarzan, swinging from ropes and leaping from tall trees. Sounds can penetrate the uterus, although the mother's voice reaches the womb more readily than other voices; of outside noises, men's voices carry better than higher-pitched women's voices. Your baby now can hear you and most of the outside racket, and may startle at a sudden noise.

Even though the organs are well developed, your baby could not survive outside the womb at four or five months because the lungs, digestive organs, and skin are not completely developed. Your baby also develops a downy coat (called lanugo), which disappears before birth, and a waxy covering (called vernix caseosa) to protect the delicate skin from the mineralized amniotic fluid in which he or she is bathed.

Your weight gain begins to pick up during the second trimester and should average about $\frac{1}{2}$ to 1 pound a week. In contrast to the first trimester, during which your baby's growth was primarily focused on developing organs, tissues, and cells, the second trimester is a time of rapid overall growth in body weight. But your weight gain also reflects changes in your body. Your blood volume increases to accommodate the increased nutrient demands of the baby and also might contribute to nosebleeds, bleeding gums, and headaches.

Your breast tissue also is increasing as it prepares for breast-feeding. In fact, your nipples might start secreting small amounts of colostrum, a yellowish fluid that will nourish your baby in the first few days of breast-feeding before mature milk is produced. (Nursing pads placed in your maternity bra will catch any leaks.) The placenta continues to grow, and your body is building fat stores to ensure that there is enough fuel for making milk after the baby is born.

Increasing body weight and an expanding tummy may change your posture as your center of gravity shifts toward your back to compensate for the baby's weight in front. The increased pressure on your lower back can cause backaches, which are best treated by sleeping on a firm mattress, wearing comfortable flat shoes, and bending from the knees, not the waist, when lifting. Leg cramps also might develop and are probably caused by the enlarged uterus pressing against the major vein, called the vena cava, that returns blood from the lower body to the heart. This squeezing effect causes the pressure in the veins of the legs to increase, which might result in leg cramps, varicose veins, hemorrhoids, and edema in the legs and ankles. The elevated pressure returns to normal when a pregnant woman lies on her side and also immediately after delivery.

In addition, the hormone relaxin now is being released to help soften your ligaments around the pelvis and hips so they will stretch more easily during labor. This effect, however, also might make rising from a chair or any sudden movement more difficult.

The Third Trimester (Weeks 28 through 40)

While you are anxious to meet your baby, you also know you're in the homestretch of pregnancy. Your baby's main job for the next three months is to gain weight at a rate of about one half to three quarters of a pound a week! By the end of the eighth month, your baby will weigh between four and six pounds. During the ninth month, weight gain averages two ounces a day! As your baby gets bigger, there is less room available in the uterus for tumbling, so the energetic quick kicks and pokes you felt during the second trimester might gradually be replaced by slow, strong turns; you may even notice a foot, elbow, or fist when the baby bumps against the wall of the abdomen. The baby also spends increasingly more time in the fetal position.

In addition to weight, your baby's brain is growing and developing, which allows the genetic blueprint for personality to express itself. For example, some babies are in constant motion, as if they can hardly wait to get out and get going; others are content to snuggle peacefully in the womb and sleep. One baby will be a "night person" and want to tumble until dawn; another might be more active in the morning. One baby will be irritated by hiccups and start kicking and thumping within minutes of a hiccup attack; another might seem unaware of the experience.

The wrinkly, reddened skin at five months now begins to smooth out as the layer of "baby fat" just under the skin begins to accumulate. This fat pad will help regulate body temperature and provide energy stores after birth. Fingernails have grown beyond the tip of the fingers and toenails have reached the end of the toes.

Your expanding tummy and the pressure of the large baby, who is three times heavier at delivery than at twenty-eight weeks, might aggravate backaches; press against your diaphragm, making breathing more difficult; limit your stomach's capacity, making big meals an impossibility; and press on the pelvic veins, possibly causing some edema in the legs and feet, as mentioned above. You may be more uncomfortable now and have to urinate more frequently, both of which interfere with a good night's sleep. Lack of sleep and the extra energy required to move might cause some fatigue and possibly some moodiness or irritability. Naps, elevating your feet, avoiding standing for long periods of time, daily exercise to keep the blood circulating, and general self-nurturing now are essential. You also may feel flushes or warmth, probably because your baby's body heat is passing through the placenta and your metabolism is working overtime during this trimester.

At twenty-eight weeks, the baby is now medically considered viable and, if born, must be registered as a birth. If a baby dies, it is considered a stillbirth, not a miscarriage. Although active and growing, a baby at seven months usually can survive outside the womb only with specialized care in a neonatal nursery. (Some infants survive at earlier ages with intensive neonatal care.) By eight months, however, a baby has a good chance of survival, even though some functions, such as the lungs and digestive tract, and the immune system, still may be undeveloped. During the ninth month, these tissues and systems mature and antibodies from your blood are transferred to the baby to provide protection against disease and infection. This passive protection continues if you choose to breast-feed.

By the ninth month, you and your baby are ready for delivery. About one to two weeks before delivery, the placenta begins to change in shape and function, becoming less fibrous and more tough, with its blood vessels beginning to deteriorate. This might be the signal to the baby that it is time to make an entry into the world. You may experience Braxton Hicks contractions, which are mild, irregular uterine cramps sometimes mistaken for labor. You will note that your baby has "dropped" or "engaged"—that is, it has settled into a head-down position and moved lower into your abdomen (a process called lightening that happens as the baby positions itself correctly for birth). This may ease some of the pressure against your stomach and lungs and make breathing and eating a little easier.

A rise in estrogen levels boosts a last growth surge in the baby, but it also causes the mother to retain more fluids. This results in some puffiness and swelling in the face, legs, ankles, and feet, a harmless condition that shouldn't be mistaken for the more serious edema of pregnancy-induced hypertension or PIH (see chapter 6). The swelling is aggravated by gravity and the pressure of the growing baby and uterus on your blood vessels. Exercise will help circulation, while elevating your feet regularly and avoiding tight shoes or stockings (if you can even reach your feet anymore!) will help reduce the pressure on your veins and lessen the fluid accumulation in your ankles and feet.

Your cervix also becomes softer and begins to thin (efface). This action may expel the mucous plug that protected your uterus or even cause your water (the amniotic fluid that has bathed your baby for the past nine months) to break before you are in actual labor. On the other hand, you may not expel the mucous plug or have your water break until you are in labor. Labor begins when you start experiencing mild, rhythmic contractions that gain in intensity, causing your cervix to experience progressive changes that ultimately lead to birth. Keep in mind, however, that leakage of the amniotic fluid, with or without labor, is an indicator that you should see your physician.

How Diet Impacts You and Your Baby

From conception to birth, your baby's body weight increases from a fraction of a gram (less than the weight of an ant) to 6½ to 8½ pounds or more. From the eighth week of pregnancy to birth, your baby's weight increases more than four-hundred-fold! (See "What Makes Up Weight Gain," page 118.) The baby's weight doubles from birth to four months and triples by the first birthday.

The diversity and rate of growth are greater during the first nine months prior to birth than at any other time of life. The first two years of life are the second

What Makes up Weight Gain During Pregnancy?

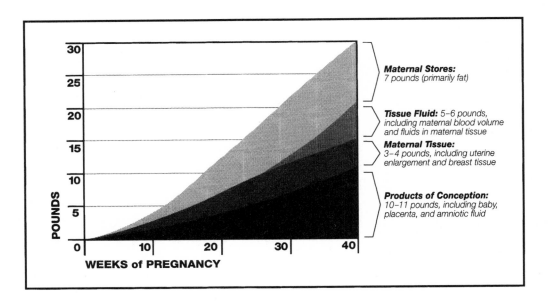

Maternal Stores:
7 pounds (primarily fat)

Tissue Fluid: 5–6 pounds,
including maternal blood volume
and fluids in maternal tissue

Maternal Tissue:
3–4 pounds, including uterine
enlargement and breast tissue

Products of Conception:
10–11 pounds, including baby,
placenta, and amniotic fluid

Source: Devan Design

fastest and most demanding growth period. Many growth processes that occur during these two critical periods happen at no other time in life; therefore, anything that interferes with this rapidly growing body could have lifelong consequences.

The development and growth of each organ, from the kidneys to the liver, and each tissue, from the muscles to the nerves, has its own pattern and timing independent of total body growth. Your baby's heart and brain are well developed in the first sixteen weeks, even though the lungs remain nonfunctional for months after that. During the first year, your baby's brain doubles in weight, but increases only 20 percent thereafter. Each organ and tissue needs the nutrients essential for growth and development during intensive growth spurts. Therefore, poor dietary intake at one point during your pregnancy might affect the heart, while at another time the nerves might be affected. Luckily, your body is very adaptable and will focus all of its efforts on building a beautiful baby, even if nausea or other pregnancy-related problems keep you from eating perfectly. Your goal during pregnancy is to eat as well as you can, when you can.

Cells and Critical Periods

Nutrition begins at the very foundation of your being: the cell. Organs and tissues are composed of specialized cells. The cells of the brain look, act, and respond differently from the cells of the muscles, liver, eyes, skin, or bones. The cells of each organ or tissue also have specific times for production and growth that do not correspond necessarily with the organ's growth cycle. For example, in the developing baby's brain there is an early stage when the cells increase dramatically in number. Each time a brain cell divides, it produces two cells that are half its original size. These two cells do not grow but, rather, divide again, producing four smaller cells. During this stage, the size of the brain does not increase, despite a substantial increase in cell numbers. It is only later, when the millions of new cells begin to grow in size while continuing to divide, that the size and number of brain cells increase and the brain grows larger and heavier.

It is during these two critical periods of development—the time of increasing cell number and the time of increasing cell size and number—that the total number of cells in the brain is determined for life. Later still, cell division stops and only the size of the existing cells continues to grow. This third stage, when the total number of brain cells is fixed and only size increases, is when the most intensive growth appears to be happening; actually, the most important events already have occurred. Because cell division is so rapid, an optimal supply of the vitamins, minerals, protein, and other essential tissue-building nutrients is needed every second during these critical periods. The importance of having all the essential nutrients available to the brain, or any other organ or tissue, during these critical periods cannot be overemphasized.

The stage of cell division in a particular organ or tissue is a "critical period" because the cell changes occurring at that time can take place *only* at that time. Poor nutrition during a critical period results in reduced numbers of cells in that organ or tissue, such as the heart, brain, or muscles. In contrast, poor nutrition throughout pregnancy results in a reduction in both number and size of cells (and possibly abnormal functioning of cells) in all the baby's organs and tissues, and in the placenta that nourishes the baby throughout the nine months.

Whatever vitamins, minerals, protein, fats, or other essential nutrients, as well as other environmental conditions, are needed during a critical period must be present and supplied in optimal amounts on time if the heart, brain, muscles, or any other organs or tissues are to reach their full potential. Granted, nausea and other pregnancy-related problems can keep you from eating perfectly every day of your pregnancy; however, if you eat an excellent diet prior to pregnancy so that you enter pregnancy with nutrient-packed tissues and then eat as well as you can throughout your pregnancy, your baby should receive all the vitamins, minerals, and other nutrients needed.

What Is an Optimal Intake?

Everyone agrees that nutrition is critical to the outcome of your pregnancy. An optimal supply of vitamins, minerals, water, protein, calories, and other essential dietary factors is needed every minute, every day, every week, throughout the nine months of your pregnancy. Determining these optimal levels of all the known vitamins, minerals, and other nutrients, however, is a more complicated matter.

The Recommended Dietary Allowances (RDAs)—suggested levels of intake for many of the vitamins and minerals—are the nutrient standards used in the United States. Established by the Food and Nutrition Board of the National Research Council, the RDAs provide dietary intake guidelines for calories; protein; the fat-soluble vitamins A, D, E, and K; the water-soluble B vitamins and vitamin C; and the minerals, including calcium, phosphorus, iodine, iron, magnesium, selenium, and zinc. An additional table of safe and adequate daily dietary intakes provides ranges of intakes for the B vitamins biotin and pantothenic acid, copper, manganese, fluoride, chromium, and molybdenum. Estimated minimal requirements also are set for sodium, potassium, and chloride. These recommendations are based on age, weight, height, gender, and whether or not you are pregnant or breast-feeding (see chapter 3).

The RDA for each nutrient is designed to meet or exceed most women's requirements for that nutrient. To ensure the nutritional needs of most people while preventing potential toxicities from overconsumption of a nutrient, the RDA for each nutrient has been set at what the Food and Nutrition Board considers a reasonable high point to meet or exceed the majority of people's nutrient needs. Theoretically, few people's requirements for any one nutrient would be above this recommendation. For example, the amount of vitamin C known to prevent scurvy is 10 mg, whereas the RDA for this water-soluble vitamin is set at 60 mg.

However, since not all functions were considered when the RDAs were set, some nutrition experts question the accuracy of some of the RDAs. For example, the role of vitamin E in heart disease was not considered when the RDA was established for this antioxidant nutrient; magnesium's roles in diabetes, hypertension, and heart disease were not included in setting the RDA for this mineral; and no RDA has been established for beta carotene alone, a potent antioxidant suspected to reduce cancer and heart disease risk. The latter is currently lumped with vitamin A, even though there is ample evidence that it often functions independent of its vitamin A activity.

The RDAs are not perfect, but unfortunately they are the only guidelines available. They were developed to aid meal planning for population groups (such as the army) and were never intended to be used as requirements for individuals or even families. They are designed to meet the known nutritional needs of a theoretical "reference" person—that is, the average woman or man with an average weight, body fat percentage, nutrient absorption and excretion rate, stress level, and heredity pattern. The reference woman is 5'4" to 5'5" tall, weighs between 128 and 138 pounds, requires about 2,200 calories per day, sleeps for eight hours, engages in two hours of light physical activity, sits for seven hours, stands for five hours, and walks for two hours each day.

No one is that reference person, since she is a composite representing an average woman in the United States. So for all practical purposes, the RDAs can be considered simply as estimates of an individual's nutrient needs. Many of the RDAs for pregnant women have been approximated from normal women's dietary intakes or from "typical" dietary intakes of pregnant women who appear healthy.

While people who are not pregnant have some room to experiment with different nutrient intakes, requirements of a woman considering or experiencing pregnancy are less flexible. The baby will be eating everything you eat, but is much more susceptible to nutrient toxicities. So during pregnancy, erring on the side of moderation is your best bet.

It is wise to strive for an average weekly dietary intake that meets about 100 percent, but no more than 300 percent, of the RDAs. While a little extra of any one nutrient won't hurt, excessive intake of several nutrients is known to be dangerous, can upset the delicate balance between nutrients, and can result in secondary deficiencies of other vitamins or minerals, even in temporary or permanent damage to your baby. Vitamins in large doses can act more like drugs than nutrients, and megadoses never should be taken if you are likely to become or already are pregnant. It is more realistic and safer to view nutrient needs as falling within a range of intakes between 100 and 300 percent of the RDA for any one nutrient. Danger zones are on either side of this range.

Beyond Nutrients

While everyone's attention is focused on which foods supply the minerals and vitamins essential for health, a much greater health benefit might come from the thousands of other nonnutritive substances called phytochemicals found in these foods.

Phytochemicals (*phyton* is the Greek word for "plant") are plants' natural protection against disease, sun damage, fungi, and bugs. But by the benevolent hand of Mother Nature, these chemicals also reduce disease risk and stimulate immunity in people. Every carrot stick, every sprig of parsley, every spear of broccoli is literally a bumper crop of disease-preventing chemicals.

Take, for example, the bioflavonoids, including rutin; the flavonones, herperidins, erioctrin, naringen, and naringenin; the flavones; and the flavonols. These phytochemicals, which are packed into citrus fruits, vegetables, and tea leaves, reduce blood clots associated with stroke and inhibit the oxidation of LDLs that turns harmless cholesterol in the blood into the sticky glue that clogs artery walls. They also stimulate the immune system, have antioxidant capabilities, and might strengthen blood vessel walls. In fact, the low incidence of heart disease in France might be caused by the high bioflavonoid content of the red wine consumed in that country.

Other phytochemicals in vegetables prevent or slow cancer growth. Broccoli is rich in sulforaphane—a compound that extradites cancer-causing compounds from cells and is linked to a reduced risk for breast cancer. Tomatoes contain two chemicals—p coumaric acid and chloragenic acid—that prevent the formation of carcinogens. Cabbage is loaded with phenethyl isothiocyanate (PEITC), which inhibits the growth of lung cancer. Ellagic acid in strawberries and grapes neutralizes carcinogens that otherwise attack the cell's DNA and initiate abnormal cell growth. Genistein in soybeans discourages the initiation and progression of cancer. The hundreds of carotenoids, of which beta carotene is only one, also have anticancer properties. The list is endless and is growing almost daily as researchers uncover more about these nonnutrients.

Other phytochemicals might protect against heart disease. Phytosterols, including beta sitosterol, stigmasterol, and campesterol, are found in wheat germ, seeds, nuts, and legumes. These compounds are plants' equivalent to cholesterol, except that they reduce, rather than promote, colon cancer risk and possibly heart disease. Plant sterols or other phytochemicals might be the reason blood cholesterol levels drop 40 percent in animals fed diets high in mushrooms.

While a clove of garlic supplies next to nothing when it comes to vitamins and minerals, it is a phytochemical gold mine. From its sulfur-containing compounds such as allicin and ajoene to the saponins and phenolic compounds, garlic has been linked to the prevention of cancer, heart disease, the common cold, and more. In garlic thirty phytochemicals alone have been isolated that help prevent cancer.

But Stephen DeFelice, M.D., chairman of the Foundation for Innovation in Medicine in New York, is cautious about making premature recommendations. "All of the research on phytochemicals is with animals. There are no clinical trials on people and without that, the entire subject remains theoretical." He also emphasizes that while eating more phytochemical-rich broccoli might help, and certainly won't hurt, it isn't a magic bullet; all the phytochemicals in the world won't neutralize the harmful effects of a high-fat diet, smoking, and other unhealthy habits. Granted, there is no scientific evidence that the phytochemicals are needed during pregnancy, but maintaining overall health by eating a wide variety of natural, wholesome foods should be a priority throughout life, especially when you are growing a baby.

Phytochemicals have spurred a wealth of new research and forced people to take a hard look at supplements. While you can get recommended amounts of any vitamin or mineral from supplements, never will a pill replace food when it comes to the phytochemicals. "All women should be taking moderate-dose multiples. Even if the only airtight proof that supplements are beneficial is with folic acid and its ability to prevent birth defects, that's reason enough to take the offensive," says Walter Willett, M.D., Dr.P.H., chairman of the Nutrition Department at Harvard School of Public Health. Of course, your best bet is to eat your broccoli, whole grains, and legumes along with a moderate-dose supplement with iron. Remember, at no other time in life does the well-being of an individual so directly depend on your well-being. When it comes to nutrition, don't settle for adequate. Go for the gold!

CHAPTER FIVE

Nutrition During the First Trimester

During the first three months of pregnancy:

1. Follow the guidelines outlined in the Baby-wise Diet as closely as possible or, in the case of serious morning sickness, eat when and what you can, but try to make it nutritious.

2. Try to limit weight gain to approximately two to five pounds (more if you entered pregnancy on the thin side, exercise intensely, or are tall, and less if you are short or were overweight and/or sedentary prior to pregnancy). Under no circumstances should you use this time to begin or continue a weight-loss diet.

3. Take a multiple vitamin and mineral supplement that contains 100 to 200 percent of the Reference Daily Intake for all vitamins and minerals plus at least 400 mcg of folic acid and 18 mg of iron each day.

4. Stop drinking alcohol, using tobacco, or taking any medication or drug not approved by your physician during pregnancy, if you have not already done so prior to pregnancy.

5. Discuss with your physician your prepregnancy exercise schedule and adjust as needed.

For some women the first trimester is a snap; for others, severe morning sickness makes it a nightmare. Most women fall somewhere in between with some fatigue, nausea, or changes in food habits. If this is your first pregnancy, you might as well enjoy the hormonal roller-coaster ride as your body generates physical and emotional cues that you may have trouble deciphering. If you've been through this first trimester before, the familiarity may help curb some of the symptoms and help you cope, but still expect some surprises.

This is a time to pamper yourself. If it feels good, do it. Take an afternoon nap, whether you are at home or at the office. Leave the dishes in the sink and relax. Let the lawn grow up to your knees while you soak in a warm (not hot!) bubble bath. Your body is adapting to an incredible upheaval in internal chemistry, so don't expect to conduct business as usual. You are producing a new life, so put your feet up when you can and revel in the process!

Weight Gain and Why

As mentioned before, pregnancy is not the time to diet. Weight gain during pregnancy is a clear and direct indicator of how you and your baby will fare, and even whether or not your baby will survive. An optimal weight gain in the mother is associated with an optimal weight gain in the baby. If you don't gain enough weight, your baby is likely to be underweight, too.

A small woman is likely to have a small yet healthy baby, so don't be alarmed by that last statement. However, usually the body weight of a full-term baby reflects nutritional health or the nutritional environment in which the baby developed. So a normal-weight baby is most likely to be a healthy baby, while an underweight baby is most likely to be a malnourished one.

Why You Should Take Weight Gain Seriously

Women who do not gain enough weight are more likely to have premature babies. In addition, birth is more likely to be complicated by problems during delivery when the baby is small than if the baby is at least 6½ pounds. Ironically, these low-birth-weight (LBW) babies (also called growth-retarded or small-for-date babies to distinguish them from premature babies) also are more likely to battle weight problems later in life, perhaps because the early malnutrition interferes with the development of that portion of the brain that controls appetite and food intake. In addition, LBW infants often have smaller organs, such as the liver, and they might have abnormal blood sugar regulation, higher blood fat levels, and elevated levels of the stress hormones. LBW babies also are more likely to develop heart disease and diabetes when they grow up.

About one in every fifteen full-term babies born in the United States is considered low birth weight, and one fourth of these babies die within the first months of life. Half of all deaths in children less than five years old are linked to low birth weight and inadequate nutrition during the developing months. Low birth weight is associated with increased risk for mental retardation, cerebral palsy, and epilepsy, probably because of the reduced availability of nutrients and oxygen to the brain during critical periods of development.

In addition, LBW babies are more frequently hospitalized for illness and have more eye and hearing disorders, more behavior problems, and more learning disabilities when they start school than do normal-weight babies. These problems are easily prevented with good nutrition prior to and during pregnancy, adequate weight gain during pregnancy, regular physician visits, and avoidance of the toxic substances also associated with low birth weight, including tobacco smoke, alcohol, and drugs.

Optimal Weight Gain

Optimal weight gain is an individual matter; however, in general, most experts agree that a normal-weight woman should gain about twenty-five to thirty-five pounds during her pregnancy. But don't get carried away. Further weight gain beyond recommended amounts will not make bigger or healthier babies; it will make regaining your figure more difficult after delivery and could increase your risk of a long-term weight problem. In fact, normal-weight women who gain more than the twenty-five to thirty-five pounds during pregnancy are more likely to struggle with five to six pounds of extra weight for months or years after the baby is born compared to normal-weight women who gain only the recommended weight.

Weight gain during the first half of pregnancy is very important to pregnancy outcome. In a study conducted at the University of Michigan in Ann Arbor, the researchers found that optimal weight gain at twenty weeks' gestation was positively related to both the length of pregnancy (these women were less likely to deliver prematurely) and birth weight. One half of the infants who weighed less than six pounds at birth were born to mothers who had gained fewer than ten pounds by the twentieth week of pregnancy, while there were no LBW infants born to women who gained at least this much weight. Thus, it is not just total weight gain but the pattern of weight gain that is important—with a slow gain in the first trimester of about two to five pounds total (more if you are thin, very active, or tall and less if you are overweight, sedentary, or short), followed by a steady increase to approximately three quarters to one pound a week in the last two trimesters.

The exercising woman might gain more. "If you are leaner to start with," says Lindsay Allen, Ph.D., professor of nutrition at the University of California, Davis, "expect to gain more weight." Weight-conscious women often are distressed when they gain what they feel is too much weight. "These women shouldn't fight it. The weight gain is perfectly natural and will drop off after a woman stops breast-feeding," says Dr. Allen. According to the National Academy of Sciences and the Institute of Medicine, underweight women should gain approximately twenty-eight to forty pounds depending on their height and degree of leanness prior to pregnancy.

Dieting is never recommended during pregnancy, even if a woman is obese. Women who are overweight (more than 25 percent of body weight is fat tissue) should gain no more than fifteen to twenty-five pounds during their pregnancies. Better yet, women who are obese should lose weight prior to conception, since obesity is associated with preterm deliveries and increased health and delivery risks for both the mother and baby. (See "Monitoring Your Weight Gain," page 129.)

When and What to Eat and Drink

The guidelines for the Baby-wise Diet are simple and easy to follow. You still can eat your favorite foods, enjoy your favorite recipes, and go to your favorite restaurants; just make sure you first eat the number of nutritious foods in the Baby-wise Diet. Basically, you should consume a diet similar to your prepregnancy diet, or at least:

> 2 servings from the Calcium-Rich Group
> 5 servings from the Vegetable Group—at least 2 servings should be folic acid–rich choices

Monitoring Your Weight Gain

The following chart allows you to compare your weight gain during pregnancy to average gains for women who are underweight, normal weight, and overweight at the onset of pregnancy. The right-hand table provides space for you to monitor your weight after each weigh-in during routine physician visits and jot down notes, comments, or thoughts about your weight-gain progress.

Prepregnancy Underweight (. . . . . .), Prepregnancy Normal Body Weight (- - - - -), Prepregnancy Overweight (— — —)

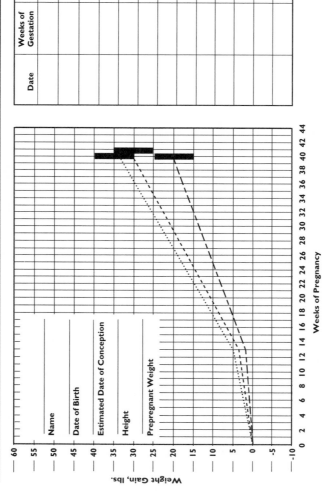

Date	Weeks of Gestation	Weight	Notes

Name _____

Date of Birth _____

Estimated Date of Conception _____

Height _____

Prepregnant Weight _____

Weight Gain, lbs.

60 — 55 — 50 — 45 — 40 — 35 — 30 — 25 — 20 — 15 — 10 — 5 — 0 — -5 — -10

0 2 4 6 8 10 12 14 16 18 20 22 24 26 28 30 32 34 36 38 40 42 44

Weeks of Pregnancy

Reprinted with permission from *Nutrition During Pregnancy and Lactation: An Implementation Guide*. Copyright 1992 by the National Academy of Sciences. Courtesy of the National Academy Press, Washington, D.C.

3 servings from the Fruit Group—at least 2 servings
   should be vitamin C–rich choices
6 servings from the Grains Group—at least 4 servings
   should be whole-grain choices
2 servings from the Extra-Lean Meats and Legumes
   Group—try to include 2 to 3 servings of fish and 4
   to 5 servings of legumes in the weekly menu
5 servings from the Quenchers Group

Now you can eat all you want, right? Not quite. It takes about 55,000 calories to complete a successful pregnancy; that's about 200 calories a day above an average woman's normal calorie intake. However, the energy costs during the first trimester are minimal. Consequently, your daily energy needs during the first trimester are the same as they were before pregnancy, and they increase by only 100 to 300 calories during the second and third trimester, with an average of 2,200 calories during prepregnancy and the first trimester and 2,500 calories for the remaining two trimesters. (Keep in mind that calorie needs vary greatly from one pregnant woman to the next.) Your best indicator of how much you can eat is the scale; if you are eating the right number of calories you will gain weight in a pattern that approximates that in the chart on page 129, while too little food means you'll gain too little weight and too much food will cause too rapid a weight gain.

National nutrition studies show that many pregnant women eat much less than the recommended 2,200 to 2,500 calories, with intakes during the first trimester averaging 1,616 calories and during the last two trimesters as little as 1,830 calories, or 73 percent of the recommended calorie intake. This might be one reason the United States rates so poorly in comparison to other countries when it comes to infant mortality rates. Women need to eat more (nutritious food, that is) and move more during pregnancy to ensure both optimal nutrition and weight gain.

While energy needs remain the same during the first trimester, vitamin and mineral needs are high from conception to delivery; consequently, during the first three months of pregnancy you must consume more nutrients for the same amount of food and calorie intake, which means making every bite count. That is why the Baby-wise Diet is packed with nutrient-dense, low-calorie foods; this ensures that every calorie supplies a whopping dose of nutrients. In contrast, a high-fat or high-sugar diet that contains too many processed foods supplies few vitamins and minerals per calorie and is called "nutrient poor."

The dietary guidelines and menus outlined in this book are just the beginning if you exercise during pregnancy. You might require calorie intakes of up to 3,000 calories or more, depending on how often and how hard you exercise. You should take extra precautions to eat enough food to maintain a steady weight gain. "If you are leaner to start with, you must eat enough and gain enough to avoid having a low-birth-weight baby," cautions Dr. Allen.

Supplements: The Right Dose During Pregnancy

For all vitamins and minerals, there are daily intakes below which symptoms of deficiency are likely to occur and above which symptoms of excess might occur. The trick is finding a happy medium. While pregnancy is no time to be experimenting with megadoses of vitamin or mineral supplements, marginal deficiencies, which are suspected to be common in many developed countries, also must be avoided.

For example, in a study conducted by the U.S. Department of Agriculture, only 6 percent of women consumed RDA levels of vitamin B6 before and during pregnancy. Babies born to mothers who did not eat well during pregnancy also were low in many nutrients, including vitamins A, E, K, and B2; folic acid; and the minerals iron, copper, calcium, and zinc. This poor nutritional status predisposes the infant to a variety of illnesses, from tumors, anemia, and poor digestive function to impaired brain function, suppressed immunity, and poor bone formation.

Although many experts avoid recommending supplements, national nutrition surveys repeatedly report that women do not get their fair share of many vitamins and minerals. Bonnie Worthington-Roberts, Ph.D., professor of nutritional science at the University of Washington in Seattle, says, "There are so many women counting calories that it often is difficult to squeeze in enough of all the nutrients, even if food choices are good. So why not play it safe and take a moderate-dose multiple vitamin and mineral?"

The stakes are even higher with folic acid. The current consensus that only high-risk women who have given birth to babies with neural tube defects (NTD) should supplement with folic acid is changing. "Many women who have NTD babies don't know they are at risk. Rather than take the chance, it is likely these recommendations will change in the future to favor a 400 to 800 mcg folic acid supplement for all women prior to and during pregnancy," says Dr. Worthington-Roberts.

Repeatedly, studies show that women who supplement sensibly have a better chance of maintaining optimal nutritional status and giving birth to healthy babies. In fact, some studies conclude that women must supplement in moderation to maintain optimal blood and tissue levels of nutrients. From early studies showing that iodine supplementation virtually eradicated the mental and physical retardation characteristic of cretinism to the more recent findings that folic acid taken prior to and following conception can dramatically reduce the risk for having a baby with a neural tube defect, responsible supplementation has proved worth more than its weight in gold.

For example, women who supplement tend to have fewer low-birth-weight infants than do women who don't supplement. In particular, zinc supplementation reduces the risk for abnormal development and pregnancy complications. Magnesium supplementation decreases pregnancy complications and improves infant development. Calcium supplementation reduces the incidence of high blood pressure and might improve skeletal development in the baby. Mothers who supplement with fluoride or drink fluoridated water have children who are resistant to dental caries throughout life. While supplementation is especially important for some women, including women who are strict vegetarians (especially with vitamin B12, calcium, vitamin D, zinc, and iron), lactose intolerant (especially with vitamin D, calcium, and vitamin B2), carrying more than one baby, who smoke, or adolescent girls who are pregnant, most women before, during, and following pregnancy probably would benefit from a well-balanced multiple vitamin and mineral supplement.

On the other hand, taking single-dose supplements or poorly balanced multiples can give a false sense of security and might do more harm than good. The minerals are a good example of why moderation and balance are key in choosing a supplement. Minerals often compete for absorption or use in the body. Supplementing with one without also increasing the intake of other minerals can result in upsets in availability and secondary deficiencies. Iron, zinc, and copper are examples of minerals that compete, so taking a supplement of one means you should also increase your intake of the other minerals.

The secret to supplementation is to do it sensibly. For a healthy woman, a multiple vitamin and mineral supplement is best. A multiple is a convenient, cost-efficient way to supply a balance of nutrients while avoiding secondary deficiencies that result when you take too much of one nutrient and crowd out another. In general, 100 to 200 percent of the Reference Daily Intake, or RDI (the nutrient standard used on supplement labels), for a nutrient is sufficient.

One exception to this rule is iron, which your physician may recommend in amounts up to 60 mg. While large doses of iron can cause constipation or diarrhea in some women, an iron supplement that contains both heme iron (iron in the form found in animal sources) and nonheme iron (plant-derived iron) might have fewer side effects. In addition, taking iron supplements in small doses throughout the day or starting the supplement program by taking a small dose and gradually increasing the amount can help offset digestive-tract problems. Ideally, take your iron supplements on an empty stomach with orange or grapefruit juice, because the vitamin C will help boost the absorption of this mineral. Do not take them with coffee, tea, or milk, which interfere with iron absorption.

Megavitamin-mineral therapy—consuming ten times or more of the RDI—implies that more is better, but it usually is a waste of money and could be harmful to your baby. The body can use only so much of any one nutrient. At best, excesses are excreted; at worst, they are stored to potentially toxic levels. In some cases, such as zinc, consuming too much can backfire. While a little zinc enhances the body's immune system and defense against disease, too much might suppress immunity.

Most one-dose multiples, however, don't contain enough calcium or magnesium. So unless you consume at least three servings daily of calcium-rich milk products and lots of magnesium-rich soybeans, nuts, and wheat germ, you might consider an extra supplement of these two minerals. If you choose to take a calcium supplement, you also should increase your intake of magnesium to a ratio of approximately 1.5 to 2 parts calcium to every 1 part magnesium (for example, 1,000 mg of calcium and 500 mg magnesium). The dose is best utilized when divided into several small doses daily, since the body can effectively digest and absorb only approximately 100 mg of magnesium at a time. When it comes to calcium, your best bets are calcium carbonate and calcium citrate. Avoid "natural" calcium sources, such as oyster-shell calcium and bone meal, since these supplements may contain lead and other toxic metals.

While a moderate-dose vitamin and mineral supplement with extra iron and folic acid might provide nutritional insurance for many women, excessive intake of nutrients is dangerous during pregnancy. Megadoses of nutrients such as vitamin A, vitamin C, selenium, or fluoride can produce numerous side effects ranging in severity from mottled teeth to birth defects. In addition, there is always the concern that a supplement will provide a false sense of security, reducing a woman's concern about her dietary practices, which could result in poor food intake and possibly marginal intake of health-enhancing substances not found in supplements. This fear has not been supported by research, however, which shows that most people tend to eat better, not worse, when they take supplements. In all cases, consult your physician before taking a supplement during pregnancy.

Of course, the best alternative is to consume a good diet plus a moderate-dose multiple vitamin and mineral, since this would cover all of your nutritional bases. The payoff is worth it. In one study, mothers whose diets were considered good to excellent gave birth 94 percent of the time to babies who were in superior health. In contrast, mothers who ate poorly during pregnancy gave birth to infants in good health only 8 percent of the time. Other studies have found the same link between diet and pregnancy outcome. According to Walter Willett, M.D., Dr.P.H., chairman of the Nutrition Department at Harvard School of Public Health, "Almost all women should be taking moderate-dose multiples. Even if the only airtight proof that supplements are beneficial is with folic acid and its ability to prevent birth defects, that's reason enough to take the offensive" (see Table 5.1).

Skin and Hair Changes: Can Diet Help?

Skin and hair are sensitive indicators of your nutritional status. Healthy hair that is shiny, lustrous, firm, not easily plucked, and with a healthy scalp and skin that is smooth, slightly moist, and has good color are outward signs of good nutrition. In contrast, dull, brittle, dry, thin and sparse, or easily plucked hair or rough, dry, scaly, pale, or bruised skin are common signals that, nutritionally speaking, something is wrong.

Although most of the physical changes during pregnancy happen deep inside your cells, tissues, and organs, other signs are only skin deep. In some cases these changes are for the better, as in the case of the pregnancy glow that some women develop, which is caused by increased blood flow to the skin. In other cases, raging hormones wreak havoc with the skin's oil-producing glands, causing the

Table 5.1   A Sample Prenatal Supplement

The following is an example of an ideal vitamin and mineral supplement. This supplement would provide all the vitamins and minerals in optimal amounts and would maximize the absorption of these nutrients. However, it must be taken in several small doses throughout the day so that three to six tablets would total the RDI amounts listed in the right-hand column. If you choose a one-a-day multiple, check the label for the amount of calcium and magnesium and consider taking a second supplement of these minerals if the multiple contains less than 100 percent of the RDI.

NUTRIENT	AMOUNT	% RDI
Vitamin A	800 RE*	100
Beta carotene	10 mg	NA
Vitamin D	10 mcg	100
Vitamin E	20 mg	200
Vitamin B1	1.5 mg	100
Vitamin B2	1.6 mg	100
Niacin	17 mg	100
Vitamin B6	2.2 mg	100
Folic acid	400 mcg	100
Vitamin B12	2.2 mcg	100
Vitamin C	70 mg	100
Calcium	1,000 mg	83
Chromium	100 mcg	**
Copper	1.5 mg	**
Fluoride	2.0 mg	**
Iodine	175 mcg	100
Iron	30–60 mg†	100–200
Magnesium	320 mg	100
Molybdenum	100 mcg	**
Selenium	65 mcg	100
Zinc	15 mg	100

*RE: Retinol Equivalents; 1 RE = 1 mcg of retinol or 6 mcg of beta carotene.
**No RDI has been set for these nutrients. Amounts given are within the range considered safe and adequate.
†Iron in amounts greater than 18 mg should be approved by a physician. The amount of supplemental iron often is high because this form of iron is poorly absorbed.

complexion to take on an adolescent look akin to acne. In addition, other skin and hair changes are a direct result of lifestyle or nutrition, such as in the case of pale skin that is a common symptom of iron deficiency or dry, scaly skin that might indicate too little linoleic acid (an essential fatty acid) in the diet. There is nothing you can do about the hormonal changes and, unfortunately, rubbing vitamin E on your skin has not proved very effective in preventing stretch marks. But you can prevent any skin or hair condition related to a nutrient deficiency and, by maintaining a healthier inside, you will automatically foster a healthier outside.

Skin from Within

All nutrients, including protein, calories, fat, vitamins, minerals, and water, play important roles in maintaining healthy skin. For example, the skin relies on the bloodstream to supply oxygen and nutrients and to remove waste products of cellular metabolism. Nutrients essential to the maintenance of red blood cells (the oxygen carriers in the blood) and other blood components include protein, iron, folic acid and other B vitamins, copper, vitamin C, selenium, and vitamin E. An inadequate supply of one or more of these nutrients essentially stops the supply of oxygen and nutrients to the skin, while allowing potentially toxic waste products to accumulate.

Other nutrients directly affect the health of the skin. For example, an essential fat in vegetable oils called linoleic acid helps maintain smooth, moist skin. Skin becomes dry and scaly when the diet is low in this fat. A linoleic acid deficiency might be one reason why women experience dry, itchy skin when on very-low-calorie diets for prolonged periods of time. The condition is reversed within days of adding linoleic acid–rich foods, such as safflower oil, nuts, and seeds, to the diet.

Another example is vitamin C. This vitamin is essential for collagen formation, the "glue" that holds the body's cells together. When vitamin C intake is inadequate, collagen is poorly formed, the body bruises easily, skin loses its elasticity, cuts heal slowly, and the skin does not produce adequate amounts of lubricating oils. A glass of orange juice and a bowl of strawberries each day provide more than the recommended amount of vitamin C, yet many national nutrition surveys report that typical American diets are low in this vitamin (see Table 5.2).

The mask of pregnancy—those patchy brown spots on the cheeks, forehead, and upper lip—is caused by an overproduction of pigment, possibly triggered by hormonal changes during pregnancy. Technically called melasma, this skin

Table 5.2   The Nutrition and Healthy Skin Connection

All nutrients are related to healthy skin. Here are a few examples why.

NUTRIENT	SKIN CONNECTION	SOURCE
Protein	Maintains underlying muscles and skin structure, elasticity, resiliency; maintains hormones that regulate skin moisture; regulates skin pigments	Milk, meat, fish, chicken, legumes
Fat	Essential fatty acid maintains skin moisture. Deficiency results in scaly, dry skin	Safflower oil, nuts, seeds, whole grains
Water	Maintains skin moisture; helps maintain normal oil secretion	Water
Vitamin B2	Deficiency causes blisters and cracks at the corner of the mouth, oily and flaky skin	Milk, dark green veggies, mushrooms
Niacin	Deficiency causes dermatitis	Chicken, peanut butter, green peas
Vitamin B6	Deficiency causes itching, dry skin; anemia	Banana, meat, fish, chicken
Folic acid	Deficiency causes anemia; pale skin	Dark green veggies; orange juice
Vitamin B12	Deficiency causes anemia; pale skin	Milk, meat, fish, chicken
Pantothenic acid	Deficiency causes dry, flaky skin	Milk, chicken, peanut butter, veggies, rice
Vitamin C	Maintains oil-producing glands, collagen, skin elasticity and resiliency; antioxidant against premature aging and skin cancer	Citrus fruits, veggies
Vitamin A (beta carotene)	Maintains outer layer of skin; protects against skin cancer and premature aging	Dark green and orange veggies

(continued)

Table 5.2   The Nutrition and Healthy Skin Connection *(continued)*

NUTRIENT	SKIN CONNECTION	SOURCE
Vitamin E	Antioxidant against premature aging and skin cancer	Safflower oil, nuts, wheat germ
Copper	Prevents anemia	Oysters, avocado, potato, fish, soybeans
Iron	Prevents anemia	Dark green veggies, red meat, legumes, dried apricots
Selenium	Antioxidant against skin cancer	Organ meats, seafood, whole grains
Zinc	Maintains collagen and elastin; might prevent stretch marks; helps heal cuts; deficiency causes dry, rough skin	Oysters, turkey, pork, wheat germ

condition affects up to 75 percent of pregnant women. Melasma that affects the outer layers of the skin, called the epidermal, is sometimes treatable with bleaching creams. Avoiding sun exposure by using hats and sunblock creams also helps prevent these dark patches.

Be good to your skin from the outside, too. Warm baths, lotions, and creams can keep your skin moist and soft. However, avoid hot tubs, saunas, and a soak in a hot bath during pregnancy, since this can raise body temperature and increase the odds of having a baby with a defect of the brain and spinal cord. In one study, researchers found that infants born to mothers who had used a hot tub were 2.8 times more likely to have these defects than babies with no heat exposure.

Healthy Hair

A low-fat, balanced diet rich in several key nutrients is essential for the growth and life of shiny, strong hair. Hair grows from follicles, which are tiny sacs imbedded in the scalp that are fed by the bloodstream. The blood provides a constant supply of oxygen and nutrients and helps remove waste products from each hair shaft and its follicle. Therefore, a diet packed with the nutrients that promote circulation and hair growth, such as protein and several vitamins and minerals, is the first step in maintaining a healthy head of hair.

Because healthy hair is a reflection of a healthy body, all nutrients are essential for maintaining hair. For example, vitamin A helps the hair stay supple and the scalp healthy. The B-complex vitamins are crucial for maintaining circulation and hair growth and color. Vitamin C is essential for strong, supple strands of hair that do not break or split. A biotin deficiency also can cause hair loss; however, this is rare and seldom seen in pregnant women.

Important minerals for healthy hair include iron, copper, and zinc. For example, the oxygen-carrying capacity of the blood depends on iron and copper. Inadequate amounts of iron can leave the hair and its follicles oxygen starved, while optimal iron intake and red blood cell levels allow a steady and ample supply of oxygen to reach all tissues, including the scalp and hair. Copper also helps in the formation of the hair pigment, while zinc is important in building proteins in the hair and preventing diet-related hair loss. All of these nutrients are supplied in ample amounts in the Baby-wise Diet.

Water is the forgotten nutrient when it comes to both skin and hair. Almost a quarter of the weight of a strand of hair comes from the water locked inside it. This moisture provides suppleness to hair and moisture to the skin. In addition, the bloodstream is a watery medium that constantly needs replenishing to ensure proper circulation of the nutrients and oxygen and to remove the waste products from the scalp, hair follicle, and skin. If you meet your quota for Quenchers in the Baby-wise Diet, you will be getting enough fluid. On the other hand, coffee, tea, and caffeinated soda pop act more like diuretics and dehydrate the skin and hair.

The health of your hair starts from within, but also depends on how the hair is treated from the surface, including washing, drying, and other daily hair-care practices. If you shampoo daily, use warm water and a gentle shampoo that does not contain detergents; use one application; and dilute the shampoo by half.

Brushing the hair stimulates circulation to the scalp, detangles the hair, and distributes beneficial oils from the scalp down the length of the hair. Avoid brushing the hair when it is wet and limit the use of hair blowers and curling irons, which can leave hair dull, dry, and brittle.

Hair is susceptible to stress. Emotional stress causes the muscles in the scalp and neck to tense and restrict blood flow, which leaves hair deprived of oxygen and nutrients and interferes with the removal of waste products from the follicle. The stress of pregnancy and the fluctuations in hormone levels may result in hair loss. Don't worry; the loss is usually temporary. Environmental stress, such as sun, wind, or salt water, can leave hair dry, split, and lackluster. Some of these stresses can be avoided, for example, by wearing a hat in the sun, protecting the hair from wind, and washing the hair after exposure to salt water. To minimize damage from unavoidable emotional or life event stresses, it is helpful to improve the blood flow and nutrients available to the hair.

A Nutritional Approach to Common Problems: From Morning Sickness to Fatigue

With the first trimester comes a unique set of problems that can interfere with making the best food choices. Nausea and vomiting sometimes surface in the initial weeks of pregnancy and can foil even the best diet intentions. Chronic or severe fatigue can make even breathing an effort, let alone sitting down to a meal. While you may not be able to avoid these problems altogether, the good news is that they usually subside by the end of the first trimester. You also can lessen their severity with a few diet and lifestyle tricks of the trade.

Morning Sickness

At a time when many women should be concerned about eating well for two, they find they cannot even eat poorly for one. The condition is called morning sickness. At best, it is a nuisance; at worst, it can disrupt your life, your health, and even jeopardize your baby. It also is a time to bag the rule book on nutrition and eat what works—that is, find foods that go down without coming back up.

Despite four thousand years of recorded reports of nausea and vomiting during pregnancy, this condition remains a mystery. Researchers estimate that between

50 and 90 percent of women experience some degree of morning sickness during at least one of their pregnancies. Each year in the United States at least 55,000 women experience morning sickness so severe it results in hospitalization.

These numbers, however, may not be accurate, according to Miriam Erick, M.S., R.D., obstetrical clinical dietitian at Brigham and Women's Hospital in Boston and author of *No More Morning Sickness*. "We record only those women who are admitted to the hospital; there are likely many more women who come into the Emergency Room or who stay home and suffer through it."

Regardless of the exact numbers, the underlying message is that a woman who experiences any degree of morning sickness, from temporary queasiness to severe vomiting, is not alone. More important, despite the discomfort and inconvenience, a woman should not be too concerned about how her bouts of nausea will affect the developing baby. The Subcommittee on Nutritional Status and Weight Gain During Pregnancy of the Institute of Medicine reports that "[morning sickness] has been associated with favorable pregnancy outcomes."

You don't need to explain morning sickness to most women who have been pregnant. Just mentioning the term brings back all the miserable sensations. The primary symptom is nausea that may or may not be accompanied by vomiting, cold intolerance, and fatigue. Despite the name, morning sickness can strike any time of the day or night. In severe cases, called hyperemesis gravidarum, the severe vomiting can cause dehydration, imbalances in electrolytes, high ketone levels in the urine, and other potentially life-threatening disorders that require hospitalization.

A woman in her first trimester is the most likely candidate, with approximately 40 percent of women reporting that morning sickness stopped suddenly toward the end of the first trimester. However, some women are still nauseated while they are in labor; and some experience nausea with all, some, or none of their pregnancies. The only absolute rule is that there are no reported cases of morning sickness lasting after delivery.

No one knows what causes morning sickness, although there are many theories. A common one is that morning sickness is brought on by changes in hormone levels, such as human chorionic gonadotropin (HCG), the hormone that indicates pregnancy in blood and urine tests. HCG levels are high during the first trimester, which correlates with the rise and fall of morning sickness in some women. Rising estrogen levels or slowed stomach emptying have also been blamed, while another theory points to the degenerative products given off by the fertilized egg implanting in the uterine lining. A research team in Sweden even postulates that it is only when the left ovary is firing that troubles arise.

Of course, emotional and psychological factors cannot be ruled out. Stress sets off bouts of morning sickness, while a restful environment often helps curb the nausea. Even hearing about an offensive food can make some pregnant women sick. Some nausea may become a learned response, an idea supported by testimonies from mothers who say they experience the same symptoms of morning sickness, but to a lesser degree, after pregnancy if they listen to music they repeatedly heard when they were pregnant. The knowledge that your body is going to change radically for several months can be distressing if you have worked hard to stay in control of your figure and fitness. For the working woman, the unpredictability and social taboo of nausea and vomiting can be devastating.

Regardless of the cause, morning sickness is real. It does not reflect a lack of control, a neurotic personality, or a woman with misgivings about her womanhood, her pregnancy, or her baby. It requires support and encouragement, and a tool kit of strategies for getting through the storm.

THE TRADITIONAL APPROACH: Most women with morning sickness turn to dry or bland foods. Lindsay Allen, Ph.D., professor of nutritional sciences at University of Connecticut, recommends that "for mild cases of morning sickness, a woman should keep crackers or dry cereal with her or by her bed and nibble before she gets out of bed in the morning and throughout the day. This will help her avoid hunger and keep something in her stomach." Dr. Allen also recommends avoiding coffee, tea, or spicy or acidic foods. Other traditional recommendations include eating small, frequent meals and avoiding fatty or overly rich foods.

Carol Archie, M.D., assistant professor in the Department of Obstetrics and Gynecology at UCLA Medical Center, says, "I don't worry about whether a woman gains weight in the first trimester, as long as she stays hydrated." Frequent, small meals that avoid overdistending the stomach might help. Eating when you can and trying to eat nutritious foods when possible also are basic survival skills recommended by all experts. (See "The Traditional Approach," page 143.)

MODERN METHODS: Although the recommendations above work for some women, they are not universal truths. Even though seven out of every ten women use crackers in an attempt to feel "less horrible," many find little solace. Miriam

The Traditional Approach

There are no hard-and-fast rules for morning sickness, since effective treatments are as diverse as the women who use them. The first line of defense is to try the traditional approach, which includes the following:

1. Keep crackers, vanilla wafers, or dry cereal (such as Shredded Wheat bite-size biscuits) by the bed and eat a few before getting up in the morning; nibble on them throughout the day; and keep them handy in an office desk drawer, a glove compartment, or a purse or briefcase. Eat breakfast after nausea subsides.
2. Eat at least every two hours to avoid hunger and keep something in your stomach at all times.
3. Eat a high-protein snack at bedtime.
4. Avoid fatigue.
5. Get up slowly (sudden movements can trigger nausea).
6. Have fresh air in the room when sleeping.
7. Avoid offensive cooking odors.
8. Have beverages and soup between meals.
9. Use fruit juices mixed with carbonated beverages to settle an upset stomach between meals.
10. Drink fluids to avoid dehydration. Eat when and what you can.
11. Have someone else cook the meals.
12. Eat before you feel queasy.
13. Take a well-balanced, moderate-dose vitamin and mineral supplement for nutritional insurance.

Always consult your physician if morning sickness is disrupting your normal routine, since some cases of nausea during pregnancy can be a symptom of other medical problems. In addition, some antinausea medications are relatively safe for pregnant women experiencing severe nausea. Consult your physician about the options.

Erick recommends a more personalized and systematic approach to morning sickness.

"I have women take a good look at what foods sound good at the time and then trust their feelings, no matter how bizarre," says Ms. Erick. During periods when the nausea is at bay (that is, no lower than 3 on a scale of 1 to 10, with 10 being feeling fine), ask yourself questions such as "What foods would make the nausea less worse—salty? sugary? liquid? dry? hot? cold? spicy? bland? soft? hard? Would a crunchy food settle my stomach?" If yes, "What color or flavor should it have? What food or beverage, no matter how silly, would have the most appeal right now?"

Also ask yourself what time of day you are most nauseated or if there is a situation, person, or place that triggers nausea. Then avoid these situations at all costs. (Don't worry about hurting someone's feelings by asking them not to wear that perfume or aftershave lotion.) Identify what places are most pleasurable to eat and eat there. Finally, when you feel your worst, what food, if presented instantaneously, would help you feel better? The results may surprise you. One woman decided that crunchy, cold, and sour foods sounded good and found she could tolerate raw carrots dipped in vinegar. Once she had eaten this "Band-Aid" food, she then could tolerate eating a few other foods. Fresh ginger also might be helpful, since it has reduced symptoms of morning sickness in some women. (See "Modern Methods," page 145.)

Although many other factors can be trigger events for a bout of nausea—such as loud noises, quick movements, bright lights, hot or humid weather, and low-level claustrophobia—the most common and powerful trigger may be smell. "I found that smells are what drive most women over the edge," says Ms. Erick. But if women use smell to their advantage, they can work with the morning sickness to find what breaks the nausea cycle.

A woman's "sniff acuity" is heightened during pregnancy, possibly because of elevated estrogen levels, a hormone that regulates smell. She can smell cigarette smoke from the car ahead of her on the freeway and "roasted dust" from the heater. The smell of boiling ham hocks, frying onions, or mildew can bring her to her knees. The best indicator of both a "hazardous" or a "safe" food is smell. If a food doesn't smell good, it probably won't settle well, while a food that smells good—or at least doesn't smell bad, no matter how unusual—may be the food that stays down. "This is where my recommendations may seem like heresy," says Ms. Erick, who gives hospitalized women with severe morning sickness whatever they want to eat. "The traditional bland foods recommended for morning sickness, such as crackers and broth, don't always work. So go with the flow. If spicy spaghetti with meatballs sounds good, give it a try." Keep in mind that what smells or sounds good to one pregnant woman may trigger nausea in another, so take all your friends' advice with an open mind and a grain of salt.

Modern Methods: Weathering Nausea

Weathering nausea during the first trimester might be as simple as identifying what types of foods sound appetizing (or at least tolerable!). The following list is a brief summary of the types of food characteristics that might soothe your upset stomach.

- *Cold:* ice cream, sherbet, Popsicles, frozen fruit juice (freeze in ice cube trays), or frozen grapes
- *Warm:* hot potato salad, mashed potatoes and gravy, soup, or cinnamon toast
- *Spicy:* Spicy Carrots (see Recipes, page 286), salsa, gingerbread, or curried dishes
- *Sour:* Lemons, limes, lemonade, grapefruit, or grapefruit juice
- *Creamy:* Whole milk, creamed soups, custard-style yogurt, or pudding
- *Crunchy:* Raw carrots, apple slices, oven-baked tortilla chips, raw celery sticks, or almonds
- *Soft:* Angel food cake, mashed potatoes, cottage cheese, or cooked carrots
- *Wet:* Milk, fruit juice, water, Jell-O, or broth
- *Salty:* Pretzels, oven-baked potato chips, chips and dip, pizza, or V-8 juice
- *Chocolate:* Pudding, milk, fresh fruit dipped in chocolate syrup, or graham crackers dipped lightly in chocolate

Another modern treatment for morning sickness that is effective for some women is the "acupressure" wrist bands that are used by passengers on planes and boats to help prevent motion sickness. A high-tech version of this, called the sensory afferent stimulating (SAS) unit, is worn like a wristwatch and delivers a continuous current directly to the site over which it is worn. Researchers at the University of California, Davis, report that 87 percent of the women they tested reported improvements in symptoms (although 43 percent of the control group who wore a placebo wristband also said they felt better). Some women also report that acupuncture significantly reduces the frequency of morning sickness.

What About Vitamin B6?

For the tens of thousands of women who battle morning sickness each year, the thought that a cure is as simple as popping a pill seems too good to be true. Since the 1940s, vitamin B6 has been called the morning-sickness vitamin, although the vitamin's effectiveness is questionable.

The early studies reported that daily doses of vitamin B6 ranging up to 100 mg curbed nausea and vomiting in pregnant women. Unfortunately, these studies were poorly designed and the effect has since been attributed to the placebo effect (an improvement in a patient's condition resulting from a belief that the treatment will work, rather than attributable to the treatment itself). Later studies showed that both vitamin B6 and a placebo reduced the symptoms of morning sickness.

Granted, the vitamin B6 status declines in the pregnant woman and it takes two to five times normal intakes to keep blood levels at prepregnancy concentrations. On the other hand, it is questionable whether the pregnancy state should match the nonpregnancy state, while the amount theorized to prevent morning sickness is fifty, not five, times the recommended amounts.

On the other hand, limited evidence shows that a multiple vitamin and mineral supplement that includes a moderate dose of vitamin B6 might help soothe nausea. Andrew Czeizel, M.D., director of the Department of Human Genetics and Teratology at the National Institute of Hygiene in Budapest, reports that women who take multiple-vitamin supplements during early pregnancy show better weight gain, report better appetite, and have fewer bouts of nausea and vomiting compared to women who don't supplement. In the research, the supplements didn't eliminate morning sickness, but they reduced the frequency and severity of symptoms.

However, the issue remains controversial. The American Medical Association's Council on Drugs found no scientific evidence that vitamin B6 is effective in the treatment or prevention of morning sickness. Some physicians disagree and find vitamin B6 somewhat useful. For example, according to Carol Archie, M.D., at UCLA Medical Center, "Vitamin B6 (given in 50 mg doses twice a day) is effective, not for your 'garden variety' nausea, but for women with severe and persistent nausea and vomiting." A woman considering vitamin B6 first should consult with her physician, since large doses taken for long periods of time can cause nerve damage and possibly affect the growing baby's nutritional status.

The most important message for all pregnant women experiencing morning sickness is this: You aren't crazy, strange, or neurotic, and, except for extreme cases, morning sickness will not hurt your baby. Although a nutritious diet is important to you and your baby, this might not be a time when you can stomach many of the foods in the Baby-wise Diet. Don't feel guilty if a bag of potato chips soothes your nausea or sniffing lemons gets you through the day. The most important thing is to feed your taste buds at the moment and worry about optimal nutrition when the dust settles and you regain control of your appetite.

Food Cravings

Don't be surprised if your taste buds during the first trimester behave as if they're possessed. As many as 85 percent of women report craving foods or combinations of foods they never would have eaten prior to pregnancy. A woman who has always eaten whole wheat noodles suddenly craves only refined egg noodles. You might swear off sugar, but find yourself possessed by a desire for fudge-ripple ice cream. Prepregnancy spinach salads may be replaced with frozen macaroni-and-cheese dinners. One woman might crave foods she ate as a child, another will eat egg-salad sandwiches at every meal. Some changes are made because of medical advice, but many more are generated by food mythology and cravings. Commonly craved foods include sweets, fruits and fruit juices, sour fruits, salty or spicy foods, and hard or chewy foods.

Cravings also might be accompanied by aversions. That delicious cup of French roast coffee now smells and tastes repulsive. You no longer can prepare your favorite bean soup because the smell sends you running from the kitchen. Italian food and pizza, once your favorite foods, now hold no appeal. A metallic taste in your mouth may make foods or beverages, such as tea, taste different and distasteful. If you found cigarette smoke annoying prior to pregnancy, you may find that during pregnancy, even a hint of smoke turns off your appetite for hours.

Occasionally, these cravings and aversions are based on an underlying nutritional need. This is true of an iron deficiency–related condition called pica, whereby a woman craves nonfood items and will eat laundry starch, clay or dirt, chalk, or ice. Cravings for salty foods—for example, pickles—may reflect increased needs for sodium as blood volume expands. Aversions often develop to foods you should not be consuming during pregnancy, such as coffee, alcohol, and cigarettes. However, more often than not the craving is driven by scrambled messages to your appetite center in the brain, caused by changing hormones.

Most cravings and aversions are more interesting than serious and, for the most part, can be indulged in moderation. A healthful diet should be one that meets your nutritional and your emotional needs, as well as your preferences. So don't fight a craving or aversion; or try to substitute a more nutritional like item for what you're craving. If you crave carbohydrate-rich donuts, try substituting more nutritious carbohydrate-rich foods such as bagels, English muffins, or apple-cinnamon muffins. If you can't stand the sight of fish or chicken, try other protein-rich foods such as tofu, or try disguising the food, such as mixing small amounts of it into a casserole or stir-fry dish. If beta carotene–rich dark green leafies are on your aversion list, try eating more beta carotene–rich fruits, such as peaches or apricots.

Other crave-control tips include eating a breakfast that includes at least one serving of grains and one serving of fruit, since skipping breakfast will escalate food cravings later in the day. If the sweet taste is your weakness, try using sweet-tasting flavorings and spices such as vanilla, nutmeg, spearmint, cinnamon, and anise. If you can, plan your cravings. Set aside a calorie allotment to accommodate a small sweet snack and make it low-fat—for example, nonfat frozen yogurt, fruit ices, vanilla wafers, or fig bar cookies. Abstinence leads to binge eating, while allowing small servings of your favorite food helps curb the crave attacks. In addition, remember to exercise daily. While couch potatoes are likely to make regular trips to the refrigerator and struggle with their weight, people who regularly exercise maintain a more constant weight and are less prone to bingeing and cravings. Finally, don't confuse emotional needs with nutritional needs. You may be more sensitive and emotional during the first trimester, and this ebb and flow of emotions can cause you to turn to food when you really need a hug.

Constipation

Before your tummy begins to bulge, your digestive tract could be doing tailspins. Along with altered taste and food preferences comes a slowing of your digestive tract and reduced digestive secretions in the intestines. The female hormone progesterone is partially to blame, since it decreases the tone and motility of the smooth muscles that line the digestive tract. Constipation is only one symptom. You also may begin regurgitating your food (heartburn becomes more common later in pregnancy) and find it takes longer to digest a meal. The relaxed muscles allow waste products to linger in the intestines, with more water being reabsorbed; constipation results. Later in the pregnancy, the enlarged uterus puts pressure on the abdominal wall and back muscles and also can contribute to constipation. Not drinking enough water, eating low-fiber foods, or not exercising daily aggravates the condition. If constipation is allowed to persist, hemorrhoids can develop.

What can you do? First, follow the Baby-wise Diet. This will ensure that you consume lots of fiber-rich fruits, vegetables, whole grains, and legumes and enough water. Use laxatives only as a last resort and then only sparingly and with medical supervision. Frequent use of these medications aggravates the condition and leads to a dependency on the laxative.

Fatigue

If during the first trimester you feel as though you are running on fumes rather than a full tank of supreme, you're not alone. Nine out of ten women feel tired to flat-out exhausted during the first few months of pregnancy. Many are tired from the moment they open their eyes in the morning, and often rest does little to energize them. Most of these women have never experienced fatigue until now. The good news is the fatigue is usually followed by a burst of energy during the second trimester.

Although the exact cause of first-trimester fatigue is poorly understood, there are a few commonsense theories. The rapid and unique storm of physiological changes that sets in within minutes to weeks after conception diverts your body's attention and probably leaves little energy for normal chores. For example, it takes a tremendous amount of energy to set up the nutritional processing plant— that is, the placenta—for your baby.

In addition, progesterone, the female hormone responsible for many of the physical changes during early pregnancy, also has a sedative effect. Finally, sleep disturbances, nausea, vomiting, and mood swings may contribute to fatigue. Granted, a wanted pregnancy and a positive attitude probably help more than they hinder energy levels, but fatigue is not necessarily caused by deep-seated confusion about having a baby. Fatigue happens to the most willing and eager mothers, while some women with unwanted pregnancies sail through the first trimester with little change in their energy level. In other words, don't let anyone tell you "it's all in your head." In fact, preliminary evidence shows that the fatigue often is related to nausea and psychological changes triggered by hormones, including depression, anger, anxiety, and confusion.

There are no magic pills for fatigue, but you can curb the energy drain by eating well, exercising when possible, and listening and responding to your body's needs. Not surprisingly, one study found that women who entered pregnancy in good physical condition and with good stamina, regardless of age, reported less problem with fatigue in early pregnancy.

To fuel your energy rather than your fatigue, avoid sugary foods and caffeinated beverages, which are a temporary quick fix and usually leave you feeling even more tired in the long run.

Instead, try to eat every four hours, include a grain and a fruit or vegetable at each meal or snack, always eat breakfast, and drink plenty of fluids. In addition, take an afternoon nap (even if you have to close your office door and take the phone off the hook), go to bed early, and pamper yourself whenever possible. If your fatigue lingers beyond the first trimester, is accompanied by pallor or dizziness, or seriously affects your daily routine, consult with your physician about a blood test for iron status (see chapter 6).

First Trimester Meals and Snacks

The calorie goal for the first trimester of pregnancy for most women is approximately 2,200 calories (or a calorie intake that maintains a desirable prepregnancy weight). While the baby's calorie needs are small during this time, the mother's nutrient needs are increasing.

Morning sickness during the first trimester may mean eating what you can, when you can. Try to stick to the menus or the guidelines for the Baby-wise Diet as closely as possible or divide the food intake into small meals that you can eat when your stomach settles. Worksheet 5.1 on page 151 will help you monitor your diet. A moderate-dose supplement will help cover your nutritional bases if food intake is too erratic during these first few weeks.

Worksheet 5.1   My First Trimester Daily Checklist

Copy this master sheet to complete daily.

FOOD GROUPS	MINIMUM SERVINGS	ACTUAL INTAKE
Calcium-rich foods	2	_____
Vegetables (at least 2 folic acid–rich choices)	5	_____
Fruits (at least 2 vitamin C–rich choices)	3	_____
Grains (at least 4 whole-grain choices)	6	_____
Extra-lean meats and legumes	2	_____
Quenchers	5	_____

Did I reach my goals? _____

What needs improvement? _____

What will I do differently next week? _____

Day 1

BREAKFAST

1 egg scrambled in nonstick pan
2 slices whole wheat toast with:
   2 teaspoons light margarine
1 cup orange juice

SNACK

6 ounces low-fat vanilla yogurt
1 banana
Sparkling water with lemon

LUNCH

South-of-the-border salad:
   2 cups chopped romaine lettuce
   $\frac{1}{4}$ cup diced red cabbage
   $\frac{1}{4}$ cup grated carrot
   1 ounce cheddar cheese, grated
   $\frac{1}{3}$ cup cooked kidney beans, rinsed
      and drained
   $\frac{1}{2}$ medium avocado, sliced
   $\frac{1}{2}$ cup salsa
1 ounce oven-baked tortilla chips
1 glass iced tea

SNACK

1/2 whole wheat bagel with:
    1 tablespoon fat-free cream cheese
1 apple

DINNER

3 ounces grilled salmon with lemon
    and dill
1 baked potato with:
    1 tablespoon light margarine
    1 tablespoon fat-free sour cream
1 cup steamed broccoli
1 whole wheat dinner roll
Water

SNACK

1 medium orange
4 graham crackers
1 cup sugar-free cocoa made with 1%
    low-fat milk

Daily totals: 2,227 calories; fat 27%;
protein 17%; carbohydrate 55%; fiber
42 grams; salt (sodium) 2.4 grams*

Day 2

BREAKFAST

1 whole wheat English muffin,
    toasted, with:
    1 tablespoon peanut butter
    2 teaspoons all-fruit jam

1 apple
1 cup 1% low-fat milk

SNACK

2 rice cakes
1 ounce low-fat mozzarella cheese
1 orange
Sparkling water with lime

LUNCH

Gardenburger:
    1 whole wheat hamburger bun
    1 veggie burger (made with
        vegetables and soybeans)
    1 tablespoon mustard
    2 tomato slices
    1 lettuce leaf
2 carrots, sliced
1/2 cup jicama sticks
1 cup 1% low-fat milk
3 fig bars
Iced tea

SNACK

1/2 cup oven-baked tortilla chips
1/4 cup salsa
1 cup pineapple juice

DINNER

1 Beef Fajita**
1 cup steamed spinach topped with:
    2 teaspoons coconut
Herbal tea

*Sodium will be higher if salt is added to foods.
**Recipes are given in the back of the book.

SNACK

1 cup warmed 1% low-fat milk
  flavored with almond extract
1 cup fresh strawberries
Water

Daily totals: 2,192 calories; fat 24%;
protein 20%; carbohydrate 56%; fiber
36 grams; salt (sodium) 2.5 grams*

Day 3

BREAKFAST

1 Currant-Date Muffin**
Fruit salad:
    1 medium orange, sectioned
    1 banana, sliced
1 cup 1% low-fat milk
Herbal tea

SNACK

½ cup cubed cantaloupe and musk
  melon

LUNCH

Turkey sandwich:
    2 ounces sliced white-meat turkey
    2 slices raisin bread
    1 ounce fat-free cream cheese
    ½ apple, sliced
½ apple (remaining from sandwich)

1 cup raw vegetables (broccoli florets,
  carrot sticks, celery sticks, etc.)
1 cup 1% low-fat milk

SNACK

2 cups air-popped popcorn

DINNER

Vegetable pizza:
    1 Boboli 4-ounce crust
    2 tablespoons spaghetti sauce
    2 tablespoons chopped green onions
    4 large olives, sliced
    3 fresh mushrooms, sliced
    1 tablespoon diced green pepper
    ¼ cup grated low-fat mozzarella
      cheese
    ½ ounce Parmesan cheese, grated
Green salad:
    2 cups chopped romaine lettuce
    ¼ cup grated carrot
    ½ cup cooked garbanzo beans
    ½ tomato, sliced
    3 tablespoons Italian dressing
Sparkling water

SNACK

1 piece angel food cake topped with:
    ½ cup fresh blueberries
    1 kiwi, sliced
    1 tablespoon light whipped topping
Water

*Sodium will be higher if salt is added to foods.
**Recipes are given in the back of the book.

Daily totals: 2,218 calories; fat 23%; protein 19%; carbohydrate 59%; fiber 34 grams; salt (sodium) 3.4 grams*

Day 4

BREAKFAST

1 cup Total wheat cereal
1 cup 1% low-fat milk
1 banana
1 cup orange juice
Herbal tea

SNACK

6 ounces low-fat vanilla yogurt with:
   $^1/_2$ cup blueberries
   1 tablespoon wheat germ
Sparkling water

LUNCH

1$^1/_2$ cups split pea soup (low-fat, canned)
1 whole wheat roll with:
   1 teaspoon margarine
1 cup raw marinated vegetables (carrots, broccoli, green beans, onions in red wine vinegar and herbs)
Water

SNACK

$^1/_3$ cup Spinach Hummus** with:
   1 tablespoon olive oil
$^1/_2$ whole wheat pita bread
1 medium apple
Sparkling water with lemon

DINNER

Hamburger:
   3 ounces extra-lean ground sirloin, broiled
   1 mixed-grain hamburger bun
   1 tomato slice
   1 lettuce leaf
   1 red onion slice
   2 tablespoons catsup
1 cup carrots and broccoli, steamed
$^2/_3$ cup corn kernels, steamed
Water

SNACK

1 slice raisin bread topped with:
   1 ounce nonfat cream cheese
1 medium orange, sliced
Water

Daily totals: 2,188 calories; fat 23%; protein 17%; carbohydrate 60%; fiber 48 grams; salt (sodium) 3.2 grams*

*Sodium will be higher if salt is added to foods.
**Recipes are given in the back of the book.

Day 5

BREAKFAST

1 whole wheat bagel, toasted, with:
  1 ounce fat-free cream cheese
1 medium apple
6 ounces orange juice

SNACK

$^1/_2$ cup 1% low-fat cottage cheese
$^1/_2$ cup grapes
Sparkling water with lime

LUNCH

Black bean burrito:
  1 8-inch flour tortilla
  $^3/_4$ cup Spicy Black Beans**
  $^1/_2$ avocado, sliced
  $^1/_4$ cup chopped tomato
  1 ounce low-fat cheddar cheese,
    grated
  $^1/_4$ cup salsa
1 carrot, sliced
$^1/_2$ cup sliced jicama
$^1/_2$ cup V-8 juice
Water

SNACK

Fruit smoothie (in blender):
  $^1/_2$ cup 1% plain low-fat yogurt
  $^1/_2$ medium banana
  $^1/_4$ cup orange juice

*Sodium will be higher if salt is added to foods.
**Recipes are given in the back of the book.

2 tablespoons wheat germ
2 ice cubes

DINNER

Chicken Parmesan**
1 baked medium sweet potato with:
  1 teaspoon margarine
Spinach salad:
  2 cups chopped spinach
  $^1/_4$ cup grated carrot
  2 tablespoons chopped red onion
  2 tablespoons Italian dressing
Sparkling water

SNACK

6 graham crackers
$^1/_2$ cup peaches canned in juice
1 cup 1% low-fat milk
Water

Daily totals: 2,208 calories; fat 26%;
protein 20%; carbohydrate 54%; fiber
39 grams; salt (sodium) 3.0 grams*

Day 6

BREAKFAST

1 cup cooked oatmeal topped with:
  1 tablespoon brown sugar
  2 tablespoons wheat germ
  1 tablespoon raisins
1 cup 1% low-fat milk
Herbal tea

SNACK

1 Currant-Date Muffin**
1 cup orange juice

LUNCH

Shrimp salad:
   3 ounces cooked small shrimp
   4 cucumber slices
   2 cups chopped mixed greens
   1 medium tomato, chopped
   2 tablespoons Thousand Island
     dressing
3 bread sticks
1 cup 1% low-fat milk

SNACK

6 graham crackers topped with:
   2 tablespoons peanut butter
   1 tablespoon raisins
1 medium orange

DINNER

3 Spinach Stuffed Shells**
1 whole wheat roll with:
   1 teaspoon light margarine
$^1/_2$ cup steamed baby carrots
$^1/_2$ cup steamed cauliflower
1 teaspoon light margarine
Water

SNACK

1 banana
1 slice raisin toast with:
   1 teaspoon all-fruit jam

Daily totals: 2,113 calories; fat 26%;
protein 16%; carbohydrate 58%; fiber
31 grams; salt (sodium) 2.1 grams*

Day 7

BREAKFAST

3 pancakes, made from mix with
   added wheat germ, topped with:
   1 tablespoon maple syrup
   1 banana, sliced
1 cup orange juice
Herbal tea

SNACK

6 ounces low-fat vanilla yogurt
$^1/_2$ cup blueberries
Sparkling water with lime

LUNCH

2 cups minestrone soup
1 slice French bread with:
   1 teaspoon margarine
Carrot-raisin salad:
   $^3/_4$ cup grated carrots
   2 tablespoons raisins

*Sodium will be higher if salt is added to foods.
**Recipes are given in the back of the book.

1 tablespoon mayonnaise
Lemon juice
Salt and pepper to taste
Herbal iced tea

SNACK

1 cup sliced crunchy vegetables, such
as broccoli, celery, zucchini,
radishes, mushrooms, or baby carrots
10 whole wheat crackers
1 ounce low-fat cheese, sliced
Sparkling water

DINNER

3 ounces halibut, grilled with tarragon
and lemon
$^2/_3$ cup steamed acorn squash
$^2/_3$ cup steamed zucchini
2 slices whole wheat bread with:
2 teaspoons margarine
Sparkling water

SNACK

1 cup fresh fruit, such as whole
strawberries, orange slices, or sliced
apple, dunked in $^1/_2$ cup apple-
cinnamon low-fat yogurt

Daily totals: 2,172 calories; fat 25%;
protein 13%; carbohydrate 62%; fiber
34 grams; salt (sodium) 4.0 grams*

*Sodium will be higher if salt is added to foods.

CHAPTER SIX

Nutrition During the Second Trimester

During the second trimester of pregnancy:

1. Follow the guidelines outlined in the Baby-wise Diet.
2. Try to limit weight gain to approximately 0.7 to 1.4 pounds a week for a total of 9 to 19 pounds (more if you entered pregnancy on the thin side, exercise intensely, or are tall, and less if you are short or were overweight and/or sedentary prior to pregnancy).
3. Take a multiple vitamin and mineral supplement that contains 100 to 200 percent of the Reference Daily Intake (RDI) for all vitamins and minerals plus at least 400 mcg of folic acid and 18 mg of iron.
4. Continue to avoid alcohol, tobacco, and any medication not approved by your physician.
5. Exercise daily, but adjust the routine, intensity, or duration as needed.

Weight Gain and Why

By the beginning of the fourth month of pregnancy, you should notice a gradual increase in weight that approaches 0.7 to 1.4 pounds a week. The average rate of weight gain during the second trimester usually is slightly greater than during the third trimester; a slowing of weight gain or even a slight weight loss is common in the final weeks before delivery. However, these weight-gain goals are merely estimates; a healthful weight gain for each woman will depend on her weight and health status prior to pregnancy, her activity level, and a rate that is natural and normal for her. In short, the experiences of many pregnant women are unlikely to fit exactly onto a standardized weight-gain grid. One concern in regard to weight is any rapid gain of more than two pounds in one week, which could signify excess fluid retention and the onset of a serious medical condition called pre-eclampsia (discussed later in this chapter).

When and What to Eat and Drink

Many women finish the first trimester still wearing their regular clothes, but by the fourth or fifth month, they are beginning to show the outward signs of baby making. While cell and tissue diversity was your baby's goal during the first trimester, increases in cell, tissue, and body size become more pronounced in the second and third trimesters. That means your baby will be demanding more energy for growth, which equates to about a 300-calorie increase in food intake above the first trimester, for a total of about 2,500 calories a day (more if you exercise).

As always, the Baby-wise Diet forms the basis of your eating plan, with the following minimum number of daily servings from each list:

> 3 servings from the Calcium-Rich Group
> 6 servings from the Vegetable Group (at least 2 servings should be folic acid–rich choices)
> 4 servings from the Fruit Group (at least 2 servings should be vitamin C–rich choices)
> 7 servings from the Grains Group (at least 4 servings should be whole-grain choices)
> 3 servings from the Extra-Lean Meats and Legumes Group (try to include 2 to 3 servings of fish and 4 to 5 servings of legumes in the weekly menu)
> 6 servings from the Quenchers Group

Why Do I Feel So Tired?
Marginal Nutrient Deficiencies

While many women report experiencing a burst of energy during the second trimester, the increased demands of pregnancy might leave other women feeling not up to par. It is easy to blame low energy or mood swings on pregnancy or the stress of a busy lifestyle, but fatigue could be a simple matter of not getting enough nutrients from your diet.

As science develops more sensitive tests for nutritional status, long-cherished beliefs about nutritional adequacy are being challenged. The stockpile of accumulating research shows that the amounts of nutrients known to prevent outright deficiency diseases, such as beriberi or scurvy, are not necessarily adequate to maintain optimal nutrition and health or prevent chronic disease. In addition, a new class of deficiency, called a marginal deficiency, is gaining acceptance even in the most conservative circles.

A person's nutritional status even a few years ago was based primarily on a visual inspection. You were considered nutritionally healthy if you looked all right, if your gums did not bleed, if your growth during childhood wasn't stunted, if your red blood cells were normal, or if you did not suffer from severe dermatitis or hair loss. The Recommended Dietary Allowances (RDAs) and the four food groups were the nutritional guideposts.

"The RDAs were derived by asking the question 'How much of a nutrient will prevent a clinical deficiency,' then adding an extra amount as a margin of safety," says Jeffrey Blumberg, Ph.D., a professor of nutrition at Tufts University. "How much calcium prevents osteoporosis, how much vitamin E prevents heart disease, or how much zinc strengthens the immune system are very different questions."

For years clinical deficiencies functioned as smokescreens. With attention focused on overt symptoms of deficiency, many of nutrition's profound, yet subtle, effects on health went unnoticed. Today, nutritional depletion is recognized to progress from mild to severe over the course of days, weeks, months, or years, much like other disorders from the common cold to heart disease. In essence, each person's nutritional status fluctuates along a continuum. Marginal deficiencies are the middle ground on this continuum, bordered by either increasingly better health on one end or advancing clinical deficiencies on the other.

The problem with a marginal deficiency is that the symptoms, if any, are vague. "The definition of a marginal deficiency is still very imprecise," says Douglas Heimburger, M.D., associate professor and director of the Division of Clinical Nutrition at the University of Alabama at Birmingham. "Often the effects of a marginal deficiency have nothing to do with how a person looks or feels." If there are symptoms, they might be something as vague as "feeling under the weather." A marginally nourished person also may feel tired, stressed, or irritable or be more prone to colds and the flu. Complications following an illness or surgery also are more common in marginally nourished people.

How a person feels and thinks is fertile ground for marginal deficiency symptoms. Insomnia, poor memory, irritability, or mood swings are common. For example, suboptimal intake of vitamin B1 produces feelings of depression or anxiety even in otherwise normal, healthy people. The nutritional demands of pregnancy can be all it takes to push a woman over the edge from adequate nutritional status to a marginal deficiency.

Researchers at the University Giessen in Germany recently reported that marginal vitamin intake is accompanied by a decrease in feelings of well-being, a heightened emotional irritability, and an increased feeling of fear. In addition, marginally deficient yet otherwise healthy subjects were more nervous, depressed, and performed poorly on memory tests compared to their well-nourished counterparts.

Fatigue can result from a host of factors, not the least of which is diet and, in particular, iron intake. As mentioned in chapter 1, iron is a component of hemoglobin in red blood cells and myoglobin within the muscles and other tissues. These iron-dependent molecules are responsible for oxygen transport and utilization from the lungs to all of the cells and within the cells. When dietary intake of iron is low or when iron absorption is poor, iron in the tissues is released to make up deficits in the blood. The cells slowly suffocate from lack of oxygen and inefficiently burn carbohydrates for energy. Consequently, a woman experiences everything from sluggishness to poor concentration. These symptoms occur as the tissue stores are drained, even when there are no signs of anemia. Symptoms worsen as the deficiency progresses to anemia. Women—especially those who exercise, are or have been pregnant within the past two years, or consume diets of fewer than 2,500 calories—are at particular risk for iron deficiency. Rather than allow your energy level to crumble or accept fatigue as a normal part of pregnancy, take the offensive by having your iron levels checked—that is, ask for a serum ferritin test rather than only the typical hemoglobin or hematocrit; consume ample amounts of iron-rich foods in the Baby-wise Diet, and request an iron supplement if your serum ferritin level is below 20 mcg/l and/or your total iron binding capacity, or TIBC, is greater than 450 mcg/l.

Recently, the impact that marginal dietary intakes have on immunity also has come to light. The immune system, the body's natural defense against everything from the common cold to cancer, is dramatically influenced by suboptimal amounts of numerous vitamins and minerals. Diminishing resistance to illness associated with aging, for example, is now suspected to be more a result of poor diet than aging genes. Consuming a little but not enough copper, iron, selenium, zinc, vitamin A and beta carotene, vitamin E, vitamin C, and/or the B vitamins, especially folic acid, vitamin B6, and pantothenic acid, can have far-reaching effects on a person's ability to fend off infection and disease.

Preventing a deficiency, or at least treating it in the early stages, is your best bet, just as identifying and treating abnormal cell changes of the cervix from a routine Pap smear has an almost 100 percent cure rate, as compared to the poor prognosis when cervical cancer has progressed to advanced stages. Even if the deficiency doesn't progress, why settle for feeling average when you could feel good or great?

While there are no inexpensive and reliable tests to assess nutritional status for every vitamin and mineral, following the Baby-wise Diet prior to and during pregnancy will improve your chances of getting everything you need to feel your best. Granted, the vague symptoms attributed to marginal deficiencies also result from a host of other factors, from the genes you were born with to the hormone storms of pregnancy. Regardless, setting your nutritional sights on the optimum improves your stamina and well-being, while a healthy body is more resilient to the problems of daily living. Consuming enough—not just a little—of all nutrients could make the difference between feeling under the weather and at your best.

A Word About Mood Swings

Granted, some mild emotional problems, from depression to irritability, can result from marginal intakes of one or more vitamins or minerals. But even more likely causes of emotional ups and downs during pregnancy are the fluctuations in hormones and the experience of pregnancy itself.

Your body is undergoing a total makeover, which is exciting and wonderful in one way, but possibly upsetting for other reasons. As your breasts enlarge, your waistline disappears, and your graceful walk transforms into a waddle, you may have mixed feelings about what is happening to your body. There will be days when you feel fat or wonder if you will ever regain your figure. These feelings are normal, so don't worry. Exercise can help you feel good about yourself, while following the Baby-wise Diet and gaining enough, but not too much, weight will help you stay healthy during your pregnancy and will make it easier to regain your "old self" after the baby is born.

The Stress of Pregnancy

Stress comes packaged in many of life's most wonderful experiences. While daily tensions or the loss of a loved one can cause negative stress or distress, even positive experiences such as a promotion at work or pregnancy can upset normal routines and increase your stress load. Muscle tightness, headaches, sleep problems, a quicker heart rate, or frequent irritability are red flags of stress.

Pregnancy adds its own set of stresses to a woman's life. Not only do the profound physical changes that accompany pregnancy require many adjustments, but the psychological and emotional changes as a woman anticipates the birth of her baby can add additional layers of stress. You also might worry about the many facets of pregnancy, from nausea, fatigue, and backaches to premature delivery, birth defects, and the pain of labor. Most of these worries can be minimized by talking to your physician, who can give you the facts about what to expect in each phase of pregnancy.

Unrelieved stress can increase a pregnant woman's susceptibility to health problems, which then affect the developing baby. For example, in studies on animals, pups born to overly stressed mothers are less active and show signs of reduced nerve and organ development. Unhealthy coping habits, such as cigarettes, alcohol, or drugs, aggravate the situation and increase the risk for birth defects. In addition, chronic high stress might increase a woman's risk for premature labor and having a low-birth-weight baby.

So you should make every effort to avoid or successfully cope with the stress of pregnancy by adopting a positive attitude, developing a realistic expectation of the pregnancy process, and taking charge of each stressful situation to find a reasonable solution. You might need to lessen the workload on the job, reduce noise at home or at work, avoid long periods of standing or sitting, take time during the day for a short nap, or let go of superwoman expectations that you can do it all. Prioritizing your time and efforts and developing an assertive communication style to effectively ask for what you need are two essential skills you must acquire. In addition, spend time with people who understand and are supportive of you during your pregnancy, and take time to exercise and rest or meditate daily.

Staying Healthy While You're Pregnant

The second trimester comes with a unique set of challenges and experiences. This is the time best suited for maintaining your exercise program, since the morning sickness and fatigue of the first trimester have waned, while your body still moves relatively easily. On the other hand, as morning sickness subsides other health issues might surface, such as heartburn, constipation, pre-eclampsia, gestational diabetes, and high blood pressure, which should be prevented when possible or closely monitored if they develop.

Exercise: How Much of What?

Earlier in this century a pregnant woman wasn't supposed to lift a finger, let alone walk a mile. Today, some women are running the entire nine months. The exercise guidelines published by the American College of Obstetricians and Gynecologists (ACOG) in 1985 were considered revolutionary and set a gold standard for exercise prescription during pregnancy. Although they acknowledged that exercise was an important part of a healthy pregnancy, they imposed strong limitations on how much of what was safe for the pregnant woman. Strenuous activities could not exceed fifteen minutes at a time and a pregnant woman's heartbeat should not exceed 140 beats per minute. Those guidelines were reasonable for a sedentary woman entering pregnancy or for less-than-active older women. However, for young women who were used to a serious exercise routine prior to conception, and who were unlikely to even break a sweat at 140 beats per minute, the guidelines were a straitjacket.

Recent evidence shows that exercise at or exceeding the levels recommended in the 1985 ACOG guidelines are beneficial to both the mother and the developing baby. A study at Columbia University School of Public Health investigated the effects of exercise on 800 pregnant women. The results showed that in fit,

Exercise Guidelines for Pregnancy*

The following guidelines are proposed by ACOG and are intended for women who do not have any additional risk factors for adverse maternal or perinatal outcomes.

1. Women can continue to exercise during pregnancy and will experience health benefits even from mild to moderate activity. Regular activity—at least three times a week—is preferable to sporadic activity.

2. After the first trimester, a woman should avoid any exercise that requires lying in the supine position (on the back). This position reduces cardiac output (blood flow from the heart). Long periods of motionless standing also should be avoided.

3. Because there is typically decreased oxygen available for aerobic activity, a woman should adapt all exercise to accommodate this shift in oxygen supply. She should stop exercising if she feels fatigued and should not exercise to exhaustion. Non-weight-bearing activities, such as swimming or cycling, help minimize the risk of injury; however, even weight-bearing activity, such as jogging, can be continued with modification under many circumstances and with physician approval.

4. Any activity that poses a threat of abdominal trauma or the loss of balance and risk to the mother or infant's well-being should be avoided.

5. Women who exercise will require up to 300 additional calories to sustain normal body functioning and a gradual weight gain.

6. To counter any increase in body temperature, a pregnant woman should drink plenty of fluids, wear appropriate clothing, and avoid exercising in hot climates.

7. Many of the physical changes of pregnancy persist six to eight weeks after delivery, so exercise routines should be resumed gradually based on a woman's physical capability.

*American College of Obstetricians and Gynecologists. Technical Bulletin 1994:189.

---

low-risk pregnant women, moderate exercise (that is, at least an hour a day, three times a week) improved pregnancy outcome and increased the birth weight of the baby by about 5 percent compared to nonexercisers; babies born to physically fit women who exercised at levels of 2,000 calories or more each week showed even greater gains of up to 10 percent in birth weights. Other studies show that women who exercise before and during pregnancy have half the risk of delivering prematurely; are better able to handle the stress pregnancy puts on the body; have fewer backaches, constipation, ankle swelling, fatigue, and excess weight gain; and report feeling better and emotionally more positive than do nonexercisers.

In 1994, the ACOG published revised guidelines that are much more flexible regarding exercise prescriptions. They acknowledge that while many women entering pregnancy might have less oxygen available for aerobic exercise and, thus, might experience a loss of exercise performance, other women do not lose their aerobic power and perform as well during as before pregnancy. In addition, most women experience a gradual drop in exercise performance over the course of pregnancy; however, women who begin non-weight-bearing sports, such as swimming or cycling, in early pregnancy actually maintain high-intensity, moderate-duration workouts for the entire nine months. (See "Exercise Guidelines for Pregnancy," page 165.)

Granted, the heart rate of the unborn baby speeds up by five to fifteen beats a minute when the mother is exercising vigorously, but there is no evidence that this is harmful. In fact, there is no evidence of an increased risk for birth defects in women who exercise at a reasonable pace, be it fast or slow. A woman entering pregnancy in good physical condition usually can maintain a higher degree of exercise performance throughout pregnancy, and she will recover from pregnancy and delivery faster than can a sedentary woman. For example, a woman who has exercised routinely at 75 percent of her maximum exertion prior to pregnancy may drop down to 57 percent by the twentieth week of pregnancy, and to 47 percent by the thirty-second week, but she is still in excellent physical shape and will return to prepregnancy fitness quickly after delivery. In short, exercise is beneficial during pregnancy as long as a woman keeps in mind the shift in gravity and weight distribution that comes in the second and third trimesters as her belly expands, and she exercises with reasonable caution.

Pregnant women, in general, cannot exercise at the same intensity and duration as they did prior to pregnancy. In addition, conventional methods for measuring exercise intensity, such as pulse, might not be accurate because of the increase in a pregnant woman's resting heart rate from the first to the third trimesters. Instead, focus on your level of exertion; exercise at whatever level makes your body feel the same as it did before you were pregnant. Don't force yourself to do anything that doesn't feel absolutely right. If running no longer feels good, try walking or swimming. (See "When Not to Exercise," page 167.)

Increased body mass, a relaxing of the ligaments around the joints, fatigue, and increased cardiovascular demands also affect the exercise performance of mothers-

When Not to Exercise

According to the ACOG, several medical or pregnancy-related conditions are contraindicators for exercise or at least will impose important limitations to an exercise program, including:

1. Intrauterine growth retardation
2. Pregnancy-induced high blood pressure
3. Premature rupture of membranes, or placenta previa
4. Persistent bleeding during the second and third trimester
5. Preterm labor, either during the current or a previous pregnancy
6. Incompetent cervix/cerclage (a surgical procedure that closes the cervix to keep the fetus intact in the uterus)
7. A history of chronic high blood pressure, active thyroid, cardiovascular or pulmonary disease, or miscarriage
8. More than one fetus—twins, triplets, etc.
9. Asthma

to-be. After the fourth month of pregnancy, you should avoid exercising while lying on your back, since the expanding uterus can compress the vena cava as it carries blood back to the heart. This could interfere with normal blood flow to the uterus. Also, don't do crunch exercises or any activity that causes you to hold your breath. Weight training is fine, but use light weights to avoid straining.

Your center of gravity has shifted, which might upset your balance. Consequently, it is best not to begin a new activity that requires balance or the risk of a fall, such as aerobic dance, roller skating, step exercises, or even cycling during pregnancy. These limitations are hardly an excuse not to exercise, but they might require some changes in how hard, or how long, or even what type of exercise you engage in during your pregnancy.

The American College of Sports Medicine (ACSM) recommends that a pregnant woman monitor her body temperature during exercise, since even a moderate elevation to 102.5° F. or higher could create problems for the developing baby. The research is incomplete on what effects elevated body temperature might have on the developing baby, while limited evidence shows that women who engage in strenuous work, prolonged standing in the third trimester, or heavy weight lifting are more prone than other women to preterm deliveries. Your body temperature may rise more rapidly during exercise than it did prior to pregnancy, so you will need to relearn your body's signals by keeping a close eye on any changes. On the other hand, body temperature, called core temperature, seldom increases more than 2.7° F. in women who exercise at a comfortable or constant moderate pace during pregnancy, so you don't need to worry if you break a sweat. To be safe, always consult your physician before either beginning or continuing an exercise program during pregnancy.

Unfortunately, a safe upper limit for exercise has not been established and probably has more to do with a woman's individual fitness and pregnancy status than a standard for all women. Some sports, however, seem to be made for pregnancy. Swimming is a perfect example.

Swimming is an aerobic activity that keeps your blood circulating, improves the flow of oxygen to your baby, increases your strength and endurance, and decreases the risk for developing high blood pressure, edema, varicose veins, and hemorrhoids. Like other sports, swimming also might help you shorten your labor and reduce overall risk for pregnancy complications. But unlike other sports such as jogging, which can cause jarring and stress your already strained back, joints, and legs, swimming and other water activities are weightless and gentle to your body. Your body is supported by the water while you exercise all the major muscle groups. It also improves your upper body strength, which is likely to be useful in the months following delivery as you tote around your bundle of joy. While you should avoid diving, water skiing, and other water sports that could be harmful to you or your baby during pregnancy, you are likely to feel much better if you enter pregnancy physically fit and stay that way for the whole nine months.

Food Additives: Which Ones Are Safe?

It's hard to believe that additives and babies can safely mix. For example, while an adult body may tolerate a little butylated hydroxytoluene (BHT) in cereal or cholic acid in dried egg whites, many women worry how the 3,000 nonnutritive substances added intentionally and unintentionally to our food supply might affect their developing babies.

For the most part, while most food additives are hardly essential nutrients, they also probably won't harm you or your baby. Because government regulatory agencies, such as the U.S. Food and Drug Administration (FDA), require stringent testing of any new substance before it enters the food supply, our food supply is safer than it has ever been in recorded history. Consequently, most additives used to preserve, treat, or improve foods are safe, including the above-mentioned cholic acid. When a substance is found harmful, such as the cyclamates and Red Dye No. 2, which produce by-products that damage the body, it is banned from the U.S. food supply.

But a few additives should be avoided if possible during pregnancy. For example, the above-mentioned preservative BHT, which is added to some ready-to-eat cereals, instant mashed potatoes, and other processed foods, produced behavioral problems in pups born to female mice who consumed this additive during pregnancy. Monosodium glutamate (MSG) is a flavor-enhancing additive that is too high in salt (sodium) to be safe during pregnancy. Some people are sensitive to MSG and develop headaches, nausea, vomiting, dizziness, or sleep disturbances after eating it. Hydrolyzed vegetable protein is another food additive that contains MSG. Avoid this additive whenever possible.

High concentrations of additives called sulfites found in some dried fruits and wines (which you aren't drinking anyway) also may cause adverse reactions in 5 to 10 percent of women with asthma who are sensitive to sulfites. In 1986, the FDA banned the use of sulfites from salad bar ingredients and now requires labeling on foods that contain sulfites, such as some processed potatoes, beer, wine, and golden raisins.

Although the sugar substitute saccharin has not been shown to cause damage to the developing baby, there is limited evidence that excessive amounts of this sweetener can cause cancer. Studies on animals show that saccharin is most likely to initiate bladder cancer when a woman is exposed to high doses before pregnancy or when the baby is exposed in the uterus and throughout life. Consequently, avoiding saccharin during the childbearing years is a good idea.

Aspartame, commonly known as NutraSweet, is a noncaloric sweetener used in a variety of foods and beverages from low-sugar yogurt to diet soda pop. It is composed of two amino acids (the building blocks of protein) that are found naturally in foods from meat to vegetables. There is no evidence that aspartame is harmful to pregnant women when consumed in moderation, since its building blocks are readily broken down in the digestive tract and are absorbed along with the other dietary amino acids. Basically, eating foods sweetened with aspartame is no different from eating other foods. In fact, the amino acids in aspartame are found in greater amounts in other foods, such as meat or milk; for example, a glass of milk had thirteen times more aspartic acid than aspartame. Methanol, another compound in aspartame, is supplied in much greater quantities in fruit juice than in aspartame-sweetened soda pop.

That is not to say that soda pop is nutritionally equivalent to orange juice, because nothing could be further from the truth. However, nutritious foods sweetened with aspartame, such as sugar-free yogurt and low-sugar instant oatmeal, can be a safe alternative to sugar for women with diabetes and are probably safe for most pregnant women when consumed in moderate amounts—that is, the equivalent of no more than one diet soft drink a day.

Waxes and pesticides in fruits and vegetables are another source of unwanted additives in the pregnant woman's diet. Waxes formulated from plants and petroleum sources are used to replace the natural waxes removed during washing and to retain moisture during shipping. They also improve the appearance of vegetables and fruits by reducing bruising and the growth of molds and other pathogens. Waxes are used on a variety of produce, including apples, peppers, cucumbers, eggplants, lemons, melons, oranges, peaches, pineapples, sweet potatoes, and tomatoes; however, these and other items are not always treated with wax.

Wax coatings have been approved by the Food and Drug Administration as safe additions to foods. However, a few wax coatings are made from animal products and would not be suitable for people following vegetarian or kosher diets. Another concern is not the wax but the pesticides and fungicides that often are sealed in with waxes. Since federal law requires wax labeling by shippers and retailers, you can ask your grocer for information on which fruits and vegetables at your store have been treated with wax.

Although the evidence is not conclusive, you probably are better off avoiding pesticides in food if possible, especially when you're pregnant. The Environmental Protection Agency (EPA) reports that approximately seventy pesticides now in use are "probable" or "possible" cancer-causing agents. Several studies suggest, but do not prove, that exposure to low levels of pesticides for long periods of time can be harmful. For example, researchers at the Mount Sinai School of Medicine and the New York University Medical Center analyzed blood samples of women with and women without breast cancer. They found that women who had the highest levels of DDE in their blood, a breakdown product of the pesticide DDT banned from use more than a decade ago, were four times as likely to develop breast cancer as women with low levels of the pesticide residue.

Regulations on pesticide use are somewhat enforced in the United States and our food supply is growing increasingly more safe. For example, potentially toxic pesticides such as DDT, dieldrin, heptachlor, and chlordane are suspended from use and other pesticides, such as alar and EDB, are tightly regulated and monitored. However, regulations, if any, in other countries may or may not be enforced. Consequently, produce coming into the United States from other countries may contain illegal residues or levels of pesticides not allowed in this country. These foods are the ones to limit or avoid, if possible.

Despite the unanswered questions about pesticides, people should be eating more fruits and vegetables. For one thing, the permissible residue levels already include hefty margins of safety, so they are likely to be protective even if studies show some produce might contain too much. To limit your pesticide exposure, purchase certified organic produce or locally grown produce when possible, peel all waxed produce, and thoroughly wash all other produce. Keep in mind that pesticide residues also are found in meat, poultry, fish, butter, grains, and other foods. You can cut down on your risk by removing the fat from meats, since that's where some pesticides concentrate. Dried beans and peas have very low levels of pesticides and are a fat-free, nutritious alternative to meat. The bottom line is that regardless of the pesticide controversy, fresh fruits and vegetables are the most nutritious foods in the diet and should be consumed in greater quantities. While most additives are safe, you should avoid a few contaminants in foods, such as heavy metals and a mold called aflatoxin. Most heavy metals, including mercury and lead, are harmful to the developing nervous system of a baby and sources of these metals, such as old plumbing, chipping old house paint, or foods sold in soldered cans, are best avoided.

Aflatoxin, a mold that may contaminate peanuts and some grains, is a potent cancer-causing substance that is harmful to both the mother and the developing baby. It is wise to avoid stale peanuts, cornmeal stored in open bins at the health food store, or rice products of questionable quality or freshness. Do not grind your own peanut butter at your local store by using their bulk nuts. Instead, purchase brand-name peanut butters and corn or rice products from well-known manufacturers.

What About Fish?

Fish is a healthful alternative to red meat and supplies hefty amounts of the type of oils needed for the development of vision and the nervous system. However, some seafood is safer than others. The biggest concerns about eating fish during pregnancy are bacterial food poisoning and chemical contaminants that come from polluted waters. While purchasing fresh fish and proper handling and cooking will reduce or kill bacteria, you have less control over chemical contaminants. Some environmental residues, such as PCBs and PBBs, have leached into rivers and lakes and accumulate in some freshwater fish. PCBs and related contaminants have been associated with reduced birth weights, neonatal behavioral problems, and poorer recognition and memory in infants.

A 1992 report published in *Consumer Reports* magazine stated that 30 percent of sampled fish were of poor quality, half the fish were contaminated by bacteria, and some samples were contaminated with PCBs and mercury. Although the sample size in this study was small and might not be representative of the total supply of edible fish, it does provide food for thought and sheds doubt on the safety of some fish for pregnant women.

So what can you do? The fish most likely to be contaminated with harmful pesticides or metals are those from freshwater sources. Marine fish, with the exception of tuna and swordfish and inshore species such as bluefish and striped bass, are relatively safe. Always check your local health department or department of fisheries about the safety of fish caught in your local lakes and streams. In addition, purchase only very fresh fish and use within twenty-four hours of purchase. Avoid tuna and swordfish during pregnancy, since these fish might be too high in mercury, a metal known to cause nerve damage.

Sushi and other forms of raw fish probably should be avoided during pregnancy, since a few people have eaten raw fish that contains parasites and developed hepatitis B. The chances are minimal, but why take the risk? (See "Fish Safety Rating," page 173.)

Avoiding Food Poisoning

Food poisoning from food eaten at a restaurant might make the headlines, but home kitchens are the worst offenders when it comes to tainted food. Since no one from the local health department inspects your kitchen, you must be your

Fish Safety Rating

In general, fish caught offshore are less likely to be contaminated by environmental pollutants, such as pesticides and PCBs, than are near-shore or freshwater fish. In addition, since most of these contaminants are stored in fatty tissue, select low-fat fish. Fish most likely to be contaminated include catfish, carp, bluefish, and striped bass. Tuna and swordfish are high in mercury and should be avoided prior to and during pregnancy.

Your safest bets, in order of safety from least likely to most likely to be contaminated, are:

FRESHWATER	NEAR SHORE	OFFSHORE
Yellow perch	Pink salmon	Cod
White perch	Chum salmon	Haddock
Brook trout	Sockeye salmon	Pollock
Rainbow trout	Flounder	Yellowfin tuna
Catfish	Sole	Swordfish
Carp		
Whitefish		

own inspector. Careless food storage and handling not only increase the risk for food poisoning but also result in loss of nutrients and good taste from foods. The four basic rules are: (1) always wash your hands in hot, soapy water before preparing food and after using the bathroom, blowing your nose, petting the dog, etc.; (2) wash your kitchen towels and dishcloths often and replace sponges regularly; (3) thaw foods in the microwave or in the refrigerator, never on the kitchen counter; (4) separate raw meats and produce—use separate cutting boards, wash the meat board in the dishwasher after use, use paper towels to wipe away blood from meats, and wash hands with soap after handling meat. In addition, the following kitchen survival skills will reduce your risk of food poisoning.

- The refrigerator door does not stay as cold as the rest of the refrigerator. Store highly perishable foods (especially milk) in the back of your refrigerator.
- Keep beverage containers closed. Orange juice loses vitamin C when exposed to air and milk loses riboflavin (vitamin B2) when exposed to light.

- The egg holders built into refrigerator doors are not cold enough to safely store eggs. Do not wash eggs before storing and throw away any eggs with cracked shells.
- Avoid soft cheeses such as Mexican-style cheeses *queso fresca* or *queso blanco*, feta, Brie, blue cheese, and Camembert. These cheeses can harbor a type of bacteria called *Listeria* that is particularly harmful to a developing baby.
- Butter and margarine absorb smells from other foods if left uncovered and turn rancid if left unrefrigerated. Rancid fats are a source of free radicals, those highly reactive compounds associated with many degenerative diseases and premature aging.
- Vegetables keep best and stay moist when stored in the crisper drawer or in plastic bags on the lower shelf of your refrigerator.
- Whole grains and wheat germ are susceptible to rancidity and insect infestation and should be kept in the refrigerator.
- Do not freeze meats, poultry, or fish in the see-through plastic wrap in which they were purchased. Rewrap them in foil or freezer wrap.
- Large containers of hot foods are breeding grounds for bacteria, since it takes hours for the center to cool enough to retard bacterial growth. Instead, divide large portions into several small freezer containers.
- Do not store foods under the sink. Cleaning products often stored there may leak. Leaking pipes can rust cans and damage boxes. Openings in the walls for pipes give insects and rodents easy access to the foods.
- Store seldom-used pots and pans above the stove. The temperature of this area is too hot for safe storage of foods, including packaged and canned foods.
- Never drink hot beverages from, store acidic juices such as orange juice in, or cook in pottery with a lead-based glaze.
- Avoid using warm tap water for drinking or cooking if it has been exposed to lead pipes (as were customary in homes built before 1930) or lead-soldered pipes (as were customary in homes built between 1978 and 1988). Have your water tested if you have any doubt about its lead content.

- Refrigerated foods should be kept at 40° F. and the freezer temperature should be at, or below, 0° F.
- Test the refrigerator and freezer doors by closing a dollar bill in the door. You should not be able to pull out the bill if the seal is tight.

A Nutritional Approach to Common Problems

Some women sail through the second trimester with hardly a care in the world while others battle minor problems. A few pregnancy-related conditions, including pre-eclampsia and gestational diabetes, can be potentially serious and the early warning signs should be taken seriously. Routine medical checkups throughout pregnancy are critical to early discovery and treatment of these conditions, which otherwise can progress undetected.

Heartburn

Heartburn is a minor grievance that can surface in the second trimester. The term is a misnomer, since this condition has nothing to do with your heart and a whole lot to do with your digestive tract. As many as 80 percent of all pregnant women struggle with heartburn or a full or burning feeling in the chest, especially after a meal. Heartburn can start as early as the first trimester, but usually is more troublesome by the fifth month and increases in frequency or severity in the third trimester.

The hormones estrogen and progesterone are responsible for much of the discomfort. For one thing, progesterone, either alone or with estrogen, decreases the tone and motility of smooth muscles that line the digestive tract and decreases the pressure of the sphincter that usually blocks the stomach contents from moving upward into the esophagus. This results in regurgitation into the esophagus, decreased emptying time of the stomach into the small intestine, and reversed peristalsis (food moves backwards instead of flowing in a constant downward motion).

In addition, the pressure of the enlarging uterus crowds the adjacent digestive tract, especially the stomach. With this crowding, the stomach contents after a meal, now semiliquid, may move up into the esophagus rather than down into the intestines, causing a burning sensation from the gastric acid mixed with the food. Increased gastric acidity during pregnancy also may contribute to heartburn.

Heartburn is aggravated by large meals, foods that produce gas such as beans and cabbage, and fatty or spicy foods. You can avoid the discomfort, or at least reduce the frequency and severity, by dividing the day's food intake into several small meals and snacks, eating a light dinner at least three hours before bedtime, and chewing and eating slowly. Other foods that might aggravate heartburn and should be avoided include coffee, chocolate, salami and other processed meats, rich pastries, fried foods, alcohol, and carbonated beverages. (See "Healthful Snacks During the Second Trimester," page 177.)

The heavier you are, the more pressure you place on the esophagus and the more likely you will experience heartburn. Consequently, a moderate weight gain of twenty-five to thirty pounds is less likely to cause heartburn than is a weight gain of forty to fifty pounds. To avoid or reduce heartburn:

- Wear loose-fitting clothes. (If your waistband or panty hose leave a ring around your growing tummy, your clothes are too tight!)
- Walk or sit after eating; avoid lying down right away.
- Keep your head elevated when in bed.
- Avoid stooping or bending.
- Avoid stress during the day and tensions when eating.
- Chew gum or suck on a sour lemon drop (this will stimulate saliva, which helps neutralize the acid in the esophagus).
- Limit fluids at meals.

Sodium bicarbonate should be avoided as a treatment for heartburn, since it can upset the normal acid-base balance in the body. Discuss the use of antacids with your physician. Overuse of antacids can interfere with iron absorption, so take supplements at opposite times of the day if you use antacids.

Constipation

Progesterone not only contributes to heartburn, it also slows the movement of food in your intestine, which leaves more time for the absorption of water and nutrients and increases the likelihood of constipation. Another hormone called motilin, which normally stimulates movement of food through the intestines,

Healthful Snacks During the Second Trimester

Cheese and crackers
Peanut butter and rice cakes
Banana bread and fat-free cream cheese
Pancake with Raspberry Sauce*
Peanut butter and raisins spread on a banana sliced lengthwise
Fat-free refried beans, salsa, and oven-baked tortilla chips
Bran muffin and applesauce or fat-free cottage cheese
Berry-Banana Salad*
Cheese and apple slices on whole wheat crackers
Whole wheat bread topped with nonfat cottage cheese and crushed pineapple
Graham crackers with peanut butter and banana slices
Tortilla filled with kidney beans, low-fat cheese, cilantro, and salsa
Raisin bagel topped with all-fruit jam
Whole wheat bread sticks and nonfat cheese
Fruit-filled crepe (premade crepes can be found in supermarket produce sections)
Soft microwave pretzel
Thin slice of angel food cake with fresh berries
Pita bread stuffed with cheese, tomato, and shredded zucchini
Cinnamon-apple–flavored mini rice cakes dipped in low-fat yogurt
Whole wheat fig or fat-free cranberry bars
Oatmeal-raisin cookies, ginger snaps, or vanilla wafers and milk
Frozen fruit juice bars and crackers
Custard-style low-fat or nonfat yogurt and fruit
Cheerios and raisins and a cup of yogurt
Baked apple topped with cinnamon and vanilla extract
Raisin bread dipped in nonfat apple-spice yogurt
Raw vegetables, such as broccoli spears, green or red bell peppers, jicama, or Chinese pea
    pods dipped in low-calorie creamy dressing
Razz 'n Blues Muffins*
Green pears, apples, cantaloupe, or watermelon dunked in vanilla yogurt

*Recipes are given in the back of the book.

also is in short supply during pregnancy. The pressure of the growing baby on your intestines and rectum can aggravate this problem. Iron supplements also cause constipation in some women. (Other women develop diarrhea as a result of iron supplementation.) Most women report improvements or even alleviation of constipation when they drink plenty of fluids and eat lots of fiber-rich whole grains, fruits, vegetables, and legumes, as recommended in the Baby-wise Diet. Daily exercise is helpful, as is avoiding caffeine, which acts like a diuretic and can cause further fluid loss. Following this dietary and exercise advice also will lessen your chances of developing hemorrhoids by avoiding constipation.

If the Baby-wise Diet does not remedy constipation, try adding a little wheat bran to the diet. Start with one teaspoon on your morning cereal and gradually increase the dose until you find a level that works for you. Too much fiber may increase intestinal gas, which can be uncomfortable at any time but especially during pregnancy. So take it slow with any concentrated fiber product. In all cases, never take a laxative unless prescribed by your physician, since frequent use of laxatives can aggravate the condition and result in a dependency on the medication.

The same diet and exercise recommendations for constipation also are useful in the prevention and treatment of intestinal gas (flatulence). In addition, eat small, frequent meals rather than gorging. Chew slowly and thoroughly and don't gulp your food, which will cause you to swallow air. This captured air forms painful pockets of gas in your intestines. Staying relaxed while eating also will lessen the chance of swallowing air and help avoid digestive-tract discomfort. Identify and eliminate from the diet any foods that continue to cause you gas, such as fried foods or sugary foods including cookies and pies. If nutritious foods, such as Brussels sprouts, broccoli, and cookied dried beans, peas, and lentils, cause more trouble than they are worth, then make sure you find other nutritious foods to take their place.

While some women struggle with constipation during pregnancy, others are troubled by diarrhea. A hormone called relaxin that is released from the placenta quiets smooth muscle contractions, which can relax the digestive tract and allow food to pass through too quickly. In addition, switching too quickly from a low-fiber diet to the high-fiber Baby-wise Diet could cause temporary discomfort from flatulence as your body adapts to the new eating style. This can be avoided by making dietary changes gradually, rather than all at once. On the other hand, diarrhea can be a sign of infection, food poisoning, or other digestive-tract disorders, so always check with your physician if symptoms are severe or persist.

Gum and Tooth Problems

More gum and tooth problems occur during pregnancy than at any other time in the childbearing years and probably result from changing hormone levels. Gingivitis is more common in the first half of pregnancy. Some women also develop reddened, fingerlike protrusions of inflamed gum tissue between teeth, called pregnancy tumors, which are not cancerous and usually disappear after the baby is born. X-rays are usually necessary if the growths do not subside, so wait until after pregnancy to have them surgically removed. You can lessen the risk or the symptoms of all gum disorders by entering pregnancy with well-cared-for teeth and rigorous dental hygiene, including frequent professional cleaning during pregnancy.

Eclampsia

High blood pressure is one of the most common problems during pregnancy, with up to 30 percent of women experiencing some elevation in blood pressure. One third to one half of these women have essential hypertension, or elevated blood pressure of unknown cause. In some women, this elevated blood pressure signals a more serious condition called pregnancy-induced hypertension (PIH) or eclampsia.

Once called toxemia, pre-eclampsia/eclampsia is a general term for a serious condition that develops in the middle to late pregnancy and is characterized by edema, protein in the urine, and high blood pressure. The condition can occur anytime after the twentieth to twenty-fourth week of pregnancy, but is most common in the later months, has an unpredictable onset, and develops in stages. This condition has nothing to do with toxins in the blood.

In the first stage, called pre-eclampsia, a woman may experience edema (swelling caused by fluid retention), high blood pressure, a sudden weight gain of two or more pounds in one week, and protein loss in the urine. In the second stage, a woman may develop vision problems, severe headaches, and abdominal pain. If allowed to progress to the final stage or eclampsia, convulsions, lapsing into a coma, and even death can result. High blood pressure prior to pregnancy or transient high blood pressure without accompanying protein in the urine or edema is not part of the eclampsia condition. Also, don't worry if your only symptom is a headache; it may be just that!

While pre-eclampsia/eclampsia is one of the most serious obstetrical complications, there is little agreement on its cause. Some physicians believe that gaining too much weight might be a factor, although there is no scientific evidence to support this theory. Others once thought eclampsia resulted from excessive salt intake, so salt-restricted diets were prescribed. A recent study showed that pre-eclampsia might be caused by abnormal attachment of the placenta to the uterine wall, which triggers widespread problems in most of the mother's major body systems. Another theory is that hormonelike compounds called prostaglandins are at the root of pre-eclampsia. It is likely that pre-eclampsia results from a variety of interconnecting factors that include age (teenage women and women over 35 are more prone to pre-eclampsia), parity (first pregnancies are more frequently associated with pre-eclampsia than subsequent pregnancies), socioeconomic factors, and nutritional deficiencies.

Other physicians do not believe diet is a factor; however, the research strongly suggests that the rate of incidence is related to low income and poor diet. For example, the greatest death rates from eclampsia are in Mississippi and South Carolina, the states with the lowest per capita incomes. While the death rate across the United States averages 6.2 per 100,000, the death rate from eclampsia in South Carolina is more than 20 per 100,000 live births and rises to 30 per 100,000 live births in Mississippi, which is an even poorer state. Pre-eclampsia/eclampsia also is less common in middle- and upper-income women, regardless of race.

The most prevalent theory today is that pre-eclampsia can be prevented, or at least the symptoms can be lessened, by improving the quality of the diet, not by salt or weight restriction. In addition, women at higher risk of developing this disorder are those with mothers or sisters who developed pre-eclampsia during their first pregnancies, those in their first pregnancy and who are less than twenty years old or more than thirty-five years old, those who have existing high blood pressure or diabetes, and those who are carrying more than one baby.

Calcium supplementation shows promise in preventing pre-eclampsia or reducing the severity of this disorder when it occurs. While calcium supplementation lowers blood pressure in both pregnant and nonpregnant women, the women who derive the greatest benefits are those pregnant women with low pretreatment blood calcium levels.

One study conducted by Dr. J. Belizan and colleagues on pregnant women who received 2 g of calcium daily compared to pregnant women taking placebos showed that calcium supplementation significantly reduced the incidence of both hypertension and pre-eclampsia. The incidence of pre-eclampsia in the placebo group was 10.7 percent versus only 7.2 percent in the calcium-supplemented group. The rate of pre-eclampsia dropped from 3.9 percent in the placebo group to 2.6 percent in the women taking calcium supplements. Favorable effects on blood pressure were noted within weeks of beginning the calcium supplements. However, pre-eclampsia rates were similar in both the placebo and supplemented women who had initially high levels of urinary calcium excretion—that is, 11 percent in the placebo group and 9.4 percent in the calcium group. Other studies have shown a similar effect with calcium intakes as low as 1 g a day.

How calcium lowers hypertension and PIH risk is poorly understood. Altered calcium metabolism has been noted in hypertensive patients, while red blood cell calcium concentrations are elevated and urinary calcium levels are low in women at risk for pre-eclampsia. Changes in how the kidneys handle sodium also might affect calcium metabolism. Regardless of the mechanism, maintaining an optimal calcium intake before and during pregnancy might be important to the prevention of pre-eclampsia.

Magnesium supplementation has been used to prevent both hypertension and the seizures associated with pre-eclampsia. However, limited evidence shows that increased magnesium intake might aggravate low calcium levels unless calcium also is increased in the diet. In other words, increasing your intake of magnesium-rich foods, such as legumes, wheat germ, green vegetables, and whole grains, or taking a moderate-dose supplement that contains magnesium should be accompanied by increases in calcium-rich foods, such as low-fat milk and dark green, leafy vegetables, or a moderate-dose calcium supplement.

If you choose to supplement during pregnancy, make sure you select a supplement that contains both magnesium and calcium in a ratio of 1:2; for example, 250 mg of magnesium for every 500 mg of calcium. You automatically will consume a diet rich in both of these minerals if you are following the Baby-wise Diet. However, never self-treat the symptoms of pre-eclampsia; this disorder is very serious, and at the first signs should be monitored and treated by a physician. Regular physician visits throughout pregnancy are the only means of early detection, since pre-eclampsia can progress unnoticed to the later, more serious stages.

If prostaglandins contribute to the onset or progression of PIH, then building blocks for these hormonelike substances might be beneficial in its treatment. Preliminary evidence suggests that evening primrose oil, fish oils, or linoleic acid (a fatty acid in safflower oil) might help prevent pre-eclampsia or edema associated with pre-eclampsia. Without conclusive evidence, however, no recommendations can be made at this time.

Women with pre-eclampsia who do not respond to nutrient-dense, moderate-salt diets plus bedrest might need to be hospitalized or their physicians might recommend antihypertensive medications, such as diuretics, as a last resort. The latter reduces the total blood volume and, with any medication, there is the risk of side effects, which are especially worrisome prior to the sixteenth week of pregnancy. However, your physician will know which medications carry the least risk while providing the greatest benefits to normalizing your blood pressure.

Hypertension

Your doctor will be keeping a close eye on your blood pressure during pregnancy, since blood pressure can be an early sign of PIH or can be a complication of pregnancy without the link to PIH. Elevated blood pressure (a systolic blood pressure of 140 mmHg or greater and/or a diastolic blood pressure of 90 mmHg or greater or a rise in systolic blood pressure of 25 mmHg or more and/or a rise in diastolic blood pressure of 15 mmHg or more before conception or in the first trimester) is an unwelcome event. In addition to its link with PIH, high blood pressure can reduce blood flow to the placenta and baby, resulting in a diminished supply of oxygen and nutrients and necessitating an early delivery. Also, as the blood pressure of hypertensive mothers rises, so does the death rate of their infants. Fortunately, most cases of elevated blood pressure during pregnancy are not related to PIH and not all women who develop hypertension during pregnancy develop complications. In most cases, with good medical attention and diet and life-style habits, women with this problem can complete pregnancy and give birth to healthy babies.

Mild to moderate hypertension usually requires that you limit your activity and rest frequently, since inactivity is one way to reduce blood pressure. In addition, while your physician might recommend limiting salt if intake is very high, in almost all cases some salt (sodium) is needed in the pregnant woman's diet.

THE SALT ISSUE: At the turn of the century, women were told to restrict salt to prevent PIH or eclampsia. While this belief has lingered, most experts now agree that a pregnant woman needs some salt in the diet. In fact, many women crave pickles, chips, or other salty foods during pregnancy, which probably reflects their bodies' need for more salt. Most people at risk for developing hypertension are told to lay off the salt shaker. However, about 60 percent of the expanding tissue in the mother's body is water, and sodium is needed to regulate this fluid in the cells and tissues.

Fluid balance in the body is maintained, in part, by how much sodium is outside and how much potassium and chloride are inside the cells. In essence, water follows sodium. Just as water moves out of the cells of a tomato when you sprinkle salt on it, sodium outside of body cells draws water out of these cells, while the potassium and chloride prevent too much fluid from escaping. It is this balance between potassium and chloride on the inside and sodium on the outside that ensures your cells do not go limp from excessive water loss and your blood does not become too concentrated from excessive water moving out of the blood and into the cells.

Some people overrespond to sodium so that a high salt intake results in too much water leaving the cells. The blood volume expands, placing greater pressure on the heart and blood vessels to pump this expanded blood volume, which results in high blood pressure. However, the blood volume naturally expands during pregnancy by up to 50 percent (even more for multiple births), so slightly more sodium, potassium, and chloride are needed to maintain the extra fluid volume. The cells also hold more water during pregnancy, so a little bit of swelling is normal starting in the second trimester and especially in the last few weeks of pregnancy. This mild edema should not be treated with salt restriction or diuretic medications (also called water pills), since you need a little extra fluid. Abnormal accumulation of fluid in the cells, however, is called edema and often is associated with a medical condition that requires physician monitoring (see below).

Pregnant women with high blood pressure fare better when they consume a normal (not excessive) salt intake, because it helps maintain the blood volume of the mother and that of the developing baby. So unless otherwise advised by your physician, continue to salt foods to taste, but avoid wasting calories on highly salted, high-fat snack foods. You will consume ample amounts of potassium if you follow the Baby-wise Diet recommendations to eat plenty of fruits and vegetables. If you struggle with cravings for salty foods, try drinking a can of V-8 juice, which will meet one serving of your vegetable needs and has some added salt.

Edema

Edema is a sign of pre-eclampsia, but not all women with edema develop the more serious disorder. In fact, as many as one out of every two pregnant women will develop some degree of edema during pregnancy without ever developing pre-eclampsia. Women with edema can gain as much as 9½ quarts of fluid and still have normal pregnancies and give birth to healthy babies. The difference between normal fluid retention and edema associated with pre-eclampsia is the rate of fluid retention. A rapid increase in fluid accumulation is a sign of pre-eclampsia, while a gradual gain in fluid weight is not abnormal.

So just because your feet and ankles swell after a long day does not mean you should worry. Sitting or lying down and putting your feet up may be all it takes to reduce the swelling. In addition, drink plenty of fluids, wear comfortable clothing, and avoid wearing tight panty hose, slips, or pants. If you have a sudden weight gain, haven't been following the Baby-wise Diet and don't feel up to par, or any unusual symptoms have developed including headaches or blurred vision, you should contact your physician immediately. Early treatment of pre-eclampsia and regular physician monitoring will reduce the seriousness of the disorder and avoid harming your baby.

Diabetes: Gestational and Insulin-Dependent

Prior to the commercial availability of insulin, virtually no infants born to diabetic mothers survived. Today, while diabetes still remains a high-risk situation, diabetic women who are closely monitored by their physicians and who take extra care and commitment during their pregnancy have a 95 percent chance of having successful pregnancies and healthy babies.

Diabetes is a disorder of the pancreas. More specifically, it is a disorder in the amount or effectiveness of insulin secreted by the pancreas. Problems with insulin activity upset the blood-sugar regulating systems in the body and involve an inability to use and metabolize dietary carbohydrates. Consequently, blood sugar levels are elevated (hyperglycemia) and there is an abnormal amount of sugar in the urine. In the diabetic, blood sugar cannot enter the cells at the normal rate. The body cells are starved for energy, while blood sugar levels reach abnormally high levels and sugar spills into the urine through the kidneys. Diabetics are at increased risk for other life-threatening diseases such as heart disease, blindness, stroke, and gangrene. Adult-onset diabetes, also known as noninsulin-dependent diabetes mellitus (NIDDM), often responds favorably to improved dietary habits and weight loss, while diabetes that begins early in life, called juvenile-onset diabetes, or insulin-dependent diabetes mellitus (IDDM), usually requires supplemental insulin therapy.

A woman may either enter pregnancy with diabetes or develop the disorder as a result of the pregnancy, a condition called gestational diabetes. In the first case, the disorder will persist after delivery, while in the latter case, the diabetes usually disappears after the baby is born. Women who are diabetic before pregnancy usually know of their condition and have made appropriate dietary changes and/or are taking insulin. Attaining a desirable weight and good metabolic control of the condition prior to conception reduces the risk for birth defects and lowers the incidence of pregnancy complications.

A physician will individualize the diabetic's pregnancy care based on her health history, existing complications, and physical needs, with the goal of maintaining tight controls on blood sugar (since both too high and too low a blood sugar can have serious effects on the developing baby) and preventing diabetes-related disorders such as hypertension, excessive fluid surrounding the baby, and premature birth. Complications of diabetes, such as eye and kidney disorders, can intensify during pregnancy, so your physician will monitor closely any changes.

Most women in the developed world experience some loss of carbohydrate (glucose) tolerance during pregnancy; however, only 2 to 3 out of every 100 pregnant women develop gestational diabetes each year. Oddly, many women in underdeveloped countries show no fluctuation or may even experience slight drops in blood sugar during pregnancy, suggesting that either genetics or life-style plays a role in pregnancy-induced changes in blood sugar.

In developed countries, gestational diabetes usually begins during the second half of pregnancy and might be related to hormones secreted by the placenta that oppose the normal metabolism of insulin. If the pancreas cannot meet the extra demands of pregnancy, gestational diabetes develops, but subsides after delivery. Since many women with gestational diabetes develop no signs of the disorder, a routine test that measures blood sugar levels in response to a test dose of sugar often is used between weeks 24 and 28 to determine the presence of diabetes. Up to 20 percent of women do not develop gestational diabetes until week 32, so be retested if there is any suspicion that hyperglycemia (high blood sugar) has developed.

While gestational diabetes is less difficult to control and is generally associated with fewer complications than insulin-dependent diabetes, it still requires careful physician monitoring and adherence to a good diet to ensure a healthy pregnancy, since it can be associated with pre-eclampsia and urinary-tract infections. The risks of congenital abnormalities and spontaneous abortion also are higher in these women. Diabetic women also often deliver large babies, which can complicate delivery and traumatize the infant or increase the risk for delivering cesarean. In addition, there is a greater risk in the baby for hypoglycemia (low blood sugar), increased bilirubin in the blood (called jaundice), and respiratory distress syndrome.

Ideally, a woman with diabetes who wants to have a baby should first achieve the best possible glucose control before conception. The diet of a pregnant woman with diabetes is similar to the Baby-wise Diet and is high in complex carbohydrate–rich foods, such as breads, pasta, legumes, and vegetables; moderate in protein (20 percent of total calorie intake); and low in fat (25 to 30 percent of total calories with fewer than 10 percent coming from saturated fat). Energy often is distributed into three meals and three snacks with 17 to 18 percent of calories consumed at breakfast, 30 percent each at lunch and dinner, and 30 grams of carbohydrate and one protein exchange (7 or 8 grams of protein) for an evening snack. These foods also will supply the added fiber, chromium, and magnesium needed to help regulate blood sugar levels, as well as the vitamin C, vitamin E, and other nutrients associated with diabetes control, whole maintaining a calorie intake that allows moderate weight gain. Snacks and spacing meals will be important, as will daily exercise and plenty of rest. Sugars and sweets should be eliminated.

While most women are discouraged from restricting calories or "dieting" during pregnancy, obese women with gestational diabetes might benefit from a moderate calorie-restricted diet of 1,600 to 1,800 calories a day. Studies show that blood sugar is maintained, excessive weight gain is avoided, and the infant's birth weight is closer to "normal" when calories are restricted in these women to less than 2,000 calories a day. Blood sugar responses to a diet and/or exercise prescription will vary from one person to the next, so all eating plans should be validated with blood glucose monitoring to ensure that the optimal mix of carbohydrates at each meal and snack is maintaining a steady blood sugar level. Your physician and a dietitian can work with you in developing a meal plan that works for you.

Second Trimester Meals and Snacks

The second trimester of pregnancy is considered by some women to be the "golden months." Often the inconveniences of the first trimester, such as morning sickness and fatigue, have subsided, yet the growing baby has not become so cumbersome as to interfere with eating or exercise. This is the time to make up for any nutritional transgressions during the early stage of pregnancy and to foster optimal eating habits that will fuel the growth of a beautiful baby. To monitor your progress, use Worksheet 6.1, below. Remember, unconventional eating can still be nutritious; feel free to have a vegetable burger with mustard or a slice of cold pizza for breakfast or a bowl of cereal for dinner.

Worksheet 6.1   My Second Trimester Daily Checklist

Copy this master sheet and complete daily.

FOOD GROUPS	MINIMUM SERVINGS	ACTUAL INTAKE
Calcium-rich foods	3	_____
Vegetables (at least 2 folic acid–rich choices)	6	_____
Fruits (at least 2 vitamin C–rich choices)	4	_____
Grains (at least 4 whole-grain choices)	7	_____
Extra-lean meats and legumes	3	_____
Quenchers	6	_____

Did I reach my goals? _____

What needs improvement? _____

What will I do differently next week? _____

Day 1

BREAKFAST

2 pancakes made with 1 tablespoon
   wheat germ, topped with:
   ¹/₂ cup fresh raspberries
   2 tablespoons raspberry syrup
   2 tablespoons fat-free sour cream
1 cup orange juice
1 cup herbal tea

SNACK

1 Currant-Date Muffin**
1 cup 1% low-fat milk
1 banana

LUNCH

Bean and cheese burrito:
   1 8-inch flour tortilla
   ¹/₂ cup fat-free refried beans
   2 tablespoons shredded cheddar
      cheese
   ¹/₃ cup chopped tomato
   ¹/₂ avocado, sliced
   Salsa to taste
1 cup Spicy Carrots** (as tolerated)
1 cup V-8 juice

SNACK

10 mini rice cakes topped with:
   1 tablespoon chunky peanut butter

1 medium apple, sliced
Sparkling water flavored with lemon

DINNER

Chicken-vegetable stir-fry:
   5 ounces chicken breast, cut into
      cubes
   ¹/₃ cup chopped onion
   3 garlic cloves
   ¹/₂ cup chopped celery
   5 mushrooms, sliced
   ¹/₂ cup Chinese pea pods
   ¹/₂ cup broccoli florets
   1 tablespoon olive oil
   1 tablespoon soy sauce
³/₄ cup cooked brown rice
1 cup 1% low-fat milk
Herbal tea

SNACK

¹/₂ cup fat-free chocolate frozen
   yogurt
3 vanilla wafers
Water or decaffeinated tea

Daily totals: 2,494 calories; fat 25%;
protein 18%; carbohydrate 57%;
fiber 43 grams; salt (sodium) 3.5
grams*

*Sodium will be higher if salt is added to foods.
**Recipes are given in the back of the book.

Day 2

BREAKFAST

2 mixed-grain frozen waffles topped
  with:
    $^1/_2$ cup canned blueberries in heavy
      syrup
    2 tablespoons fat-free sour cream
6 ounces grapefruit juice
1 cup 1% low-fat milk
Herbal tea

SNACK

1 whole wheat English muffin, toasted
  and topped with:
    1 tablespoon fat-free cream cheese
$^1/_2$ cup thinly sliced cantaloupe
Sparkling water

LUNCH

Turkey and Swiss sandwich:
    3 ounces turkey breast, sliced
    2 slices Swiss cheese
    2 slices whole wheat bread
    1 large lettuce leaf
    1 tablespoon low-fat mayonnaise
10 baby carrots
1 cup German potato salad
Water

SNACK

6 ounces apple-cinnamon low-fat
  yogurt
1 banana
2 celery stalks filled with:
    1 tablespoon peanut butter
    1 tablespoon raisins
Sparkling water

DINNER

5 ounces halibut, grilled with lemon
  and dill
4 broccoli spears, steamed
1 sweet potato, baked
1 whole wheat dinner roll
Water

SNACK

1 slice angel food cake topped with:
  $^1/_2$ cup strawberries
2 tablespoons light whipping cream
Water

Daily totals: 2,513 calories; fat 27%;
protein 20%; carbohydrate 53%;
fiber 39 grams; salt (sodium) 4.0
grams*

*Sodium will be higher if salt is added to foods.

Day 3

BREAKFAST

6 ounces pineapple juice
1 cup cooked oatmeal with:
    2 tablespoons wheat germ
    1/4 cup raisins
1 cup 1% low-fat milk
Herbal tea

SNACK

1 whole wheat bagel, toasted, topped
with:
    1 tablespoon fat-free cream cheese
1 medium orange
Sparkling water flavored with lime

LUNCH

2 cups minestrone soup
Tossed salad:
    2 cups chopped romaine lettuce
    1/3 cup grated carrots
    1/3 cup bean sprouts
    3 tablespoons low-calorie Italian
      dressing
1 slice French bread
1 cup 1% low-fat milk
Water

SNACK

4 graham crackers topped with:
    1 tablespoon peanut butter

1 medium peach
Water

DINNER

5 ounces sirloin steak, trimmed and
    broiled
1 baked potato topped with:
    2 tablespoons fat-free sour cream
    2 teaspoons butter
1 cup sliced zucchini, steamed
1 cup raw, crunchy vegetables, such as
    carrots, broccoli, jicama, or
    cauliflower
1 piece cracked wheat bread topped
with:
    1 teaspoon butter
Water or herbal tea

SNACK

1 piece mixed-grain bread, toasted and
topped with:
    1 teaspoon butter
    1/2 teaspoon cinnamon sugar
1 cup sugar-free cocoa made with low-
fat milk

Daily totals: 2,454 calories; fat 25%;
protein 20%; carbohydrate 55%;
fiber 40 grams; salt (sodium)
4.1 grams*

*Sodium will be higher if salt is added to foods.

Day 4

BREAKFAST

1 cup Shredded Wheat, small
  biscuits
1 cup 1% low-fat milk
1 slice whole wheat toast with:
  1 teaspoon butter
  ¼ teaspoon cinnamon
1 cup fresh strawberries
1 cup orange juice
Herbal tea

SNACK

1 cup low-fat plain yogurt with:
  ½ cup sliced peaches
  ¼ cup toasted wheat germ
Sparkling water

LUNCH

Spinach salad:
  2 cups chopped spinach
  4 fresh mushrooms, sliced
  1 hard-boiled egg, diced
  2 tablespoons grated Parmesan
    cheese
  ¼ cup chopped tomato
  ½ cup cooked kidney beans
  2 tablespoons Italian dressing
1 piece French bread with:
  1 teaspoon butter
Iced tea with lemon

SNACK

1 medium banana
5 fat-free whole wheat crackers topped
  with:
  1 tablespoon chunky peanut butter
Sparkling water

DINNER

1 chicken breast, broiled with lemon,
  garlic, and tarragon
1 medium baked potato with:
  2 teaspoons butter
1½ cups steamed broccoli
1 whole wheat roll
Herbal tea

SNACK

2 cups air-popped popcorn
1 cup sugar-free cocoa made with 1%
  low-fat milk

Daily totals: 2,507 calories; fat 26%;
protein 20%; carbohydrate 53%; fiber
52 grams; salt (sodium) 2.3 grams*

Day 5

BREAKFAST

1 cup sliced cantaloupe
Breakfast burrito:
  1 10-inch flour tortilla, warmed
  1 egg scrambled in nonstick pan

*Sodium will be higher if salt is added to foods.

¼ cup chopped green pepper,
   steamed
¼ cup grated zucchini, steamed
¼ cup chopped tomato
2 tablespoons salsa
1 cup orange juice
Herbal tea

SNACK

1 cup fat-free cottage cheese
1 cup pineapple chunks
1 tablespoon shelled sunflower seeds
Water or tea

LUNCH

Grilled cheese and tomato sandwich
   (grilled in nonstick pan):
   2 slices whole wheat bread
   2 ounces cheddar cheese, sliced
   1 tomato slice
   Mustard to taste
Raw vegetables:
   10 baby carrots
   ½ cup cauliflower florets
   ½ cup broccoli florets
¼ cup low-calorie sour cream dip
Iced herbal tea

SNACK

Orange-cranberry bread topped with:
   1 tablespoon fat-free cream cheese

1 medium apple
Sparkling water

DINNER

2 cups split pea soup made with:
   ½ cup cooked carrots
2 pieces cornbread
1 cup 1% low-fat milk

SNACK

2 celery stalks filled with:
   1 tablespoon peanut butter
   2 teaspoons raisins
½ cup canned mandarin orange slices,
   drained

Daily totals: 2,484 calories; fat 29%;
protein 17%; carbohydrate 54%; fiber
41 grams; salt (sodium) 5.3 grams*

Day 6

BREAKFAST

1 cup granola
1 cup 1% low-fat milk
1 medium banana
Herbal tea

SNACK

1 medium orange
Sparkling water

*Sodium will be higher if salt is added to foods.

LUNCH

Spaghetti:

    1 cup cooked spinach spaghetti

    1/2 cup meat sauce

Tossed salad:

    1 cup chopped romaine and other
       leaf lettuce

    1/4 cup grated red cabbage

    3 cherry tomatoes

    1 1/2 tablespoons French dressing

1 sourdough roll with:

    1 teaspoon butter

1 baked apple

Water

SNACK

1 medium tangelo

1/2 cinnamon-raisin bagel, toasted,
    topped with:

    2 teaspoons all-fruit jam

6 ounces low-fat vanilla yogurt

DINNER

2 cups tomato-based fish chowder

15 oyster crackers

Carrot salad:

    3/4 cup grated carrots

    1/4 cup diced apple

    1 tablespoon raisins

    4 teaspoons fat-free mayonnaise

Water or tea

SNACK

1 cup frozen fresh blueberries

Daily totals: 2,532 calories; fat 27%;
protein 17%; carbohydrate 56%; fiber
42 grams; salt (sodium) 3.1 grams*

Day 7

BREAKFAST

1 toasted whole wheat English muffin
    topped with:

    2 tablespoons peanut butter

    2 tablespoons wheat germ

    1 tablespoon honey

1 cup honeydew melon cubes

1 cup pineapple juice

Tea

SNACK

2 pieces pumpernickel bread filled
    with:

    4 teaspoons fat-free cream cheese

    4 cucumber slices

1 1/2 cups sparkling water mixed with
    1/2 cup orange juice

LUNCH

Baked potato filled with (reheat in
    oven):

    1/4 cup low-fat ricotta cheese

*Sodium will be higher if salt is added to foods.

1 tablespoon grated Parmesan
   cheese
¼ cup chopped broccoli, steamed
1 cold roasted chicken drumstick
1 medium apple
10 baby carrots
1 cup 1% low-fat milk
Water

SNACK

½ cup black bean dip (from mix)
10 oven-baked tortilla chips
1 cup orange juice

DINNER

Shrimp and vegetable medley (sautéed
   in 1½ tablespoons safflower oil):
   4 jumbo shrimp
   1 cup broccoli florets
   1 cup sliced carrots
   5 mushrooms, thickly sliced
   3 tablespoons grated cheddar cheese
1 cup pasta spirals, cooked
Water or tea

SNACK

1 frozen fruit juice bar

Daily totals: 2,509 calories; fat 25%;
protein 16%; carbohydrate 59%; fiber
44 grams; salt (sodium) 1.9 grams*

*Sodium will be higher if salt is added to foods.

CHAPTER SEVEN

Nutrition During the Third Trimester

During the third trimester of pregnancy:

1. Follow the guidelines outlined in the Baby-wise Diet.
2. Try to limit weight gain to approximately 0.7 to 1.4 pounds a week for a total of 9 to 19 pounds. Don't be surprised if weight gain drops slightly in the final two to three weeks.
3. Continue to take a multiple vitamin and mineral that contains 100 to 200 percent of the Reference Daily Intake (RDI) for all vitamins and minerals plus at least 18 mg of iron each day.
4. Continue to avoid alcohol, tobacco, or any medication not approved by your physician as safe during pregnancy.
5. Exercise daily, but adjust the routine, intensity, or duration as needed.
6. Rest. Put your feet up and take an afternoon nap.

Weight Gain and Why

During the third trimester your baby gains a considerable amount of weight, stretching your abdomen to its maximum. Some women eat less during this time because their stomachs cannot find room for large meals. Others cut back on their food intake because they think they look or feel heavy. However, this is not a time to limit weight gain.

Weight gain in the last trimester is just as critical, if not more so, than during the previous six months. Women who restrict calories at this time could be jeopardizing the birth weight, health, and mental development of their babies. The placenta, head circumference (a measurement of brain development), and birth length are reduced when food and calorie intake are not sufficient. In fact, some evidence shows that the mother's weight gain in the third trimester is the most important indicator of the baby's birth weight.

Interestingly, a woman born to a mother who restricted calories in the third trimester and so was a low-birth-weight baby at birth also can pass on that heritage to her baby. Consequently, your mother's weight gain throughout, and especially in the third trimester, might affect your baby's birth weight, just as your weight gain during pregnancy might influence the birth weight of your grandchildren! It cannot be overemphasized, however, that the sins of our ancestors can be, to a great extent, corrected by taking good care of ourselves before, during, and after pregnancy.

Of course, encouraging weight gain during the last trimester does not give you a license to gorge! (Excessive weight gain, or more than two pounds a week, could be a sign of pregnancy-induced hypertension, or PIH, and should be checked by your doctor.) Also, limit the number of times you weigh yourself to once a week. Your weight is likely to vary during this last trimester because of water retention and fluctuations in weight gain, so daily weigh-ins could give you a false reading.

While much of your weight gain in the second trimester was caused by your expanding tissues, including the placenta, your fat stores, breast tissue, and blood volume, in the third trimester it is your baby, and to a lesser extent the placenta and amniotic fluid, that is causing the gain. Your baby will double in size during the last three months of pregnancy. In addition, your breast tissue and other body tissue are gearing up for breast-feeding. That means you'll be gaining between nine and nineteen pounds during the last three months of pregnancy, with an emphasis on pacing the gain—that is, about one pound per week. Women who entered pregnancy already overweight should gain about a half-pound a week during this last trimester, while women who were underweight prior to pregnancy may gain as much as five pounds per month. However, these weight gains are averages; some women will gain more, others less, and still give birth to healthy babies.

If you are having trouble eating enough, try dividing your food intake into several small meals and snacks so that you eat every three hours. Drink liquids between meals rather than at mealtime, so that you can save every bit of your small stomach for food. If you aren't gaining enough weight, reevaluate your eating habits. Are you following the Baby-wise Diet guidelines or are you falling short of one or more essential servings? Are you forgetting to include several nutritious snacks throughout the day? If you are eating only three meals a day, chances are you aren't consuming enough calories or nutrients.

If you are gaining too much, check with your physician to make sure there are no health issues related to your weight gain. Next check your fat intake. Have extra salad dressing, fried foods, gravies, creamy desserts, or other hidden fats crept into your menu plans? Also, choose foods that give you the most nutrient "punch" for the least calories. That means concentrating on nonfat milk, not whole milk, for your calcium-rich servings; strawberries, not dried apricots, for your fruit servings; and broccoli, not corn, for your vegetable. Also, don't cheat. Even an extra 100 calories can add an extra pound in one month, so stick to the Baby-wise Diet. Finally, review your daily exercise. Have you stopped walking every day or cut back? Although the intensity and duration of your exercise may decrease in the third trimester, you can still exercise in several short sessions during the day to maintain a good level of fitness and burn extra calories.

When and What to Eat and Drink

While your baby is putting on the pounds (at a rate of an ounce or two a day in the ninth month!) during this trimester, the infant brain also is developing rapidly. The brain increases in size and in the number of mature nerve cells it contains. These metabolically active cells account for only 2 to 3 percent of body weight, but are now consuming up to 20 percent of the baby's entire energy intake. Your baby also is storing nutrients, in particular iron and calcium. You will be transferring more calcium to help calcify your baby's bones and iron to help build his or her iron stores and protect against anemia in the first few months of life. So you must make sure you eat enough or the supply will go to the baby, leaving you feeling tired and mentally sluggish. (See "Sneaking More Calcium into Your Diet," page 198.)

Sneaking More Calcium into Your Diet

Tired of drinking four glasses of milk every day? Does the thought of another cup of yogurt put a damper on your appetite? You can obtain ample amounts of calcium without even knowing it. Try the following tricks for adding calcium to your diet:

1. Make creamed soups and cream sauces with evaporated nonfat milk instead of cream.
2. Cook your brown rice, oatmeal, or noodles in milk instead of chicken stock or water.
3. Add nonfat dry milk to recipes for muffins, breads, pancakes, milkshakes, or even meatloaf.
4. Drink calcium-fortified orange juice or use calcium-fortified bread.
5. Substitute low-fat cheese for meat in lasagna, ravioli, or stuffed shells.
6. Use undiluted evaporated nonfat milk in mashed potatoes.
7. Use canned salmon with the bones.
8. Blend milk with fresh fruit to make a fruit shake.

Your calorie intake should average approximately 2,500 calories a day (more if you exercise). As always, the Baby-wise Diet forms the basis of your eating plan, with the following minimum number of servings from each list:

> 3 servings from the Calcium-Rich Group
> 6 servings from the Vegetable Group (at least 2 servings should be folic acid–rich choices)
> 4 servings from the Fruit Group (at least 2 servings should be vitamin C–rich choices)
> 7 servings from the Grains Group (at least 4 servings should be whole-grain choices)
> 3 servings from the Extra-Lean Meats and Legumes group (try to include 2 to 3 servings of fish and 4 to 5 servings of legumes in the weekly menu)
> 6 servings from the Quenchers Group

This is the time to keep cheating in check. A piece of chocolate cake might taste good, but it is a poor source of vitamins and minerals, which your baby needs right now. So make sure you've eaten your quota of nutritious foods before diving into the cheesecake! Be a shrewd cheater. If you want a cookie, make it a more nutritious oatmeal-raisin rather than a chocolate sandwich cookie. Angel food cake topped with raspberries might satisfy the sweet tooth and is more nutritious than pound cake with icing, and frozen fruit ice may satisfy a craving for something sweet and cold without spending the extra calories on ice cream.

Your diet should continue to be rich in carbohydrates, such as fruits, vegetables, grains, and cooked dried beans and peas. These foods help avoid constipation and fatigue and supply ample amounts of all the vitamins and minerals, while being low in fat and thus helping regulate weight gain.

Protein requirements also are at an all-time high in the last trimester. Protein is the building block for the baby's muscles and tissues, which are growing at record rates. Extra protein also is needed as you gear up for labor, delivery, and breast-feeding. However, typical American diets are already high in protein, so unless you are following a strict vegetarian diet or are eating few protein-rich foods, your intake of this nutrient is probably more than adequate. The Baby-wise Diet supplies at least 70 grams of protein daily, which is more than the 60 grams recommended for pregnant women. In addition, your protein needn't come from expensive cuts of meat, such as lamb chops, steak, or roast prime rib. Cooked dried beans and peas, tofu, chicken without the skin, low-fat milk, and fish also are sources of quality protein.

Other nutrients that become increasingly more important as you approach labor and delivery are those related to immune function, including vitamin A, copper, zinc, and the B vitamins; the antioxidant system, including beta carotene, vitamin C, vitamin E, and selenium; and circulation, including protein, iron, and calcium. These are also needed in moderate amounts for optimal healing of tissues after delivery. In addition, several of these nutrients function directly in the healing process.

Vitamin C is especially important in wound healing and recovery from delivery. Skin, blood vessel walls, and all body tissues are "glued" together by connective tissue, of which collagen is a major component. Repairing tissues includes producing and laying down new connective tissue and collagen, and vitamin C is a critical factor in collagen formation. Slow wound healing and poorly formed scars that break open, scaly skin, and tender joints are symptoms of vitamin C deficiency.

Zinc, vitamin E, and several B vitamins, including pantothenic acid, are important in healing wounds and speeding recovery after surgery. Vitamin A is essential for maintaining and repairing the delicate tissue that lines the vaginal and uterine walls, called epithelial tissue. Optimal intake of this vitamin helps restore these tissues after the baby is born. Marginal intake of these nutrients has been reported in pregnant women, while deficiencies are common during times of stress, illness, or hospitalization.

By following the Baby-wise Diet, you are assured of obtaining all the nutrients you need to meet the added stress of the third trimester and of labor and delivery. If you have chosen to take a vitamin and mineral supplement, keep in mind that moderation is the rule. For example, although increased intake of zinc either through dietary or supplemental sources is recommended for helping improve healing and recovery from injury, caution should be used in overdosing with this trace mineral. Intakes in excess of 50 mg could result in secondary deficiencies of other trace minerals, such as copper.

Water: The Most Important Nutrient

Water is one of the most important nutrients in your diet, and it can undermine your energy and mood during pregnancy if consumed in short supply. Water constitutes half of your body weight, or ten to twelve gallons. You need this essential fluid to digest and absorb other nutrients, remove waste products from the body, regulate body temperature, and perform the millions of metabolic processes essential to life. You also lose about two to three quarts of water every day through perspiration, urination, and other wastes. Consequently, dehydration can set in quickly if you aren't replacing these fluid losses.

Weight gain during pregnancy and milk production during breast-feeding place an added demand on your body's fluid supply; you must consume ample amounts of water and other fluids to meet this need. Unfortunately, many women fall far short of optimal when it comes to drinking enough water. Since thirst is a poor indicator of need, your best bet is to drink at least twice as much water as it takes to quench your thirst, with a minimum of at least six to eight glasses of fluids each day. If you exercise regularly, you'll need even more.

Food and Mood Changes

There is nothing quite so permanent as having a baby. You can change jobs, move to a new city, and get a divorce, but you can't stop being a parent. So it's not surprising that while pregnancy is one of the best of times in a woman's life, it also can have its not so good moments when fears, worries, or doubts surface. Don't worry if you have a few mixed feelings as the due date approaches; most women experience at least a little ambivalence, although until recently many women kept their feelings to themselves. Many women also report problems with memory loss during pregnancy. One study found that recall, recognition, and memory were impaired in pregnant women as compared to nonpregnant women; however, there is no evidence that any loss of memory persists longer than a few weeks after the baby is born.

First, view your mood swings as natural, not pathological. In fact, emotional ups and downs might result from changes in hormones, such as prolactin, a hormone that stimulates milk production and mood swings, and is produced in increasing amounts. Second, recognize that any emotional high or low is probably a phase that will pass. So revel in the highs and wait out the lows. Third, share your feelings with someone you can trust and who can provide understanding: a spouse, a friend, a parent, or even your physician. A support network is critical for getting the help, advice, and hand-holding that every mother-to-be needs. Be honest with yourself about your fears. (Will I be a good parent? Can I juggle work and a family?) Also, be realistic; you don't have to be perfect to be a good parent. In addition to the normal emotional ebb and flow of pregnancy, what a woman eats, even at a single meal, could affect whether she is happy, sad, irritable, calm, absentminded, or clear-thinking.

It is no coincidence that people turn to pasta, desserts, and other carbohydrate-rich foods when they feel down in the dumps. Carbohydrates have a profound effect on numerous body chemicals that regulate how a woman feels and acts.

According to Richard Wurtman, M.D., professor of brain and cognitive science at Massachusetts Institute of Technology (MIT), carbohydrates stimulate the release of the hormone insulin from the pancreas, which in turn lowers blood levels of all amino acids except tryptophan. Normally, tryptophan must compete with other amino acids for entry into the brain, but with reduced competition, tryptophan levels rise. The brain then converts tryptophan into serotonin, a neurotransmitter that sends messages between nerve cells. Serotonin helps regulate sleep, reduces pain and appetite, alleviates irritability, and elevates mood.

Interestingly, several conditions associated with depression and fatigue also are linked to increased cravings for carbohydrate-rich foods, suggesting that people unknowingly self-regulate their moods with the foods they eat. Dr. Wurtman reports that the carbohydrate-rich snack alters brain chemistry and provides temporary relief from mild depression or tension. In contrast, a high-protein diet, by supplying more of the competing amino acids, reduces tryptophan and serotonin levels in the brain. Consequently, carbohydrate-sensitive people who eat high-protein breakfasts might experience fatigue or mood swings and crave carbohydrate-rich midmorning snacks in an effort to raise brain serotonin levels and "feel better."

Often people are less alert, have trouble concentrating, make more mistakes, and feel sleepier after carbohydrate-rich meals as compared to protein-rich meals. Consequently, the time of day you grab a bagel or chow down on a plate of pasta also could affect your mood. Pasta for dinner might leave you feeling relaxed, while the same meal for lunch could make you sluggish.

Research conducted by Larry Christensen, Ph.D., chairman of the Department of Psychiatry at the University of Southern Alabama, adds fuel to the carbohydrate-mood controversy. Dr. Christensen's research shows that depression and fatigue often vanish when sugar (and caffeine) are removed from the diet. In essence, using sugar to self-regulate mood is a temporary fix. In the long run, it could create a vicious cycle. "The person suffering from depression who turns to sugary foods might relieve the fatigue and feel better for a short while, but the depression and fatigue return," says Dr. Christensen. The person then must either reach for another sugar fix or seek help elsewhere. As opposed to the temporary sugar high, eliminating sugar and caffeine from the diet is a permanent solution.

So what can you do? First, carbohydrate cravers cannot "will away" their cravings, so work with them instead. Make sure every meal contains some complex carbohydrate–rich foods, such as bread, cereals, crackers, or other starches. In addition, carbohydrate cravers should plan carbohydrate-rich snacks during that time of the day when they are most vulnerable to snack attacks, and they should choose whole-grain breads and cereals. People who know they are sensitive to sugar should avoid sweets or eat them in small doses and always with other, more nutritious foods.

Second, any dramatic change in normal eating patterns can alter brain chemistry. Cutting calories, bingeing on sweets, skipping meals such as breakfast, or other unusual eating habits affect neurotransmitter levels and, consequently, mood and behavior. In contrast, the Baby-wise Diet that contains at least 2,200 calories from fresh fruits and vegetables, whole-grain breads and cereals, cooked dried beans and peas, nonfat milk products, fish, poultry, and extra-lean meats provides ample amounts of all the nutrients associated with mental and physical health. Consuming several small meals or snacks throughout the day, rather than two to three big meals, helps maintain steady blood sugar and neurotransmitter levels.

Regular exercise, effective coping skills, and a strong social support system also are important considerations. Chronic depression and fatigue can be symptoms of other problems and might affect the outcome of your pregnancy, so always consult a physician if emotional problems persist or interfere with the quality of your life and your pregnancy.

Gearing Up for Delivery

In the game of life and birthing, there are no guarantees. Every woman's experience giving birth is different and even varies from one pregnancy to the next. Even a pregnancy nourished on whole grains, dark green leafies, and brisk walks cannot promise a two-hour, pain-free labor. However, a growing body of evidence does show that good nutrition prior to and during pregnancy and exercise during pregnancy might improve your odds for an easier pregnancy, delivery, and speed your return to prepregnancy weight and fitness levels. Feeling good and fit also pumps up your self-esteem, helps you tolerate labor pains, and boosts your endurance during the hard work of birthing a baby. Having a support person by your side throughout labor also might shorten the labor process and help speed recovery.

The fluid and nutrition needs of a woman in labor have been compared to the needs of a competition athlete. Consequently, depriving yourself of food and fluids before or during labor could affect the labor progress and outcome. Researchers at St. Louis University Medical School speculate that consuming ample amounts of carbohydrate-rich foods or carbohydrate loading the week before labor onset—the same dietary practice used by athletes prior to a marathon—might increase tissue glycogen stores and help supply extra energy for labor and delivery.

Some physicians recommend restricting food and/or fluids during labor because of the possibility of vomiting or problems with aspiration if anesthesia is required. On the other hand, not eating throughout a lengthy labor might mean fasting all day. Blood sugar and muscle glycogen (energy) stores, the major sources of energy for both the laboring mother and the baby, are depleted during a fast, and this could affect the baby's well-being. Babies of mothers who did not eat anything for several hours prior to and/or during labor are less active than babies born of mothers who periodically replenished energy stores by drinking fruit juice or eating small snacks. When blood and muscle stores of sugar are depleted, the body turns to fat tissue. As a result, large quantities of fat fragments, called free fatty acids or ketones, are partially broken down for energy, causing an increase in blood levels of ketones. The accumulation of these fat fragments is called ketosis. It is unclear whether or not ketosis is harmful to the mother or infant. There is some evidence that ketosis is associated with prolonged labor, but it is uncertain which comes first.

Evidence shows that as ketone levels rise in the mother, they cross the placenta and rise in the baby's blood, increasing the acidity of the blood. Babies apparently have a relatively high tolerance for this fluctuation in the normal acid-base balance. On the other hand, women who consume some carbohydrates, in the form of juice or food, during labor lower their ketone levels and decrease their babies' exposure to these breakdown products as well. Levels of essential amino acids, the building blocks of protein, also drop after only twelve hours of food deprivation.

Despite the lingering belief that women should not eat during labor, more recent evidence shows that eating something periodically could be beneficial. In one study of forty laboring women, those women who ate light meals of toast, ice cream, yogurt, or fresh fruit required less pain relief and their labors were shortened by an average of ninety minutes, as compared to women who were allowed only toast and tea at the onset of labor and sips of water thereafter. In addition, Apgar scores (an indicator of a baby's physical condition a few minutes after birth) of babies in the well-fed group were higher than in the food-restricted group.

In the weeks prior to your due date, you should discuss all of your labor plans with your physician, including how you will nourish yourself prior to and during the birthing process.

Premature Labor and Delivery

Premature labor is when labor begins more than three weeks before the due date. Uterine contractions cause the cervix—the mouth of the uterus—to open sooner than normal, which can result in the birth of a premature baby who is at high risk of developing serious complications, including problems with breathing, eating, and body temperature regulation. Understanding the early signals of premature labor can help you prevent your baby from being born too soon.

Premature labor often is not painful, but might be accompanied by uterine contractions that occur every ten minutes or more often. You might experience some menstrual-like cramping in the lower abdomen that might come and go or stay constant. These cramps are your uterine wall tightening, and you can feel it tighten or harden during the contraction and soften after the contraction stops. While most women experience some "false alarm" contractions during pregnancy, called Braxton Hicks contractions, these cramps are irregular, while more than five contractions an hour might signal premature labor. Other symptoms of premature labor include intermittent or constant dull aches and pains in your lower back below the waistline, some pressure in the pelvic area as if the baby were pushing down, and a sudden increase in vaginal discharge. Call your doctor right away if you experience more than five contractions in one hour with or without any of the other symptoms. Medications are available that can stop premature labor if it is caught in the early stages.

A Nutritional Approach to Common Problems

The last trimester comes with its own set of ups and downs. Some you may have encountered in the second trimester, such as constipation; others, such as insomnia or leg cramps, might develop for the first time in the last months or weeks of pregnancy. In many cases, there is something you can do to prevent or at least lessen the symptoms.

Constipation

If constipation and/or hemorrhoids weren't a problem during your second trimester, they might develop now. Hemorrhoids are varicose veins that swell in small lumps around the anus. They usually develop from the uterus's putting pressure on these veins or from straining associated with constipation.

Try drinking plenty of water—at least six to eight glasses of water and other fluids every day. If you are following the Baby-wise Diet, your intake of fiber-rich fruits, vegetables, legumes, and whole grains should be sufficient to keep constipation at bay. Try prunes, prune juice, or figs, or add a little extra bran to your breakfast if you need an added fiber boost. Eating regularly also might help, since it keeps your body on a schedule that might help regular bowel movements. Daily exercise also is important. As mentioned before, do not take laxatives without physician approval.

Frequent Urination

The expanding baby and uterus will put pressure on your bladder, especially after the baby drops lower into the pelvic space in preparation for delivery. This might increase the need to urinate during the day and throughout the night. Even though your bladder might be almost empty, the pressure gives the same sensation of fullness as if the bladder were filled to capacity. Do not cut back on your fluid intake! However, you may want to drink most of your fluid allotment in the early part of the day and cut back in the evening hours. When you are resting, lie on your side so that the uterus is not pressing on the kidneys and bladder, interfering with their proper function.

If the pressure of the uterus on the bladder causes urine to leak between visits to the bathroom, you can practice Kegel exercises to strengthen the muscles that surround the urethra (the tube that carries urine from the bladder out of the body). Your doctor or nurse can help you learn the proper technique for doing Kegels correctly. Basically, you contract the muscles in the vaginal, urethra, and anal areas as if you were stopping the flow while urinating. Contracting these muscles for three seconds, then relaxing and repeating this exercise twelve to fifteen times in a row, at least six times a day, should help you hold your urine and will help strengthen the vaginal walls after delivery.

Hemorrhoids

As mentioned in chapter 6, hemorrhoids can develop in the later stages of pregnancy. Although the pressure of the expanding uterus and weight of the baby alone can cause hemorrhoids, often these painful, swollen veins around the rectum develop as a result of constipation. Straining during bowel movements and having very hard stools only make the situation worse. Always check with your physician before self-medicating with over-the-counter preparations. In addition, the Baby-wise Diet contains plenty of fiber-rich foods to help prevent constipation and, combined with daily exercise and at least six to eight glasses of water a day, can go far in preventing hemorrhoids. Warm baths, ice packs, and lying down periodically can help relieve hemorrhoids. The associated itching and burning can be treated with topical ointments or a physician-approved safe suppository.

Insomnia

Irregular sleep habits, an inability to fall or stay asleep, and frequent awakenings are all symptoms of insomnia, which can develop in the last trimester of pregnancy. Your abdomen has grown so large that a comfortable position is hard to find, plus the anticipation of the new baby might keep you awake at night. Pregnant women are most likely to have trouble falling asleep and are likely to wake up more frequently in the middle of night, often because of the increased need to urinate. In contrast, after the baby is born, new mothers report they have no trouble falling asleep, but either do not sleep soundly or are awakened frequently in the middle of the night by you-know-who. Either way, many women yearn for mornings when they awaken refreshed, energized, and free from fatigue.

Many people assume that insomnia refers only to chronic sleeplessness. They're wrong. Insomnia is any sleep problem, from occasional difficulties falling asleep or waking up in the middle of the night to awakening too early or sleeping too lightly. While insomnia is a complex issue with numerous causes, sometimes the answer to your sleep problems might start at the dining table.

While most women cut back or eliminate coffee and other caffeinated beverages during the early months of pregnancy, they sometimes resume drinking colas later in pregnancy. Not only are these soft drinks a source of caffeine, but they could contribute to sleep problems. "People eat chocolate or drink a caffeinated soda pop during the day and then wonder why they can't sleep at night," says Robert Sack, Ph.D., professor of psychiatry and director of Adult Sleep Disorder Medicine at the Oregon Health Sciences University in Portland. "Even small amounts of caffeine can affect sleep architecture, especially in caffeine-sensitive people."

What and how much you ate for dinner could be at the root of your insomnia. Big dinners make you temporarily drowsy, but they also prolong digestive action, which keeps you awake. Instead, try eating your biggest meals before mid-afternoon and eat a light evening meal of 500 calories or less. Small, low-fat meals also will help curb the heartburn that might trouble you during the last trimester. Include some chicken, extra-lean meat, or fish at dinner to help curb middle-of-the-night snack attacks.

Spicy or gas-forming foods also might be contributing to your sleep problems. Dishes seasoned with garlic, chilies, cayenne, or other hot spices can cause nagging heartburn or indigestion, while the flavor-enhancer MSG (monosodium glutamate) causes vivid dreaming and restless sleep in some people. Gas-forming foods or eating too fast cause abdominal discomfort, which in turn interferes with sound sleep. Try avoiding spicy foods at dinner time. Limit your intake of gas-forming foods to the morning hours and thoroughly chew food to avoid gulping air.

The evening snack might be the best alternative to sleeping pills. A high-carbohydrate snack, such as crackers and fruit or toast and jam, triggers the release of a brain chemical called serotonin that aids sleep. "According to our preliminary studies," comments Gary Zammit, Ph.D., director of the Sleep Disorders Institute at St. Luke's Hospital in New York City, "a light carbohydrate-rich snack [before bedtime] may not influence how fast you fall asleep, but it may help some people sleep longer and more soundly." On the other hand, the glass of warm milk, a protein-rich beverage, probably doesn't affect serotonin levels, but the warm liquid soothes and relaxes and provides a feeling of satiety, which might help facilitate sleep.

The stress of pregnancy or the anxiety associated with the approach of labor and delivery can cause insomnia. Often, solving tensions and anxieties eliminates sleep problems. In addition, a major difference between good sleepers and poor sleepers is not what they do at bedtime but what they did all day. Good sleepers exercise and use every opportunity to move. Physical activity helps a woman cope with daily stress and tires the body so it is ready to sleep at night. In addition, try a warm bath before bedtime, and when sleeping, try lying on your side with a pillow supporting your abdomen and another supporting your legs.

Muscle Cramps

Some women suffer from leg cramps, especially at night when they are tired, during the last trimester. In the past, some people mistakenly thought that too little calcium caused muscle cramps; however, there is no evidence that dietary calcium is a factor in pregnancy-related leg or muscle cramps. Many cramps probably develop because of poor circulation and the pressure of the growing baby on your bladder, ribs, lungs, blood vessels, nerves, stomach, and intestines.

Pain in the pubic area and in your thighs could be caused by the baby's pressing against the nerves or by the pelvic joints as they soften in preparation for labor. Women who carry their babies low are most prone to twinges and cramps in the pelvic area that might be relieved by wearing maternity support panty hose or an elastic maternity belt that helps brace and support this area.

Although the exact cause of leg cramps is unknown, often moderate exercise, such as walking, and flexing your feet toward your knees is helpful. In addition, stretching your legs before going to bed can help relieve cramps, but avoid pointing your toes while stretching or exercising, since this added tension might trigger a toe cramp. Wearing support hose during the day and elevating your legs several times throughout the day can help eliminate leg cramps.

Fatigue

The renewed zest you felt during the second trimester might begin to wane as your due date approaches. As mentioned in chapter 5, diet alone cannot wipe out that burned-out feeling. Fueling your body with all the nutrients and calories it needs to function at its best will, however, minimize unnecessary fatigue and help you cope with the stresses of pregnancy.

Make sure you exercise daily, get enough rest (including an afternoon nap), and follow the guidelines outlined in the Baby-wise Diet. Don't turn to candy bars and doughnuts for a quick energy fix; they'll only aggravate your fatigue in the long run. Turn instead to nutritious snacks that include at least one whole grain, fruit, or vegetable and one protein-rich selection, such as low-fat milk or yogurt, beans and peas, a slice of chicken breast, or peanut butter. Don't try to push through the fatigue; rather, take advantage of these last few weeks before your baby is born to nurture yourself.

Third Trimester Meals and Snacks

The biggest obstacles to eating well in the third trimester are a limited capacity, caused by the enlarged uterus pressing against the stomach, and heartburn. If you cannot eat large meals, especially in the evening, try dividing your food intake into several small meals and snacks so that you eat approximately every three hours. This means your snacks will be more like mini-meals and your meals will be more like large snacks. Also, drinking enough fluids remains very important, but try drinking fluids between meals to save more room in your crowded stomach for food. You can watch your diet by using Worksheet 7.1, below.

Worksheet 7.1   My Third Trimester Daily Checklist

Copy this master sheet and complete daily.

FOOD GROUPS	MINIMUM SERVINGS	ACTUAL INTAKE
Calcium-rich foods	3	_____
Vegetables (at least 2 folic acid–rich choices)	6	_____
Fruits (at least 2 vitamin C–rich choices)	4	_____
Grains (at least 4 whole-grain choices)	7	_____
Extra-lean meats and legumes	3	_____
Quenchers	6	_____

Did I reach my goals? _____

What needs improvement? _____

What will I do differently next week? _____

Day 1

BREAKFAST

¹/₂ cup Grape-Nuts cereal
1 cup 1% low-fat milk
1 banana
Herbal tea

SNACK

10 fat-free whole wheat crackers
1 ounce low-fat mozzarella cheese,
  thinly sliced
1 medium orange, sliced
Sparkling water

LUNCH

Chicken salad sandwich:
  ¹/₃ cup chicken salad with celery
  2 slices seven-grain bread
  1 lettuce leaf
6 tomato slices
¹/₂ cup cauliflower florets
1 medium pear
Water or tea

SNACK

Carrot-apple-raisin salad:
  ³/₄ cup grated carrots
  1 tablespoon raisins
  ¹/₄ cup diced apple
  1¹/₂ tablespoons fat-free mayonnaise
2 bread sticks

3 fig bar cookies
1 cup 1% low-fat milk

DINNER

5 ounces salmon, broiled with lemon
  and dill
1 medium sweet potato with:
  2 teaspoons butter
1 whole wheat dinner roll with:
  1 teaspoon butter
Water or decaffeinated coffee

SNACK

1 baked apple seasoned with
  cinnamon, nutmeg, and vanilla
5 cinnamon-apple mini rice cakes with:
  1 tablespoon calorie-reduced peanut
    butter
Water

Daily totals: 2,492 calories; fat 27%;
protein 17%; carbohydrate 55%; fiber
43 grams; salt (sodium) 2.4 grams*

Day 2

BREAKFAST

2 whole wheat pancakes made with:
  1 tablespoon wheat germ
1 cup blueberries
¹/₂ cup nonfat sour cream
1 cup grapefruit juice
Herbal tea

*Sodium will be higher if salt is added to foods.

SNACK

1 corn muffin
1 medium orange
Sparkling water

LUNCH

1 bean and cheese burrito (with salsa if
    tolerated)
1 cup lightly steamed sliced carrots
    (Spicy Carrots** if tolerated)
1 cup 1% low-fat milk
Water

SNACK

⅓ cup raisins
1 whole wheat bagel with:
    2 tablespoons calorie-reduced
        peanut butter
Sparkling water

DINNER

3 ounces chicken breast, roasted with
    seasonings
½ cup spinach noodles, cooked
1 cup steamed peas
Salad:
    1 cup chopped romaine lettuce
    2 tablespoons grated Parmesan
        cheese
    1½ tablespoons Italian dressing
Water or tea

SNACK

2 cups air-popped popcorn
1 cup crunchy vegetables
1 cup 1% low-fat milk, warmed and
    flavored with almond extract

Daily totals: 2,536 calories; fat 26%;
protein 19%; carbohydrate 56%; fiber
50 grams; salt (sodium) 2.8 grams*

Day 3

BREAKFAST

1 large poached egg
2 slices whole wheat toast with:
    1 teaspoon butter
    2 teaspoons all-fruit jam
1 cup fresh orange juice
Tea

SNACK

6 ounces nonfat yogurt with:
    2 tablespoons wheat germ
    ¼ cup fruit salad canned in juice
1 banana
½ toasted English muffin with:
    1 teaspoon butter
Sparkling water flavored with lime

LUNCH

Roast beef sandwich:
    3 ounces sliced lean roast beef

*Sodium will be higher if salt is added to foods.
**Recipe given in the back of the book.

2 slices whole wheat bread
2 teaspoons fat-free mayonnaise
1 lettuce leaf
1 cup steamed green beans
1/2 cup fat-free cottage cheese with
    1/2 cup sliced pear
Water or herbal iced tea

FIRST MIDAFTERNOON SNACK

1 ounce cheddar cheese
5 fat-free whole wheat crackers
1 cup cole slaw made with cabbage,
    pineapple chunks, and 2 tablespoons
    fat-free mayonnaise
6 ounces tomato juice
Water

SECOND MIDAFTERNOON SNACK

1 cup vanilla ice milk
1/2 cup fresh raspberries
Water

DINNER

1 cup split pea soup with 1/4 cup
    steamed diced carrots
1 piece cornbread made with:
    2 teaspoons wheat germ
Tossed salad:
    1 cup chopped butterhead lettuce
    3 tablespoons grated carrots
    2 tablespoons ranch dressing
Water, tea, or decaffeinated coffee

SNACK

25 oyster crackers
2/3 cup cocoa made with 1% low-fat
    milk

Daily totals: 2,488 calories; fat 27%;
protein 18%; carbohydrate 55%;
fiber 37 grams; salt (sodium) 6.1
grams*

Day 4

BREAKFAST

2/3 cup multigrain cereal, cooked with:
    1 tablespoon raisins
    1 cup 1% low-fat milk
1 banana
Herbal tea

SNACK

4 graham crackers
1 nectarine
1 tangelo
3 vanilla wafer cookies
Sparkling water

LUNCH

Peanut butter and jam sandwich:
    2 slices whole wheat bread
    2 tablespoons reduced-calorie
        peanut butter
    1 tablespoon all-fruit jam

*Sodium will be higher if salt is added to foods.

1 medium orange
1 cup 1% low-fat milk
Water

SNACK

1 cup vegetable soup with kidney beans
4 fat-free whole wheat crackers
10 baby carrots
Water

DINNER

1²/₃ cups spaghetti with meatballs
  (made from extra-lean meat)
1 cup steamed cauliflower
½ cup steamed green peas
2 teaspoons butter
Tea or water

SNACK

1 piece angel food cake topped with
  ½ cup peeled and sliced peaches
Water

Daily totals: 2,513 calories; fat 25%;
protein 15%; carbohydrate 60%; fiber
51 grams; salt (sodium) 4.3 grams*

Day 5

BREAKFAST

2 pieces whole wheat toast with:
  2 teaspoons butter
  1 tablespoon all-fruit jam

*Sodium will be higher if salt is added to foods.

1 medium orange
1 cup 1% low-fat milk
Herbal tea

SNACK

1 cup cubed cantaloupe
6 ounces low-fat vanilla yogurt
Sparkling water

LUNCH

1½ cups black bean soup
6 whole wheat saltine crackers
2 tablespoons fat-free cream cheese
2 cups broccoli spears
Sparkling water

SNACK

1 soft pretzel
2 carrots, sliced
1 pear, sliced
Water

DINNER

3 ounces London broil, trimmed and
  broiled
²/₃ cup linguini cooked mixed with:
  2 tablespoons olive oil, basil, garlic,
    and salt to taste
1 cup lima beans with:
  1 teaspoon butter
Water

SNACK

1 cup hot chocolate
1 medium apple

Daily totals: 2,522 calories; fat 25%;
protein 18%; carbohydrate 57%; fiber
61 grams; salt (sodium) 2.3 grams*

Day 6

BREAKFAST

1 cinnamon-raisin bagel, toasted and
   topped with:
   1 tablespoon fat-free sour cream
1 medium orange
1 cup 1% low-fat milk
Herbal tea

SNACK

Fruit smoothie (in blender):
   1 cup nonfat plain yogurt
   1 banana
   $\frac{1}{3}$ cup apricots, canned in light
      syrup
   2 tablespoons wheat germ
   6 ounces pineapple juice
3 graham crackers

LUNCH

1 hot dog (97% fat-free) on 1 hot dog
   bun
Cole slaw:
   1 cup grated cabbage

$\frac{1}{4}$ cup chopped apple
   2 tablespoons fat-free mayonnaise
6 ounces tomato juice
Water

SNACK

1 slice orange-cranberry bread
6 ounces vanilla yogurt
2 celery stalks filled with:
   2 tablespoons calorie-reduced
      peanut butter
Sparkling water

DINNER

4 ounces turkey breast with
   1 tablespoon gravy
$\frac{2}{3}$ cup mashed potatoes made with 1%
   low-fat milk
$\frac{1}{2}$ cup steamed green peas
1 slice whole wheat bread with:
   1 teaspoon butter
Herbal tea

SNACK

$\frac{1}{2}$ whole wheat English muffin, toasted
   and topped with:
   1 teaspoon butter
   1 teaspoon jam
Water

Daily totals: 2,524 calories; fat 25%;
protein 20%; carbohydrate 55%; fiber
28 grams; salt (sodium) 3.9 grams*

*Sodium will be higher if salt is added to foods.

Day 7

BREAKFAST

1 cup puffed cereal with:
    1 tablespoon raisins
    1 tablespoon wheat germ
1 cup 1% low-fat milk
1 slice whole wheat toast with:
    1 teaspoon butter
Herbal tea

SNACK

1 cup frozen grapes
1 cup frozen blueberries
1 cup fat-free cottage cheese
1 multigrain rice cake
Sparkling water

LUNCH

Black bean and couscous salad:
    1/2 cup cooked black beans
    1/2 cup cooked couscous
    1/2 cup chopped green, yellow, and
       red peppers
    1 tablespoon olive oil
    2 tablespoons chopped fresh parsley
    2 garlic cloves, crushed
1 whole wheat roll
1 cup 1% low-fat milk
Water

SNACK

10 baby carrots
5 whole-grain, fat-free crackers
1 ounce cheddar cheese, sliced
Water

DINNER

Chicken-vegetable stir-fry:
    4 ounces chicken breast, cut into
       cubes
    2 tablespoons dry-roasted, unsalted
       peanuts
    4 cups chopped assorted fresh
       vegetables
    1 tablespoon safflower oil
2/3 cup cooked brown rice
1 cup mandarin orange slices
Water or herbal tea

SNACK

1 frozen banana
1/2 cup sherbet
3 vanilla wafers
Water

Daily totals: 2,500 calories; fat 26%; protein 18%; carbohydrate 55%; fiber 49 grams; salt (sodium) 1.9 grams*

*Sodium will be higher if salt is added to foods.

CHAPTER EIGHT

Nutrition and High-Risk Pregnancies

Every woman's dream is to have a problem-free pregnancy and give birth to a healthy, bright baby. Most women's dreams come true as far as having a healthy baby, although they might have a few minor ups and downs, such as nausea or heartburn, on their way to delivering. Even girls and women in high-risk situations who battle the odds against having a healthy baby often can reach their goals with medical attention, good nutrition, and a healthful lifestyle.

Some of the factors that contribute to a high-risk pregnancy are beyond a woman's control, including age; teenagers and women more than thirty-five years old are at higher risk of pregnancy complications and health problems in the newborn than are other women. Multiple births—that is, having twins, triplets, or more—also have their own set of complications. Certain medical conditions, such as diabetes (discussed in chapter 6) or certain infections, also can stack the odds against a pregnant woman. However, just because you are in a high-risk category does not mean you will have problems, especially since you can control most of the other contributing factors, including what you eat, when and how often you exercise, and the quality of your medical attention before, during, and following your pregnancy.

Pregnant Teenagers

Approximately one in every five girls has sexual intercourse by the time she is sixteen years old, and more than one third of these girls become pregnant by the time they are nineteen years old. Consequently, teenage pregnancies account for more than 500,000 births each year, including the 10,000 infants born to mothers younger than fifteen years old.

Biologically speaking, a "mature" woman is at least eighteen years old. By this age, her body has matured enough to handle the physically demanding job of building and delivering a healthy baby. Realistically, however, women younger than twenty-five years are in an in-between zone, since the most successful time statistically for pregnancy is between twenty-five and thirty-four years old.

Five out of every hundred births in the United States are to mothers who are between fifteen and nineteen years old; birth rates are on the increase in girls younger than fifteen years old. These teenagers are taking on one of life's most serious and important tasks at a time when their own bodies are teetering between childhood and adulthood. For example, often the uterus is not structurally or functionally fully developed and does not respond to ovarian hormones in the same way as does a mature organ. So teenage pregnancy comes with its own set of challenges.

A mother less than fifteen years of age who does not eat well or obtain regular medical care is twice as likely to have a preterm or low-birth-weight infant compared to a woman in her mid to late twenties. Babies born to teenage mothers often weigh less at birth than babies born to older women and are more likely to require intensive care or die at birth or within the first twenty-eight days of life. For those babies that live, low birth weight increases the risk for numerous complications, from infection to reduced intelligence. Many of these babies never catch up as they mature and require special attention, schooling, and health care.

To complicate the issue, many health problems are related to insufficient nutrient intake. The nutritional needs of a teenager's body are at an all-time high. To support the accelerated growth during this stage of life, teenagers need as much as 50 percent more calcium, iron, magnesium, protein, and zinc compared to other people. Because of the increased energy demands, the recommended intake for the B vitamins increases. Vitamin D is important in the formation of longer bones, and the recommendation for many nutrients, such as folic acid and vitamins A, C, E, and B6, reach the levels recommended for adults.

Couple these high nutrient needs with the added nutritional demands of pregnancy and you have a situation where the mother's growing body fights with the baby's developing body for every calorie and nutrient. Often, both end up getting less than they need. For example, the competition for nutrients can result

Daily Food Guide for the Pregnant Teenager

FOOD FAMILY	SERVINGS EACH DAY
Calcium-rich group	4–5
Vegetables	6–7
Fruits	4–5
Grains	8–9
Extra-lean meats and legumes	4–5
Quenchers	6–8

SAMPLE MENU

- *Breakfast:* ½ cup oatmeal cooked in nonfat milk and sprinkled with sugar and wheat germ; 1 cup 1% low-fat milk, ½ cantaloupe, and 1 glass orange juice
- *Snack:* 1 cup low-fat fruited yogurt, 1 bagel with peanut butter, 1 apple, and water
- *Lunch:* Cheeseburger, milkshake, 1 cup carrot-raisin salad, and tomato juice
- *Snack:* 1 cup baby carrots, grilled chicken drumstick, and 1 cup 1% low-fat milk
- *Dinner:* 2 bean-and-cheese burritos, 1 cup cooked brown rice, 1 cup tossed salad with low-calorie dressing, 1 cup steamed broccoli, and fruit juice or water
- *Snack:* ½ cup ice cream topped with ½ cup fresh berries, and water

in decreased uterine blood flow during the period of maximum growth in the baby (the third trimester), reduced availability of nutrients in the mother's blood, and limited transmission of nutrients from the mother to the baby, all of which can interfere with infant development and birth weight (see "Daily Food Guide for the Pregnant Teenager," above).

In contrast to older women, teenagers are more susceptible to peer pressure. They are more likely to fill up on soda pop, French fries, and snack foods than on nonfat milk, steamed broccoli, and grilled chicken. One study reported that pregnant teens nibbled primarily on sweets, desserts, soda pop, chips, and other snack items while watching television (for up to five hours) each day. Teens also are likely to have irregular eating habits: as many as one in five skips breakfast and another 50 percent eat nutritionally poor breakfasts. So when the needs of her and her baby's body are at their nutritional peak, the pregnant teenager is eating at her worst.

In fact, national nutrition surveys show that the diets of most teenagers fail to meet even their own nutritional needs, let alone the added needs during pregnancy. Adolescent girls typically consume suboptimal amounts of most vitamins and minerals; in one study, the only nutrient supplied in recommended amounts was protein. Half of all teenage girls consume less than two thirds of the RDA for calcium and up to 70 percent have depleted tissue iron stores; 30 percent are in the final stages of iron deficiency and are diagnosed as anemic. (Iron-deficiency anemia escalates to 55 percent of teenagers after the baby is born.) Magnesium, zinc, vitamin C, vitamin A, and other nutrients also are low. These marginal intakes are likely to affect the outcome of pregnancy, while teenagers who eat nutrient-packed diets and/or supplement their diets with well-balanced vitamin and mineral supplements show improvements in their health and the health of their babies.

Young mothers can eat well and can give birth to healthy, full-term, robust babies. It just takes planning and dedication. If you are less than eighteen and pregnant, you must eat enough nutrient-packed foods to fuel both your growth and the growth of your baby. Both your body and your baby's body are growing twenty-four hours a day, so you must space your food intake so that you eat at least every four hours in order to ensure a constant supply of nutrients and calories. If you skip meals you are more likely to come up short nutrient-wise and are more likely to deprive your baby of essential nutrients needed for growth and development.

A teenager who is normal weight should gain approximately thirty-five pounds during pregnancy; more if she entered pregnancy underweight and less (approximately twenty pounds) if she entered pregnancy overweight. It also is important to space the gain. Teens who gain little weight in the first six months of pregnancy (less than ten pounds by week 24) are more likely to give birth to low-birth-weight babies, even if they make up the weight gain by delivery time. Gaining less than a pound a week in the last trimester also increases the chances of having a premature baby or a low-birth-weight baby. So put aside the "thin is beautiful" beliefs and think more about having a healthy baby. Don't worry; most teenagers return to their prepregnancy weight within forty weeks after (and many well before this) having their babies.

If you are eating all the foods outlined on page 219 and still are having trouble gaining sufficient weight, boost your calorie intake by snacking on ice cream, milkshakes made with Instant Breakfast, cheese, and other high-calorie snacks.

Table 8.1   Vitamins, Minerals, and Other Nutrients in the Pregnant Teenager's Diet

NUTRIENT	RECOMMENDED AMOUNT
Calories	at least 2,400
Protein	76 grams
Vitamin A	5,000 IU
Vitamin D	15 mcg
Vitamin E	10 mcg
Vitamin B1	1.5 mg
Vitamin B2	1.6 mg
Niacin	16–17 mg
Vitamin B6	2.4–2.6 mg
Folic acid	800 mcg
Vitamin B12	4 mcg
Vitamin C	70–80 mg
Calcium	1,600 mg
Iodine	175 mcg
Iron	30–60 mg
Magnesium	450 mg
Selenium	200 mg
Zinc	20 mg

Avoid high-calorie junk foods, such as potato chips, candy, and French fries. Instead, nibble on dried fruits, baby carrots, cherries, frozen grapes, and other nutrient-packed snack foods.

Keep in mind that even if you are pressed for time, preparing a nutritious meal can take no more than five minutes. For breakfast, you can put two slices of cheese in a flour tortilla and microwave it for one minute. Peanut butter mixed with honey and wheat germ and spread on whole wheat bread takes five minutes at most. Even nutritious convenience foods, such as fruited yogurt, a granola bar, oven-baked tortilla chips, and cold pizza, are worthwhile snacks. Take nutritious quick fixes with you, such as fresh fruit, bagels, boxed fruit juice, or packaged cheese and crackers (see Table 8.1).

The challenges of teen pregnancy aren't done when the baby is born; the quality of the baby's life is now a consideration. A teenage mother faces numerous conflicting issues, including social, financial, legal, educational, vocational, and other difficulties. An unplanned or unwanted baby is at even higher risk for problems related to mental, emotional, and physical development. Optimal nutrition continues to be essential, but adopting a healthful diet is most successful only if these other lifestyle issues also are addressed.

The Mature Woman and Pregnancy

While the pregnancy rate has dropped for women in their twenties, it has skyrocketed for women past the age of thirty-five. Today, it is common for a woman to have her first baby or start a second family when she is in her forties. While the risks associated with pregnancy and childbirth are higher in this age group than for younger women, at the same time these women often have planned their pregnancies and are more willing and ready to accept the responsibilities of parenthood than they would have been in earlier years. Limited evidence shows that these women are more mature, better educated, financially more secure, and more settled and patient—all factors that make for good parenting. In short, they are willing to accept the slight increases in risks for the even higher benefits that having babies will add to their lives.

The first challenge faced by the mature woman is becoming pregnant, since infertility increases with age. This results possibly from the aging reproductive system's reduced efficiency, the increased frequency of disorders such as endometriosis and pelvic inflammatory disease, or the escalating risk of diabetes and obesity in this age group. Uterine function and receptivity as well as ovarian hormone levels also decline with age, while the risk for spontaneous abortion rises (see chapter 1 for more information on fertility).

Once a woman has conceived, the next hurdle is avoiding other health risks. The mature woman who becomes pregnant is slightly more likely to develop high blood pressure (especially if she is overweight), diabetes, and other pregnancy-related conditions than a younger woman, and she is at a slightly greater risk for miscarriage. Older women are at even higher risk of delivering low-birth-weight babies if they smoke cigarettes. However, most of these conditions are not related to postponing pregnancy until late in the reproductive years but are linked to preexisting conditions that worsen with age. There is no evidence that low-birth-weight rates, premature delivery, or the labor and delivery experience are any different for the younger or older woman, although there is a higher rate of cesarean section in older women. Other health conditions of concern to the mature pregnant woman are an increased risk for having a Down syndrome baby and the possibility of finding a breast lump while pregnant. These issues should be discussed with your physician, but are not directly related to diet and nutrition.

The importance of lifestyle cannot be overemphasized when it comes to having an uncomplicated pregnancy and a healthy baby in the middle years. In essence, advanced age does not automatically place a woman at high risk, while a lifetime of smoking, drinking alcohol, eating poorly, being sedentary, having chronic stress, and maintaining other unhealthful habits does take a toll. An older mother who eats well, exercises regularly, avoids tobacco and limits alcohol, and takes good care of herself cuts years off her pregnancy profile and can reduce her risk of pregnancy complications to that of a younger woman. Numerous studies show that women past thirty-five who take good care of themselves have no more serious maternal complications than women between twenty and thirty-four years of age. In fact, one study showed that their babies had lower rates of prenatal death and were less likely to have a low birth weight. In essence, women in their thirties and forties who want to get pregnant should:

1. Avoid using birth control pills, since these drugs might delay conception even after they are discontinued.
2. Avoid cigarette smoking and alcohol consumption before and during pregnancy, since these can increase the rate of miscarriage and birth defects.
3. Undergo an amniocentesis (a routine screening test for all mothers-to-be who are more than thirty-five years old) to detect early the presence of Down syndrome or other congenital abnormalities.
4. Seek professional assistance if pregnancy does not occur within six months or so, since the sooner you or your partner begin treatment for infertility the better.

The dietary recommendations for mature pregnant women are the same as for women in their twenties and thirties. See the Baby-wise Diet recommendations for gearing up for pregnancy (chapter 1), during the three trimesters (chapters 5, 6, and 7), and after pregnancy (chapters 9 and 10).

Multiple Births

More women today are having twins and triplets than ever before. In 1992 alone, 92,916 twin births were reported in the United States and they represent up to 2 percent of the live births in other countries such as Canada. This increase is partly due to the use of ovulation-inducing drugs. (The reported incidence of multiple births while using these drugs is as high as 66 percent.) The growing number of women older than thirty-five who are becoming pregnant also is a factor in the increased rates. Regardless of cause, triplets and "higher order" births occur only once in every 1,411 births. The incidence of quintuplets is only one in 20 million deliveries! (Interestingly enough, more than fifty intact quintuplet sets live in the United States alone.) So while all pregnant women are special, there is something superspecial about a multiple birth.

The causes of naturally occurring multiple births (that is, those that cannot be explained by the use of drugs) are poorly understood. A woman may produce multiple eggs, a condition called superovulation (producing fraternal twins), or the fertilized egg may undergo one or more cleavages (producing identical twins or triplets).

Although advances in pre- and postnatal medical care in the last ten years have improved the outcome of these pregnancies, multiple births still remain a high-risk condition that can result in premature labor and delivery and low birth weights. These babies have higher risks for disease and death than do single births and are more likely to show delayed growth while in the uterus, called intrauterine growth retardation (IUGR), especially from week 32 to term. IUGR is partially related to inadequate calorie and nutrient intake and/or tobacco use, but also is strongly related to reduced blood supply to the placenta and the degree to which the uterus can expand, as well as genetic makeup and the woman's prepregnancy condition and age.

A woman carrying twins or triplets is less likely to have a full-term pregnancy (the averages are 37 weeks for twins, 33.8 weeks for triplets, and as little as 31 weeks for quadruplets versus the normal 40 weeks). Women carrying more than one baby are thirty-three times more likely to give birth to preterm, low-

Bed Rest Survival Kit

Remember the old adage, "Be careful what you wish for; you might get it." While most women dream of the chance to put up their feet, lie in bed all day, and enjoy a little stress-free time, for the woman carrying triplets or quadruplets assigned to her bed for months during the second and third trimester, bed rest can be as stressful as cabin fever.

A physician will prescribe bed rest for a variety of reasons, including pregnancy-induced hypertension, multiple fetuses, premature labor, or IUGR. Whatever the reason, a woman assigned to bed for more than a few days needs to develop some strategies for making it a pleasant experience.

1. Set up your makeshift bedroom in an area of the house where you can live and visit with family, such as a family room or a room off the kitchen. (One woman even had a hospital bed brought to her office and continued working from bed until her eighth month!)
2. Surround yourself with the essentials—soft pillows; a telephone; a television with a remote control; a mini-refrigerator or ice chest filled with fruit, chopped vegetables, ice water, fruit juice, and other nutrient-packed items; a table with nutritious snacks, such as rice cakes, peanut butter, nuts, and dried fruit; an intercom system; and any medications for constipation, heartburn, or other pregnancy-related problems.
3. With the help of your physician, identify exercises you can safely do, such as arm exercises using weights (even soup cans will work) or isometric exercises, and do them regularly.
4. Be creative. Take this time to read, keep a diary, write letters, balance your checkbook, write shopping lists for your family, complete puzzles or crossword puzzles, take up knitting or cross-stitch, listen to books on tape, or give yourself a facial.
5. Be industrious. Volunteer to do phone work for a fund-raiser. Call elderly shut-ins to check on their health. Take a correspondence course. Learn a foreign language. Plan your finances or retirement. Start your Christmas shopping by using catalogs. Plan a flower or herb garden.

birth-weight, and very-low-birth-weight infants. For example, the average birth weight for triplets is a little more than 4 pounds, with an average hospital stay of twenty-nine days. The average weight of quadruplets may be only 3¼ pounds. This high incidence of low birth weight is a major contributing factor to the increased risk for disease and death in these babies. Consequently, the most important contributing factor in producing healthy twins and triplets is reducing the rate of low-birth-weight births.

Triplets and higher-order multiple births also are more prone to nervous system problems, including cerebral palsy and mental retardation. The good news is that healthy twins and triplets that do not have a very low birth weight at delivery show little or no differences in nerve and sensory development by one year of age and at school age compared to single-birth babies.

Complications for the mother include postpartum hemorrhage, probably because of the inability of the overdistended uterus to contract effectively after delivery; increased risk for developing pregnancy-induced hypertension (PIH); and an increased risk for birth trauma if the babies are born vaginally. (See "Bed Rest Survival Kit," page 225.)

Diet, Weight Gain, and Multiple Births

If you are carrying more than one baby, you can improve your chances of having bigger, healthier babies by careful selection of what and how much you eat. For one thing, how much weight you gain has a lot to do with how much weight your babies will gain. You need more food, more calories, more protein, and more vitamins and minerals than a woman carrying a single baby. However, one study found that women carrying more than one baby ate about the same amount of food as women with just one baby. In short, they were eating for two rather than three or more, so the babies were forced to split their meals.

Unfortunately, no guidelines have been developed for women with twins, triplets, or higher-order pregnancies. A woman carrying two babies does not need twice as many calories or twice as many nutrients and a mother carrying triplets doesn't need three times the nutrition, but these women do need more than a woman carrying only one baby. The recommendations for multiple births are at best guestimates based on the increased weight gain, with a proposed 50 to 100 percent increase in the Recommended Dietary Allowances (RDAs) advised for normal pregnancies. To ensure optimal nutrient intake, a woman carrying

Table 8.2   Nutrient Needs for a Woman (At Least Age 25) Carrying Twins

NUTRIENT	NORMAL PREGNANCY	TWIN PREGNANCY
Calories	2,500 calories	3,000 calories
Protein	60 mg	90–120 mg
Vitamin A	800 mcg	1,000 mcg
Vitamin D	10 mcg	15 mcg
Vitamin B1	1.5 mg	3.0 mg
Vitamin B2	1.6 mg	3.0 mg
Niacin	17 mg	25 mg
Vitamin B6	2.2 mg	4.0 mg
Folic acid	400–800 mcg	800 mcg
Vitamin B12	2.2 mcg	3.0 mcg
Vitamin C	70 mg	150 mg
Calcium	1,200 mg	1,800 mg
Iodine	175 mcg	300 mcg
Iron	30–60 mg	50+ mg
Magnesium	320 mg	450 mg
Selenium	65 mcg	100 mcg
Zinc	15 mg	30 mg

more than one baby should seriously consider taking a moderate-dose multiple vitamin and mineral supplement, if she is not already taking one (see Table 8.2).

Additional babies mean additional weight gain, not only from the baby but because the placenta(s), the amniotic fluid surrounding the babies, the blood volume, the uterus, and other support tissues also expand. An approximate weight gain of thirty-five to forty-five pounds above the prepregnancy weight (unless already overweight) or about 50 percent more than a normal pregnancy has been recommended for women carrying twins. The rate of gain in the second and third trimesters should be approximately 1.7 pounds a week.

There is not enough research on triplets and higher-order pregnancies to establish an ideal weight gain. One study from Rush Medical College and Johns

Hopkins University School of Medicine reported that the "ideal" twin pregnancy was thirty-five to thirty-eight weeks gestation, and the mothers gained more weight during the early months of pregnancy than did mothers who experienced more complications during their pregnancies. Limited evidence shows that a weight gain of fifty pounds, with at least thirty-six pounds gained by week twenty-four, is needed to ensure higher birth weights and optimal outcomes for triplets.

Researchers at the Higgins Nutrition Intervention Program at the University of Sherbrooke and McGill University in Quebec report that a high-calorie, nutrient-packed diet can dramatically improve a woman's chances of having healthy twins. The 177 women in this study consumed an additional 500 calories (for a total of 2,700 to 3,200 calories) and an additional 25 grams of protein (a normal pregnancy requires 60 grams so the total for a twin pregnancy would be at least 85 grams) after week 20. These well-nourished women gave birth to bigger babies, they had lower rates of having low-birth-weight and very-low-birth-weight infants (25 and 50 percent lower, respectively), and were less likely to have preterm infants compared to the group of women carrying twins who did not eat the higher calorie and protein diets. In addition, the well-nourished mothers had lower incidences of pre-eclampsia and gestational diabetes.

Iron also is a concern for multiple pregnancies. The extra demands on the mother's iron reserves from the larger placenta and the need to provide greater blood volume to the two or more babies increase the likelihood that the mother will develop anemia. In fact, studies show that up to 35 percent of these mothers are anemic, which implies that many more are iron deficient (the stage prior to anemia). These women must combine an iron-rich diet with iron supplements to make sure they maintain their tissue iron stores and should continue this regimen for at least one year after the babies are born. Even with the best diet, babies born prematurely usually have not had time to accumulate iron in their tissues and are more susceptible to anemia in the first few months of life. Your pediatrician can help monitor your babies' iron status and may recommend supplements if iron levels drop below normal.

A diet of 3,000 calories or more may seem like a lot and you may wonder how you could eat this much food. First, follow the Baby-wise Diet, which forms the foundation for your nutrition plan. Second, to make up the extra 500 to 1,000 calories, you can add more of the same foods, such as more milk (some evidence shows women carrying more than one baby should drink the equivalent of six glasses of milk each day), fruits, vegetables, or grains; or you may choose to splurge and add a few calorie-dense items to make up the difference in energy without adding too much bulk. Adding a little butter to your toast, choosing whole milk instead of nonfat, or snacking on a few cookies in the evening may be all it takes to pump up your calorie intake. Third, divide your food intake into five or six meals and snacks throughout the day, so that you eat at least every three to four hours during waking hours.

AIDS and Pregnancy

Estimates indicate that by 1991 as many as 988,000 Americans were infected with the human immunodeficiency virus (HIV), with an additional 55,000 to 70,000 new cases each year thereafter. HIV infection is in epidemic proportions in many countries around the world. Heterosexual intercourse is now the leading mode for the spread of HIV in women in the United States. In New York City, AIDS is now the leading cause of death in women between the ages of twenty-five and thirty-four, and one in every eighty births is to an HIV-infected woman. Consequently, prior to pregnancy, any woman considering pregnancy should be tested for HIV, which is responsible for the AIDS complex. (Keep in mind that an antibody test for the virus might show up negative for up to three months after infection and no test is 100 percent accurate, although the Western Blot test has an accuracy rate of approximately 96 percent.)

More than likely there will be no symptoms of infection in the first few years after exposure to HIV; however, since pregnancy affects the immune system, it might trigger the onset of AIDS in a woman who is antibody-positive to HIV but previously has had no symptoms. It also is possible to become infected with HIV during pregnancy or for symptoms of AIDS to develop soon after the baby is born.

HIV infection can be transmitted from the mother to the baby and is associated with high rates of disease and death in infants and children. In fact, AIDS in children represents 2 percent of all AIDS cases; AIDS is now as prevalent as cancer in children and is in the top ten leading causes of death in children under the age of 18. In babies, 80 to 90 percent of the time the HIV infection is caused by transmission of the virus from the mother to the developing baby or newborn. Transmission of the virus to the unborn happens 13 to 50 percent of the time in infected mothers, and might occur during pregnancy, at birth, or after birth if the baby is breast-fed. Babies born to HIV-infected women always have antibodies to the virus. However, a baby born to a healthy HIV-infected woman might lose the antibodies after six to eighteen months. But it may take a year or more of repeated testing before it is certain a baby is or is not carrying the virus. Slightly fewer than one in four HIV-positive newborns actually develop AIDS. The incidence climbs to 66 percent in women who already have given birth to an infected infant. The risk is even higher for a woman with AIDS. A baby infected in the womb might have birth defects and have a characteristic facial appearance of a very small head, box-shaped forehead, flat nose, blue, widely spaced eyes, and full lips.

Several studies report that babies born to HIV-positive women are more likely to have low birth weight, and a recent report from Baltimore concluded that babies who are infected with the virus are small for gestational age compared to noninfected infants born to infected mothers. However, many of these women used illicit drugs during their pregnancies, so the low birth weights could have resulted from exposure to drugs or a combination of the HIV infection and drug exposure.

The bottom line? Women who test HIV-positive should think seriously about pregnancy and the potential harm to the baby if the virus is transferred. Women who discover they are HIV-positive after they have become pregnant should make sure they maintain excellent diets. In addition to the immunological consequences of HIV infection, there are several nutritional deficiencies associated with AIDS, including poor intake and low blood levels of vitamin A, beta carotene, vitamin E, vitamin C, vitamin B6, vitamin B12, calcium, magnesium, selenium, and zinc. Preventing these deficiencies could help slow the progression of the disease and help protect the developing baby.

These women also should avoid tobacco, drugs, and alcohol; get plenty of rest and avoid becoming overly stressed; discuss the condition with their physicians and obtain regular medical checkups and monitoring; and generally obtain and maintain their highest levels of health. They also will be advised to formula-feed their infants rather than breast-feed.

The Follow-Up

Women who have experienced complications during pregnancy and have delivered healthy babies sometimes have new issues to face after the babies are born. Researchers at Yale University and Johns Hopkins University report that women who had complications such as diabetes or pregnancy-induced hypertension during pregnancy were more likely to be overprotective and overly concerned about their children's health and safety for years after delivery compared to women who had normal pregnancies. They were more likely to keep their children indoors, call the doctor more often, or worry about daily nuisances such as the sniffles. If you find yourself overly worried about your child, discuss your concerns with your physician to make sure you are not dragging past worries into the present.

III.

After Pregnancy

CHAPTER NINE

Nutrition and Nursing Your Baby

Pregnancy is more than the nine months of developing a baby. The baby-making process began months before you ever conceived, and if you choose to breast-feed, plan on having another baby, or want to regain your prepregnancy figure, it can continue for up to a year after the baby is born. For women who choose to breast-feed their babies, the nutritional link between mother and child remains as important as it was during pregnancy. While the mother provides her baby with the best that nature can offer, she also must make sure she eats a good diet to replenish her body's nutrient stores.

Why Breast-feed?

- "The most tender moments of my life were those first three months when I stayed home with my baby and we'd while away the afternoons snuggled on the couch nursing."
- "I still get a tear in my eye when I remember how my baby would look up at me while nursing and break into a sweet, contented grin."
- "Even though I love my sleep, I wouldn't give up those peaceful middle-of-the-night nursings. Often my baby and I fell asleep while nursing and woke up in the morning rested and ready to nurse again."

Breast-feeding is the ideal option when it comes to feeding your baby. Fortunately, almost all women can breast-feed their babies, regardless of age, breast size, or work schedule. Even health conditions such as diabetes or lupus are not deterrents to nursing as long as the woman consults a physician. The only exceptions are women who take street drugs or who are HIV-positive (in these cases, the possibility of transferring the drug or the infection to the infant is too high to justify nursing); whose babies are lactose intolerant or have a congenital disorder called phenylketonuria, or PKU; or who have a debilitating illness such as kidney disease. However, breast-feeding is a learned skill, not a natural one, so make sure you locate a breast-feeding specialist at the hospital or contact the LaLeche League, a certified lactation consultant, or a local breast-feeding agency as soon as you arrive home to ensure you get off to the right start!

Not only is breast milk the closest thing to "the perfect food," providing all the nutrients in the right proportion and amount for your baby, but it also supplies many vital factors not found in formulas, including essential omega-3 fatty acids (see below for information on DHA) for normal development of vision and the nervous system. Breast milk stimulates the growth of "friendly" bacteria in the infant's digestive tract and reduces the incidence of stomach upsets, diarrhea, or colic. It also might reduce the risk of sudden infant death syndrome (SIDS), obesity, and diseases such as heart disease, lymphoma, and diabetes later in life. Granted, bottle-fed infants grow faster than breast-fed babies; however, this may predispose them to greater risks for obesity later in life. In addition, the slower growth rates observed with breast-feeding might be beneficial for normal nerve development.

Breast milk does something else that formulas cannot: it provides the newborn with a natural defense against colds, infections, allergies, and disease during the early months before the baby's own immune system is fully developed. For example, breast-fed infants are much less likely to develop otitis media, or inner ear infections, not only while breast-feeding but for months after they have switched to solid foods and/or bottles. With more than 60 percent of children suffering from at least one inner ear infection during the early years of life, and since this infection can cause permanent hearing defects and subsequent problems with language development, the potential benefits of breast-feeding cannot be overemphasized.

While the breast-fed baby is physically healthier than a bottle-fed infant, he or she also may benefit intellectually. Children who were breast-fed in the early months of life score higher on IQ tests later in childhood. This effect might be dose-dependent; that is, the longer a baby breast-feeds, the higher are his/or her intelligence scores, with the greatest effects observed on verbal skills. Although inconclusive, these findings suggest that breast milk contains many beneficial substances not found in formulas.

Breast-feeding also benefits the mother. She is more likely to regain her prepregnancy weight than is a woman who chooses not to breast-feed, although the last five pounds may not drop off until after she stops nursing. Breast-feeding also has been linked to a lower risk for developing breast cancer and osteoporosis later in life.

While breast-feeding may be a natural form of birth control, it is not a reliable one; as many as 57 percent of women become fertile again while nursing and almost 80 percent of women begin menstruating within four weeks after they stop nursing. So make sure you use a proven method of birth control, even when nursing your baby.

Nursing mothers are often concerned that their babies aren't eating enough. Unlike bottle-feeding, whereby you can gauge how much your baby is getting, your only clue with breast-feeding is whether or not your breast feels "emptied" and your baby appears satisfied after a feeding. Nursing mothers also express concern that their milk looks diluted or "watery," and worry that their baby isn't getting enough to eat. One way to be assured your baby is eating well and thriving is to check the diapers. A newborn baby who nurses about ten times a day and wets six or more diapers every day is probably getting plenty to eat. Weight and height checks at your regular physician visits also will give an indication of how well your baby is doing. Finally, how your baby acts often is an indicator of how well he or she is eating. Good indicators that a baby is healthy and eating well are if he or she is happy and alert. (See "Overcoming Obstacles to Breast-feeding," page 238.)

Nutrition and Nursing

Women who choose to breast-feed are still eating for two, much as they did when they were pregnant. The same concerns about what you eat and how it will affect your baby apply. Should you drink coffee? Is it safe to celebrate the new arrival with a glass of champagne? Could pesticides in foods find their way into breast milk and harm your baby? Can you breast-feed and still lose weight?

Overcoming Obstacles to Breast-feeding

Many women have the best intentions about breast-feeding but stop soon after starting. In one study, half of the women who had chosen to breast-feed had switched to formula after twelve weeks. Another study concluded that most women breast-feed for only one month. In some cases, early termination of nursing is associated with younger working mothers or mothers suffering from postpartum depression. While you are most likely to continue nursing if you are older, well-educated, relatively affluent, or live in the western United States, there is every reason to believe that any woman can nurse. Since many of the obstacles to nursing can be overcome, including a lack of support at the hospital, at home, or in the workplace, breast-feeding is a possibility for every woman.

Hospital practices are oriented toward bottle-feeding, as are the public displays of infant formula advertising in hospitals, public health programs, and doctors' offices. At the workplace, a lack of flexibility, role models, and privacy (to express milk) further complicate the nursing process. Coupled with self-doubts, lack of motivation, and lack of support from friends and family, these challenges can become obstacles to continuing nursing. Choosing a physician who supports your decision to breast-feed and selecting a hospital that allows "rooming in" (having the baby in the room with you) and provides breast-feeding guidance during your hospital stay can greatly improve your chances of sticking with it after you get home.

By far the greatest factor influencing a woman's decision to breast- or bottle-feed is her motivation and support at home. Granted, it is difficult to combine a career with nursing; however, the overwhelming majority of women who successfully accomplish both report that it is worth the trouble, that they recommend it to other women, and that they had done something special for their babies. In essence, they have adopted an attitude that nursing is important, they are proud of what they are doing, and they figure out a way to keep doing it. They get up a little earlier to express milk at home or express at the office. They develop a sense of humor to get them through days when their milk leaks all over a new silk blouse. They surround themselves with the support of other women who have breast-fed. They overcome obstacles to nursing in public by draping a baby blanket over the shoulder to cover the nursing baby.

Women who decide to breast-feed and continue for more than a few weeks usually have partners who are supportive of their decision. Fathers also can help their nursing partners by taking over some of the household work, making sure the mother has plenty of nutritious food to eat, helping care for the newborn, protecting the mother from people who don't understand breast-feeding, and being patient with her emotional ups and downs.

Whatever the cause, a woman should never feel guilty for deciding to stop nursing. Repeatedly, the research shows that women who stop nursing and those who nurse their babies for months are equally good parents, love their children, and do not differ in their perceptions of themselves as parents. They both report enjoying parenthood and view their babies as "easy" to manage.

In most cases the nutrient needs of a woman who is breast-feeding are even higher than during pregnancy. The plus side to this increased nutrient demand is that breast-feeding "burns" an additional 500 to 700 calories a day; that's the equivalent of running five or more miles without putting on your running shoes!

Unfortunately, the nutritional status of breast-feeding women has not been adequately studied. Limited evidence suggests that, like other women, most breast-feeding women's diets fall short of optimal. One study reported that breast-feeding mothers consume only 59 percent of their calcium requirements, 70 percent of their magnesium needs, 48 percent of their zinc needs, and less than 100 percent of required folic acid, vitamin B2, and vitamin B1. Low dietary intake increases the risk that a mother's nutritional reserves will be depleted to meet the nutritional needs of the infant.

Fortunately, a dietary slipup here and there, such as not drinking enough milk or falling short of your broccoli quota for any given day, has little impact on the overall quality of your breast milk. On the other hand, frequently skipping meals, making poor food choices, or repeatedly consuming less than optimal amounts of one or more nutrients could have far-reaching effects on the health of you and your baby.

Weight, Dieting, and Breast-feeding

Breast-feeding is a natural way to lose weight after the baby is born. You have stored added fat during pregnancy in preparation for breast-feeding. Studies on animals show that if the mother nurses her pups, all this stored fat is "burned" by the end of the nursing period. In contrast, the fat remains if the mother is not allowed to breast-feed. Even more fat is likely to be stored if the animal becomes pregnant shortly after the first baby. In studies on humans, researchers report that women who nurse their babies are more likely to regain their prepregnancy weights than are women who bottle-feed their infants. In short, women who do not breast-feed are more likely to stay "fatter" for a longer period of time than those who do breast-feed.

On the other hand, breast-feeding women require more calories than at any other time in their lives; consequently, this is no time to adopt a strict diet. Unfortunately, weight loss often is a concern for women after the baby is born. They have watched as their figures changed and their bellies grew, and now they are anxious to fit back into their jeans. It is not surprising, therefore, to find that many women do not consume enough calories during lactation, thus placing themselves and their infants at nutritional risk. In many cases, daily energy intake falls to 1,562 calories or fewer—far short of the recommended 2,700 calories they should be consuming. Women who did not gain enough weight during pregnancy and continue to follow low-calorie diets after their babies are born are at particularly high risk of compromising their health and the current and future health of their babies.

For example, cutting calories while breast-feeding can result in fatigue, poor milk supply, and a reduction in the immune factors in breast milk that provide the newborn with a resistance to colds and infections. Several studies have shown that women who try to lose too much weight too fast by severely restricting calories may jeopardize the health and well-being of their babies. Dieting also may be an underlying reason why some women are unable to produce enough milk.

A hidden concern about losing too much weight while breast-feeding is the potential for chemical contaminants to migrate into the baby's milk supply. The breakdown of fat tissue could release other fat-soluble contaminants, such as PCBs, that are stored in this tissue. This concern is theoretical, since there has not been research to test the contaminant levels in the breast milk of women who are dieting. However, since severe weight loss is not recommended, this adds one more argument against strict dieting while breast-feeding.

Weight management and breast-feeding can coexist; however, new moms shouldn't worry about losing weight until at least six weeks after delivery. Instead they should use those first few weeks to focus solely on the care of themselves and their babies. After the first six weeks and when breast-feeding is established, a mild calorie restriction that allows gradual weight loss of no more than two pounds a month is possible. The key word here is *gradual*, since prior to pregnancy the weight-loss goal could have climbed to as high as two pounds a week, while now it is only two pounds per month. Keep in mind that it took nine months to gain the weight and it may take as long or longer to achieve a desirable weight after the baby is born.

Another key to weight loss while breast-feeding is timing. The first four to six months are the most calorie-intensive period for breast-feeding, since during these early months the baby is exclusively drinking breast milk. However, milk production gradually decreases as solid foods are added to the diet in later months. Consequently, the nursing mother must decrease her food intake or she is likely to gain weight. The best indicator of your varying calorie needs is the scale. If you are gaining weight, your calorie intake is too high (or your exercise is too low).

First-time mothers often lose more weight in the first few months after the baby is born than do women who already have children. However, mothers with two or more children often lose more weight between the third and sixth months after delivery. In most cases, weight loss begins to level off by the sixth month. Black mothers also are twice as likely as white mothers to retain more weight, often because they gained more weight during pregnancy. An additional five pounds usually drops off when you stop nursing. According to Lindsay Allen, Ph.D., professor of nutrition at the University of Connecticut, "breast-feeding stimulates a woman's appetite, but once she stops producing milk, her weight drops off." Consequently, whatever your weight is at six months postpartum, minus five pounds if you are breast-feeding, is approximately where you need to start in your weight-management goals.

A breast-feeding mom requires an additional 500 calories above the 2,200 quota for pregnancy. That means she can eat an additional three slices of bread, three ounces of lean chicken, serving of a fruit or vegetable, and a cup of nonfat yogurt for a total of 500 calories. It doesn't mean she can order an extra cheese-burger, French fries, and a soda pop, which would add more than 1,000 calories and far fewer vitamins and minerals. In short, breast-feeding gives you some extra calories to work with, but you need to use them wisely.

While 2,700 calories is optimal, an average calorie intake of 2,200 calories is associated with adequate milk production and appropriate infant growth and allows most women to lose about one to two pounds a month. The extra 36,000 or more calories stored in fat reserves during pregnancy can help make up the energy difference. In fact, most women will gradually lose weight (on average about 1.3 to 1.6 pounds monthly for the first four to six months) without even trying. How do you know if you are getting enough to eat? The most obvious signs are your hunger and the scale. If you are hungry all of the time or if you are losing more than one pound a week, you're not eating enough.

About 20 percent of women will maintain their weight or even gain a little weight after pregnancy. One study found that women who had gained little weight during pregnancy and who had returned to their prepregnancy weight very rapidly—that is, within three months after the baby was born—actually gained weight during the next three months. In contrast, women who had gained the recommended weight or slightly more continued to lose weight during the same amount of time. The researchers speculate that as the extra fluids that accumulated during pregnancy are lost, some women put on fat and so they do not notice the normal postpartum weight loss. In the overly thin woman, the weight gain is probably the body's attempt to stockpile the added fat needed for breast-feeding. For the normal or overweight woman, the postpartum weight gain could result from inactivity and inappropriate eating (see below for more information on the nibbling syndrome).

Another rule to remember is that no woman, especially one who is nursing, should lose weight to please anyone else or even consider trying to achieve unrealistic, and potentially harmful, fashion-model thinness. A new mother's greatest and most important task is to love and nourish both her baby and herself. She should be proud of herself and her accomplishment and should never feel apologetic or guilty about a few extra pounds.

Exercise and Breast-feeding

Daily exercise is an excellent alternative to dieting. Moderate physical activity helps mobilize fat from the mother's fat stores and burns calories, creating a calorie deficit, which is what you need to lose weight. Staying fit also helps avoid the postpartum blues that many women experience in the first few weeks after delivery. It also helps a woman feel livelier and boosts confidence. In fact, women who exercise during pregnancy and resume a modified exercise plan after delivery report they get their "lives back in order" in half the time—that is, in approximately two weeks, compared to women who haven't exercised postpartum (or thirty-four days).

Limited research has been done on exercise during breast-feeding; however, the information that is available supports the benefits to both the mother and the baby. For example, women who exercise are leaner, have higher fitness levels, and produce more milk than do couch potatoes. They burn more calories, so they can eat more food while still losing weight; consequently, they are more likely to eat optimal diets. Breast-feeding women who exercise have the best of all worlds. "Research shows that these women consume more calories, lose weight more consistently, and their milk production is better than sedentary women," says Bonnie Worthington-Roberts, Ph.D., professor of nutrition at the University of Washington in Seattle. So get moving!

Women who have exercised throughout their pregnancies often resume physical activity sooner and will be capable of doing more than women who remained sedentary during those nine months. If you plan to exercise during lactation, the same guidelines apply as during pregnancy, which include obtaining medical clearance, exercising at least three times a week, beginning and ending the session with a warm-up and cool-down period, and gradually increasing the frequency and intensity. In addition, avoid any jarring or bouncing movements and maximal exertion until your pelvic area is completely healed, which usually takes at least six weeks postpartum. Always consult your physician before beginning any exercise program.

Probably the biggest challenge to exercise after the baby is born is time. You may need to set aside a half hour or hour and arrange child care ahead of time. Gyms and health clubs often have baby-sitting services, or you can purchase a baby jogger or a backpack and bring the baby on your walks. Some mothers get together and share child care or take turns watching the children so they can exercise. You will need to decide how you will take time for yourself, while staying realistic about how much you can take on while caring for a new baby. Keep in mind that your exercise program will be in transition during the first few months after the baby is born. Some days you will find time to exercise for an hour; other days you may be lucky if you fit in a walk around the block. Don't let a slip progress to a relapse; just do it—exercise, that is—when and where you can!

Water, Water Everywhere

The most important determinant of how much milk is produced is the infant's demand for milk; in essence, the more you nurse, the more milk you will have. However, the mother's diet has a significant effect on the quality and, in some cases, the quantity of that milk. First, drinking enough fluid is paramount. A nursing mother is losing considerably more fluid, up to 23 ounces or more daily. This fluid drain will automatically make you thirstier. However, thirst is not always a good indicator of fluid needs. A general rule of thumb is to drink twice as much water or fluid as it takes to quench your thirst, or at least six glasses of water in addition to other drinks daily.

While you need more fluid, it is a myth that drinking large quantities of water will increase your milk supply. In one study, nursing women increased their fluid intakes by 30 percent but produced no more milk than before the study. You may tax your kidneys to produce more concentrated urine or develop constipation when fluid intake is too low and you are likely to feel fatigued and thirsty, but ignoring the need for water will not jeopardize your baby's nutrition.

The Big Guys: Fat, Protein, and Carbohydrate

The fat, protein, and carbohydrate content of milk varies little with the mother's intake; however, the type of fat in breast milk is a direct reflection of her diet now and while she was pregnant. Whether a woman is eighteen or eighty, active or inactive, healthy or ill, she should be following a low-fat diet that derives no more than 30 percent of its calories from fat. That recommendation also holds for the breast-feeding woman; however, there is more to the fat issue than just total fat. The type of fat in the nursing mother's diet also is critical.

The composition of fats in milk is controlled primarily by the mother's diet during pregnancy (which established the type of fat built up in her fat stores) and during lactation. If her diet is high in vegetable oils (polyunsaturated fats), her breast milk also will be high in these fats. If she is dieting, her breast milk will be higher in the saturated fats that have been stored in her fat tissue.

A type of fat found in fish oils called the omega-3 fatty acids, and in particular docosahexaenoic acid, or DHA, accumulates in the eyes and brain of the infant during the last trimester of pregnancy. Breast milk also contains DHA, especially when the mother includes a few servings of fish in the weekly diet. Mother Nature wasn't fooling around when she included this fat in breast milk. Recently, researchers have identified a fundamental role for this fat in the development of vision and possibly behavior.

The link between DHA and vision first was studied in young monkeys. Those fed a DHA-free diet performed poorly on vision tests and the defect persisted even into adult life. Next, the evidence showed that premature human babies were at higher risk for vision problems when fed infant formulas, which are typically low in or devoid of DHA. These studies showed that increasing the infant's intake of DHA improved visual activity at four months and possibly beyond. The research now shows that even full-term infants need DHA and are most likely to obtain enough from breast milk, especially if the mother includes a few servings of fish in the weekly meal plan.

In contrast to fat, the amounts of protein and carbohydrate (that is, lactose) are relatively constant in all human milk, regardless of the mother's diet. But that does not mean they can be taken lightly. Protein is your body's basic building block for muscles, organs, bones, cartilage, enzymes, skin, hormones, and numerous other body components. You need it, your baby needs it, and you lose quite a bit of it in breast milk. Consequently, your protein needs are higher during breast-feeding than at any other time in your life. Fortunately, this requirement is easily met by increasing your intake of low-fat milk. In addition, most diets already supply more than enough additional protein, so there is no reason to start ordering 8-ounce steaks or drinking protein-fortified milkshakes. The chicken, fish, milk products, beans and peas, peanut butter, and even grains in the Baby-wise Diet will more than meet your protein needs.

Carbohydrates continue to be the mainstay of your energy needs. If you are feeling fatigued, look first to how much bread, cereal, starchy vegetables, and fruit you are consuming and how often. The Baby-wise Diet supplies 50 percent or more of its calories from complex carbohydrates, which is the perfect mix to help fuel your energy stores and your health.

The Vitamins

When it comes to vitamins, what you eat is what your baby receives. The vitamin content of breast milk reflects the mother's diet. If your diet is rich in the B vitamins, vitamin A, or vitamin D, your milk will be high in these vitamins and your baby will receive ample amounts to sustain growth and health. In contrast, as the vitamin intake of the mother's diet decreases, so does the vitamin content of her milk and the baby's nutritional status suffers as well.

While some is good, excessive dietary intake of the fat-soluble vitamins, such as vitamin A and vitamin D, can result in too high a concentration of these vitamins in breast milk. For example, women who supplement their diets with 20,000 IU of vitamin A produced a sevenfold increase of vitamin A in their milk. No harmful effects have been noted in these cases, but the potential for toxicity remains. Consequently, a nursing mother's goal is optimal, not excessive, when it comes to vitamins and minerals.

B VITAMINS: Nowhere is the relationship between the mother's diet and the newborn's milk supply more pronounced than with vitamin B6. In one study, women who consumed less than 2.5 mg of vitamin B6 daily produced milk that also was significantly low in this B vitamin. A low intake of vitamin B6, in turn, jeopardizes the infant's neurological development. As the mother's intake of B6 increases, so does the B6 concentration in her breast milk—up to two times the current Recommended Dietary Allowance of 2.2 mg. In another study conducted at the University of Maryland, women who supplemented with 4.0 mg of vitamin B6 increased their blood levels of this vitamin, while their breast milk levels of vitamin B6 also increased significantly. In contrast, the babies of women with low vitamin B intakes were more drowsy and less alert than babies nursing from well-nourished mothers. To compound the problem, the vitamin B–deficient mothers provided less stimulation and care to their less-alert babies.

The intricate bond between the mother's and the infant's diets does not stop with vitamin B6. The mother's dietary intake of other vitamins, such as vitamin B1, folic acid, and vitamin C, directly influences the concentration of these nutrients in her milk. Breast-feeding women who follow strict vegetarian diets that exclude all foods of animal origin are likely to produce milk that is low in vitamin B12, unless they take supplements or consume vitamin B12–fortified foods. Babies fed vitamin B12–deficient breast milk are at risk for developing nerve problems, anemia, and metabolic disorders associated with insufficient supply of this vitamin. A diet rich in water-soluble vitamins will produce breast milk that contains optimal levels of these nutrients.

The Baby-wise Diet supplies optimal amounts of all the B vitamins. However, if your diet frequently falls short of perfect when it comes to these guidelines, it would be wise to consider a moderate-dose multiple vitamin and mineral supplement that provides approximately 100 percent and no more than 300 percent of all the B vitamins, including vitamin B1 (thiamin), vitamin B2 (riboflavin), niacin, vitamin B6 (pyridoxine), folic acid, vitamin B12 (cobalamine), biotin, and pantothenic acid.

VITAMIN C: Vitamin C will be important to your baby throughout life. This water-soluble nutrient is essential in the formation of the body's most abundant tissue—connective tissue, which supports and strengthens all other tissues, from the gums to the blood vessels. The vitamin C content of breast milk varies somewhat depending on your dietary intake, so your baby will consume between 24 and 40 mg each day. The nursing mother should consume at least 95 mg of vitamin C daily during the first six months of nursing and 90 mg after that. This amount is easily obtained by including the recommended ten servings of fruits and vegetables in the Baby-wise Diet. Especially good sources of vitamin C include citrus fruits, dark green leafy vegetables, and green or red peppers.

VITAMIN D: Vitamin D helps maintain your bones and builds your baby's bones by enhancing calcium absorption and aiding in the transportation of calcium into the bones and teeth. Children who do not receive enough vitamin D develop bowed legs when they begin to walk because the poorly calcified bones cannot withstand the weight of the body. Limited evidence suggests that vitamin D in breast milk is not affected by the mother's diet. Infant vitamin D status is more affected by sunlight exposure than by the mother's nutritional status.

Consequently, breast milk is a minor source of vitamin D during periods of adequate sunlight exposure, but during periods of reduced sunlight exposure, the vitamin D from milk becomes increasingly important. The baby who is not in the sun and who is breast-fed by a mother who consumes a vitamin D–deficient diet is at highest risk for deficiency.

While there is no evidence that breast-feeding women need any more vitamin D than other women, in general women often don't get enough of this vitamin. The only reliable dietary source is vitamin D–fortified milk (not yogurt, cheese, or other dairy products unless made from vitamin D–fortified milk). A breast-feeding women should consume at least three servings of milk daily to ensure optimal intake of vitamin D, unless she is regularly out in the sun.

VITAMIN K: Vitamin K is unusual as nutrients go, since most of a person's requirements are obtained from bacterial synthesis in the intestines rather than from the diet. However, babies don't have well-established bacterial colonies in their intestines and are at risk for developing vitamin K deficiencies. In fact, newborn infants have low blood levels of this fat-soluble vitamin and are at elevated risk for developing hemorrhage, since vitamin K is essential in the normal blood-clotting mechanisms that stop a bruise or a cut from progressing into a hemorrhage. Consequently, the American Academy of Pediatrics recommends that all newborns get a onetime injection of vitamin K, which usually is administered at the hospital or soon after birth.

Typical dietary intakes or amounts found in supplements (that is, 88 mcg/day) do not significantly affect milk concentrations. However, Frank Greer, Ph.D., at the University of Wisconsin at Madison, reports that daily supplemental intakes of 2.5 mg for the mother can increase vitamin K in her breast milk to a level that approaches that found in commercial formulas and that helps avoid the risk for deficiency in breast-fed infants. Dr. Greer cautions, however, that this research is preliminary and further studies are needed before nursing mothers should self-medicate with vitamin K supplements. In the meantime, it is wise to consume a vitamin K–rich diet that contains several servings of dark green leafy vegetables, Brussels sprouts, nonfat milk, fruit, and cereal, as outlined in the Baby-wise Diet.

The Minerals

CALCIUM: Calcium is the main mineral in bones and teeth and an important mineral in nerve transmission and muscle contraction. No one can do without it, especially a nursing mother who loses 200 to 300 mg of calcium in breast milk every day. If the nursing mother's diet does not supply enough calcium to replace these losses, either the growth of the baby during breast-feeding will be affected or the mother's risk for later osteoporosis increases, since the body will rob the mother's bones to obtain calcium for the infant.

Consequently, optimal calcium intake remains a priority during breast-feeding. A woman should consume at least 1,200 mg of calcium—the equivalent of four glasses of nonfat or low-fat milk. A woman who consumes adequate amounts of calcium-rich foods, such as nonfat milk and milk products, broccoli, and dark green leafy vegetables, can give birth and breast-feed one or many children throughout her life with no harm to her bones. In fact, breast-feeding can have a protective effect against osteoporosis if calcium intake remains optimal.

CHROMIUM: Chromium may be of particular concern for breast-feeding mothers. Insufficient intake of chromium is a problem for most adults, with only one in every ten people consuming enough of this essential mineral. However, chromium might be an even greater problem for breast-feeding women because of the increased demands for this mineral owing to milk production. The research supports this link. For example, nursing women have lower levels of chromium in their hair than do women who don't breast-feed. Hair chromium levels decrease after both pregnancy and lactation, and it takes four months or more between pregnancies to raise hair chromium levels back to prepregnancy levels.

While the baby can concentrate chromium from the mother and thus is protected to a certain extent from deficiency, research conducted by Richard Anderson, Ph.D., research chemist at USDA Vitamin and Mineral Nutrition

Laboratory in Beltsville, Maryland, shows that breast-fed babies may consume as little as 2 percent of their recommended levels of chromium. Insufficient intake of this trace mineral also can increase a woman's risk for developing high blood sugar and even heart disease.

To consume optimal amounts of chromium during breast-feeding, select several servings daily of chromium-rich foods such as wheat germ, whole-grain breads and cereals, fish, cooked dried beans and peas, spinach, and orange juice.

IRON: Both you and your baby need iron to build hemoglobin, the protein in red blood cells that carries oxygen to all the body's tissues. Although the mother's iron intake has little effect on the iron concentration in breast milk, iron remains a primary concern for women after the baby is born. Even with iron supplementation, many women's iron reserves are depleted as a result of pregnancy. Breast-feeding delays the return of menstruation and so gives a woman a chance to replenish herself if she is eating an iron-rich diet. On the other hand, a nursing mother who also is menstruating has an even higher iron requirement because she is losing iron during her period and in her breast milk.

All women should continue eating iron-rich diets and possibly continue taking iron supplements for three months to one year after pregnancy to restock tissue iron stores. In addition, consult your physician about iron supplements for your nursing baby, since some research shows that breast-fed infants are more prone to iron deficiency after the fourth month than are bottle-fed infants.

SELENIUM: Selenium is another mineral of particular concern to breast-feeding women. The nursing baby's selenium status reflects the mother's intake, which should be higher during lactation than at any other time in a woman's life. To add to the risk of developing a deficiency, the selenium content of most foods of plant origin—from fruits and vegetables to legumes and grains—is dependent on the selenium content of the soil in which the food is grown. Consequently, maternal selenium status often reflects the region in which the woman lives. Because of increased needs and suboptimal intakes, breast-feeding women often are low in selenium.

Poor selenium status is easily reversed by increasing consumption of selenium-rich foods, such as seafood (for example, salmon, shrimp, oysters, and trout), extra-lean meat, cooked dried beans and peas, and chicken. A moderate-dose supplement that contains 50 to 200 mcg of selenium also raises blood selenium levels in breast-feeding women and improves the selenium content of breast milk.

Just because some is good does not mean more is better. Selenium is one nutrient that can be toxic if taken in large amounts. So limit intake from supplements to the above-mentioned dose. The "organic" forms of selenium, such as selenium-rich yeast and selenomethionine, are particularly effective in raising selenium levels and might not be as potentially toxic as the inorganic forms, such as selenite.

ZINC: Several studies have reported that breast-fed infants don't get enough zinc, a trace mineral essential for growth and development. Granted, the zinc content of mother's milk is not high and babies often receive as little as 10 percent of their recommended intake when exclusively breast-fed. However, the zinc in breast milk is very well absorbed, while limited evidence shows that the mother's diet has little effect on the zinc concentration of breast milk. Unless a child shows delayed growth or a low resistance to colds and infections, there is little evidence that low zinc intake from breast milk is harmful.

Consequently, while a woman should consume ample amounts of zinc from dietary sources to ensure her health and the health of her baby, there does not appear to be any reason to take extra zinc as supplements while breast-feeding. Infants who are breast-fed for more than four months and who show symptoms of delayed growth might be suffering from marginal zinc intake. Discuss with your physician the need to supplement your baby's diet with zinc under these conditions.

OTHER MINERALS: All other minerals, from magnesium and manganese to iodine and copper, are important for the health of both the mother and her baby. Unfortunately, there is little or no research on how the mother's dietary intake of these minerals affects the baby's food supply. It is safe to say that a diet of fewer than 2,200 calories daily is unlikely to supply all the minerals in optimal amounts, which is yet another reason why every bite counts when you are breast-feeding. The Baby-wise Diet supplies at least the recommended amounts of all the known minerals and, if followed closely, will guarantee optimal nutritional health for you and your baby.

Garlic, Beer, Toxins, and Other Concerns

Wives' tales flourish when it comes to breast-feeding. A woman is told to drink more beer because it will boost her milk supply. She is told to avoid eating onions and garlic because they cause colic. While some of these recommendations have some merit, many are more fiction than fact. For example, salt doesn't increase the sodium content of your breast milk and pepper won't make your milk "spicy." A bowl of beans may give you gas, but it won't affect your milk or your baby's health. Citrus fruits or tomatoes are thought to be acidic foods, but they have no effect on your blood or the acidity of your milk. While you may hear that a baby will develop diarrhea, irritability, or eczema if you eat chocolate, there is no scientific evidence that this is true.

GARLIC: Garlic is often avoided by breast-feeding mothers, who fear it will cause colic in their newborns. However, research shows infants actually nurse longer and suck more overall, with no apparent discomfort, when there is a hint of garlic in the milk.

However, an infant who is sensitive to certain foods, such as cow's milk protein, might develop an allergic reaction or colic when these foods are included in the breast-feeding mother's diet. While cow's milk and soy products are commonly associated with colic, no one food can be said to cause colic in all children, so a mother must be her own sleuth and eliminate those foods in her diet that seem to be causing her baby discomfort. A mother should be cautious, however, when avoiding too many foods, since limiting variety in the diet can mean restricting essential nutrients. Always talk with your physician before eliminating a major food group, such as milk products or products made from wheat.

BEER AND ALCOHOL: For centuries women have been told that alcohol, in particular beer, would increase their milk supply and strengthen their nursing babies. In the early 1900s, beer companies advertised their products as "tonics" to stimulate appetite and enhance milk yield.

Granted, beer consumption does increase blood levels of prolactin, a hormone necessary for milk production, in men and non-breast-feeding women. However, whether or not beer has a similar effect in breast-feeding women is unimportant, since regardless of the milk supply, babies prefer nonalcoholic breast milk and drink less milk (up to 23 percent less) after their mothers have consumed beer than they do after their mothers have consumed a nonalcoholic beverage.

Beer apparently flavors the milk and makes it less appetizing to the infant. In general, the Subcommittee on Nutrition During Lactation of the Food and Nutrition Board and the Institute of Medicine recommends that mothers who want to drink while breast-feeding should consume no more than 2 to $2\frac{1}{2}$ ounces of liquor, 8 ounces of wine, or two cans of beer a day.

Wine drinkers might be exposing their babies to lead. A foil-wrapped wine bottle can leave a lead-salt deposit on the bottle's rim. Unless the drinker carefully wipes the rim and the exposed cork before pouring, these deposits can dissolve when the wine is poured and raise the lead content of the beverage. Better yet, choose wines that do not have this type of wrapper.

CAFFEINE: After the baby is born, some women mistakenly think they can resume their prepregnancy coffee intake. Granted, caffeine stimulates milk production; however, a nursing baby does an even better job of increasing the milk supply by suckling. Although one cup of coffee, tea, or cola, or a small amount of chocolate or other caffeinated food or beverage appears to be harmless, by the second serving the caffeine is accumulating in breast milk to levels that might affect the baby.

Babies eliminate caffeine from their systems more slowly than do adults, so accumulation can occur in the infant, prolonging the effects of this drug. Although poorly researched, anecdotal reports include irritability, wakefulness, and poor eating habits following maternal consumption of caffeine. In addition, coffee and tea inhibit iron absorption and anemia is common in countries where there is heavy coffee consumption. At a time when a woman needs to be stockpiling iron, coffee may undermine her efforts.

PESTICIDES: Pesticides are another concern for the breast-feeding mother. It is virtually impossible to avoid these environmental contaminants, and almost all women carry contaminants such as PCBs and dioxin in their bodies. Dioxin is a by-product of chemical manufacturing and is most commonly remembered as the contaminant in Agent Orange, the defoliant used in Vietnam. This chemical has accumulated in the soil and in our food since the 1940s and is stored in fat tissue of all animals, from fish to humans. The best a woman can do is limit her intake of fatty meats and lose weight slowly so as not to concentrate too much of these stored contaminants in her system too rapidly. To minimize your baby's exposure to harmful chemicals:

1. Eat a variety of wholesome, minimally processed foods so that you limit your exposure to any one food.
2. Avoid fatty cuts of meat, trim all meats, and skin poultry before cooking.
3. Purchase foods in season and local produce (or at least produce grown in the United States) when possible.

4. Wash produce, peel waxed foods such as cucumbers or apples, discard outer leaves on vegetables, and peel any suspect fruits or vegetables.

5. If you purchase "organic" produce, verify that the food really is grown without the use of pesticides.

DRUGS, MEDICATIONS, AND TOBACCO: As with pregnancy, drugs of any kind, from the chemicals in cigarettes to prescription or street drugs, should be viewed with concern. Tobacco smoke could increase your child's risk for asthma, respiratory infections, and possibly even lung cancer. If you or someone in your household smokes, now is the time to quit. (See chapter 1 for more on smoking.)

Many prescription and over-the-counter medications can be absorbed into breast milk, thus exposing the infant to unwanted and potentially harmful substances. A partial list of medications is found in "The Dos and Don'ts of Medications When Breast-feeding," page 254. If you must take one of these drugs, always check with your physician and your pharmacist about safer alternatives. To relieve pain, for example, your physician might recommend acetaminophen rather than aspirin, since the former medication is not absorbed into breast milk. Another way to minimize your baby's exposure is to take a medication just after breast-feeding or just before your baby takes a long nap. This will allow time for the drug to be metabolized and reduce its accumulation in your milk.

Can You Eat to Avoid Colic?

For no apparent reason, approximately 20 percent of healthy, happy babies develop colic. They start crying, usually in the evening and usually between three weeks and three months of age—their fists clench, their faces turn red, their legs pull up to their chests, and they howl in pain for up to an hour or more. Then as quickly as they started, those babies stop crying and start to smile again. Granted, most babies have fussy periods, especially later in the day, but they usually are comforted by the breast when they are tired, bored, lonely, or uncomfortable. The difference between normal fussiness and colic is that the colicky baby has periods of intense crying that are difficult to soothe.

There are as many folk remedies for colic as there are parents who have survived colicky babies. Holding the baby in a sitting position on your lap and

The Dos and Don'ts of Medications When Breast-feeding

Even if a medication is listed as safe, always check first with your physician. According to the American Academy of Pediatrics, the following medications may be safe:

Acetaminophen, codeine, ibuprofen (painkillers)
Amoxicillin, streptomycin (antibiotics)
Birth control pills
Lidocaine (anesthetic)
Loperamide (antidiarrhea medication)
Naproxen (anti-inflammatory)

The following medications are not recommended:

Aspirin
Clemastine (antihistamine)
Diazepam (antianxiety medication)
Ergotamine (antimigraine medication)
Caffeine
Sulfasalazine (antiulcer medications)

pulling the baby's knees up to his or her chest may help. Some parents find ingenious ways to soothe the troubled baby. They place the infant in a baby seat on top of the washer during the spin cycle. They go for a car ride. They pace up and down the hallway singing whatever song seems to work.

No one knows exactly what colic is; it is more than likely an umbrella term for a variety of troubles. The most common belief is that colic is related to the baby's immature digestive tract and the pain caused by spasms, cramps, or gas. Limited evidence shows that some cases of colic might be remedied by the mother's avoiding cow's milk in her diet for the first few months of the baby's life; as many as one third of colicky babies improve when the mothers adopt milk-free diets. One study showed that mothers of colicky babies have higher levels of cow antibodies in their breast milk than do other mothers, suggesting that some component of cow's milk actually passes into the mother's breast milk.

This does not mean all breast-feeding mothers should give up cow's milk, especially since this is the best dietary source of calcium, vitamin D, and other essential nutrients. However, if you have a colicky baby, try avoiding cow's milk for a week to see if your baby's symptoms improve. If so, avoid cow's milk for the baby's first few months and look to other dietary sources of calcium, such as spinach, turnip greens, broccoli, canned salmon with bones, tofu, and collard greens, or take a calcium supplement. If not, there is no reason to avoid this nutritious food.

Breast-feeding Twins or Triplets

Common sense alone tells you that if you are feeding more than one baby you will need to consume more nutrient-packed food than the average nursing mom. You will be secreting daily 420 to 700 calories per child, which means you will need an additional 500 calories for each baby. For twins, the average nursing mother should consume 2,200 calories plus 1,000 calories for a total of 3,200 calories daily. For triplets, the total intake is approximately 3,700 calories. You will need more fluids, protein, calcium, trace minerals, and vitamins, which means additional servings of whole grains, nonfat milk products, protein-rich beans or animal products, and more fruits and vegetables.

When and What to Eat and Drink
If You Are Nursing

Your calorie intake should average 2,200 to 2,700 calories a day (more if you exercise). As always, the Baby-wise Diet forms the basis of your eating plan, with the following minimum number of servings from each list:

> 3 to 4 servings from the Calcium-Rich Group
> 6 servings from the Vegetable Group (at least 2 servings should be folic acid–rich choices)
> 4 servings from the Fruit Group (at least 2 servings should be vitamin C–rich choices)
> 9 servings from the Grains Group (at least 4 servings should be whole-grain choices)

3 servings from the Extra-Lean Meats and Legumes
Group (try to include 2 to 3 servings of fish and 4 to
5 servings of legumes in the weekly menu)
8 servings from the Quenchers Group

You have a little more leeway because of the extra 500 calories needed to produce breast milk. If you want to splurge every so often, now's the time to do it.
That is, unless you are trying to gradually lose weight, in which case you still can
eat more than ever but should limit your choices to nutritious foods within the
Baby-wise Diet.

The Postpartum Blues

Eight out of every ten women experience "the blues" after the baby is born. For
some, the transient weepiness, mood swings, anxiety, and irritability are only a
minor nuisance that lasts a few days. For others, the depression is more serious or
lasts for weeks. Defining the problem is difficult and the causes are unknown.
Some researchers theorize that fluctuations in hormones or other brain chemicals
called endorphins might underlie the mood swings, while others believe that
feelings of anxiety or depression are a normal phase everyone experiences during
major life changes.

Mild depression or mood swings are normal and temporary. As with many
other adjustments during the early weeks of parenthood, ride the storms and
revel in the tender moments. Your moods should start stabilizing within a few
months. However, you should consult with your physician if you are experiencing severe depression, whereby you feel very down day after day.

Finally, forget the rules when it comes to adjusting to parenthood. The recommendation that you should be back to normal in six weeks is now recognized
to be outdated and downright sexist. The ovaries may have recovered, but your
body and emotions may still need some tender loving care. Some women take
from three months to up to one year to start feeling like their old selves again.
Many suffer from colds, sinus trouble, earaches, bronchitis, hair loss, acne, poor
appetite, memory loss, and loss of sexual drive for months, without feeling tired
or depressed. Pregnancy and delivery may not be categorized as a sickness, but
they are major stresses to the body, so give yourself plenty of time to heal, physically and emotionally.

Quick-Fix Snacks

Fruit Ices*

1/2 cantaloupe filled with nonfat cottage cheese and fresh blueberries

Whole wheat bagel topped with melted cheese

Whole wheat pita filled with pinto beans, grated cheese, chopped tomatoes, and diced green chilies

Warmed flour tortilla filled with leftover diced meats, beans, grated vegetables, and/or cheese

Naughty Nachos*

Slice of sourdough bread topped with fat-free cream cheese and cucumber slices

Newfangled Potato Skins*

Slice of whole wheat toast topped with peanut butter and a sliced banana

1 cup plain nonfat yogurt topped with low-fat granola and 1/2 banana

Papaya with lime juice

Water-packed fruit

Graham crackers and Fruity Spritzer*

Cucumber Toss-Up* and bread sticks

Dried fruits, such as raisins or dried pears

Baked apple with cinnamon and nutmeg

Whole wheat raisin bagel dipped in nonfat apple-spice yogurt

Bran muffin with apple butter

Savory Potato Salad*

Angel food cake with fresh raspberries

*Recipes are given in the back of the book.

Nursing Meals and Snacks

A new mother has a difficult time trying to feed herself and keep up with the new commitment of caring for a baby. Women with small children and a new baby have even more trouble taking time to eat well. At the same time, there is almost nothing more important than to make sure you follow the Baby-wise Diet for at least a year after the baby is born.

Eating well doesn't need to take time, but it does mean planning ahead and listening to your body's needs. A bowl of cereal and a glass of orange juice for breakfast; a turkey sandwich, baby carrots, an apple, and milk for lunch; cold chicken, a salad, and lots of steamed vegetables for dinner; and several nutritious snacks in between are all it takes. Each of these meals takes less than ten minutes to prepare. (See "Quick-Fix Snacks," page 257.)

The following menus are based on the 2,200 to 2,700 calorie recommendation for nursing mothers. Use Worksheet 9.1 below to monitor your progress.

Worksheet 9.1   My Postpregnancy Daily Checklist (for the Breast-feeding Mother)

Copy this master sheet to complete daily.

FOOD GROUPS	MINIMUM SERVINGS	ACTUAL INTAKE
Calcium-rich foods	3–4	_____
Vegetables (at least 2 folic acid–rich choices)	6	_____
Fruits (at least 2 vitamin C–rich choices)	4	_____
Grains (at least 4 whole-grain choices)	9	_____
Extra-lean meats and legumes	3	_____
Quenchers	8	_____

Did I reach my goals? _____

What needs improvement? _____

What will I do differently next week? _____

Day 1

BREAKFAST

2 bran muffins
1 ounce cheddar cheese
1 cup fresh berries
1 cup orange juice
1 cup 1% low-fat milk

SNACK

1 banana, sliced into:
    6 ounces low-fat vanilla yogurt
10 almonds
Water

LUNCH

Grilled chicken salad:
    3 ounces grilled skinless and
        boneless chicken, sliced
    2 cups chopped romaine lettuce
    1 tomato, sliced
    ½ cup sliced mushrooms
    1 tablespoon poppyseed dressing
2 slices French bread
1 cup nonfat milk
1 nectarine
Water

SNACK

1 corn tortilla filled with:
    ½ cup canned kidney beans

1 ounce low-fat cheese, shredded
2 tablespoons chunky salsa
Water

DINNER

Chinese vegetable medley:
    2½ cups chopped broccoli florets,
        mushrooms, celery, carrots,
        onions (optional), and zucchini
    3 ounces shrimp, stir-fried in
        2 teaspoons canola oil and
        seasoned with soy sauce
1 cup cooked cellophane noodles
1 cup nonfat milk

SNACK

1 slice angel food cake with:
    ½ cup sliced peaches sprinkled with
        nutmeg
Water

Daily totals: 2,622 calories; fat 26%;
protein 19%; carbohydrate 54%; fiber
40.6 grams; salt (sodium) 3.5 grams*

Day 2

BREAKFAST

2 whole wheat toaster waffles topped
    with:
    1 cup blueberries
    ¼ cup fat-free sour cream
1 cup honeydew melon chunks

*Sodium will be higher if salt is added to foods.

1 cup orange juice
Tea or water

SNACK

1 can sliced peaches, canned in own
   juice
1 cup fat-free cottage cheese
Water

LUNCH

Quick pizza:
   1 small prepackaged pizza crust
      (6-inch round) topped with
   4 tablespoons tomato sauce
   ¼ cup sliced mushrooms
   1 can artichoke hearts, canned in
      water, drained
   1 tablespoon chopped onion
      (optional)
2 cups chopped raw vegetables
   (broccoli, carrot sticks, zucchini
   sticks, etc.)
1 cup 1% low-fat milk
2 oatmeal cookies

SNACK

2 slices whole wheat bread topped
   with:
   2 tablespoons peanut butter
   1 banana, sliced
1 small box of raisins
Water

DINNER

Chicken-vegetable kabobs (skewer,
   drizzle with 2 teaspoons sesame oil,
   and grill):
   5 ounces skinless and boneless
      chicken breast, cut into 2-inch
      cubes
   6 mushrooms, sliced
   1 zucchini, cut into 1-inch slices
   6 cherry tomatoes
   6 pearl onions (optional)
¾ cup cooked basmati rice, sprinkled
   with:
   2 tablespoons chopped fresh cilantro
1 cup 1% low-fat milk

SNACK

½ cup vanilla ice cream
Water

Daily totals: 2,712 calories; fat 24%;
protein 19%; carbohydrate 58%;
fiber 60 grams; salt (sodium) 3.5
grams*

Day 3

BREAKFAST

1 whole wheat bagel, toasted and
   topped with:
   2 tablespoons fat-free cream cheese
2 kiwis, sliced
1 cup pineapple juice

*Sodium will be higher if salt is added to foods.

Coffee supreme:
  1 cup warmed 1% low-fat milk
  1/4 cup decaffeinated espresso or
    strong coffee
  1 teaspoon sugar

SNACK

2 rice cakes topped with:
  2 tablespoons peanut butter
1 banana
1 cup fresh cherries
Water

LUNCH

Turkey sandwich:
  2 slices whole-grain bread
  3 ounces smoked turkey breast
  2 teaspoons Dijonnaise
  1 romaine lettuce leaf
1/2 cup three-bean salad
1 cup baby carrots
1 cup 1% low-fat milk

SNACK

10 fat-free, whole wheat crackers
1 ounce low-fat cheese, sliced
1 cup V-8 juice

DINNER

1 1/2 cups cooked linguini topped with:
  3 ounces grilled scallops

2 cups chopped and lightly steamed
  vegetables, including broccoli,
  celery, carrots, mushrooms, green
  onions (optional), and bok choy
  (seasoned with 1 tablespoon olive
  oil)
  2 tablespoons grated Parmesan
    cheese
1 cup chopped leaf lettuce with:
  1 tablespoon creamy ranch dressing
1 cup 1% low-fat milk

SNACK

1 cup frozen grapes

Daily totals: 2,602 calories; fat 23%;
protein 20%; carbohydrate 57%; fiber
44 grams; salt (sodium) 3.9 grams*

Day 4

BREAKFAST

1 cup cooked oatmeal (cooked in 1 cup
  1% low-fat milk), topped with:
  1/4 cup wheat germ
  1/4 cup 1% low-fat milk
  1 tablespoon brown sugar
1 slice raisin toast with:
  1 teaspoon all-fruit jam
1 cup orange juice

SNACK

Fruit and yogurt mix:
  1 orange, peeled and sliced

*Sodium will be higher if salt is added to foods.

1 kiwi, peeled and sliced
6 ounces lemon-flavored low-fat
    yogurt
Water

LUNCH

1½ cups lentil soup
1 piece cornbread
1 cup carrot-raisin salad
1 medium apple
1 cup 1% low-fat milk

SNACK

1 cup oven-baked tortilla chips dipped
    into:
    ½ cup fat-free refried beans
    ¼ cup salsa
6 ounces tomato juice

DINNER

3 ounces salmon, broiled with lemon
    and dill
1 cup cooked instant brown rice
1 cup steamed broccoli
1 cup crunchy raw vegetables, such as
    jicama, carrot sticks, cauliflower
    florets, and cherry tomatoes
Water

SNACK

1 cup cocoa made with 1% low-fat milk
3 vanilla wafers

*Sodium will be higher if salt is added to foods.

Daily totals: 2,606 calories; fat 24%;
protein 18%; carbohydrate 58%; fiber
48 grams; salt (sodium) 4.4 grams*

Day 5

BREAKFAST

Strawberry banana shake (in blender):
    1 cup fresh strawberries
    1 banana
    1 cup 1% low-fat milk
    ¼ cup wheat germ
    Vanilla extract to taste
2 slices raisin toast with 2 teaspoons
    all-fruit jam

SNACK

4 graham crackers with:
    2 tablespoons peanut butter
1 cup 1% low-fat milk
1 plum

LUNCH

Thai salad with beef:
    2 cups chopped mixed greens
    2 tomatoes, sliced
    ¼ cup sliced mushrooms
    3 ounces extra-lean beef, sliced in
        thin strips
Sauce:
    1 tablespoon soy sauce
    1 tablespoon sesame oil

1 tablespoon lime juice
$^1/_4$ cup chopped cilantro
Coarsely ground pepper to taste
2 whole wheat rolls
1 nectarine
Water

SNACK

1 barbecued chicken drumstick, cold
6 ounces nonfat strawberry yogurt
Water

DINNER

$1^1/_2$ cups tomato soup (made with
  1 cup nonfat milk)
Grilled cheese sandwich:
  2 slices whole-grain bread
  2 ounces low-fat cheese
  $^1/_2$ tomato, sliced
  1 teaspoon mustard
$^1/_2$ cup baby carrots
Water

SNACK

$^1/_2$ cup cantaloupe cubes
20 frozen blueberries

Daily totals: 2,527 calories; fat 30%;
protein 20%; carbohydrate 51%;
fiber 36 grams; salt (sodium) 4.8
grams*

Day 6

BREAKFAST

2 scrambled eggs cooked in a nonstick
  pan with:
  $^1/_4$ cup diced green pepper
  $^1/_4$ chopped tomato
  1 ounce low-fat cheddar cheese
2 slices whole wheat toast
1 cup orange juice

SNACK

1 slice banana bread with:
  1 tablespoon fat-free cream cheese
1 cup fresh pineapple chunks

LUNCH

Ham and cheese sandwich:
  2 slices rye bread
  2 ounces lean ham
  1 ounce low-fat cheese
  1 teaspoon mustard
  1 lettuce leaf
1 cup cabbage coleslaw made with:
  2 tablespoons low-fat coleslaw
    dressing
1 cup nonfat milk
1 tangerine

*Sodium will be higher if salt is added to foods.

SNACK

6 ounces low-fat vanilla yogurt mixed
  with:
  $\frac{1}{4}$ cup low-fat granola
5 dried apricot halves
Sparkling water flavored with lemon

DINNER

3 ounces pork chop, broiled
1 large sweet potato, baked, with:
  1 teaspoon butter
1 cup steamed green peas
2 dinner rolls with:
  1 teaspoon butter
1 cup nonfat milk

SNACK

$\frac{1}{2}$ cup vanilla frozen yogurt topped with:
  $\frac{1}{2}$ cup fresh berries

Daily totals: 2,588 calories; fat 30%;
protein 20%; carbohydrate 50%; fiber
32 grams; salt (sodium) 3.8 grams*

Day 7

BREAKFAST

1 cinnamon-raisin English muffin,
  toasted, with:
  1 tablespoon peanut butter
  2 teaspoons strawberry jam
1 cup cantaloupe cubes
1 cup 1% low-fat milk

SNACK

4 sesame bread sticks
1 ounce cheddar cheese
1 medium apple
Water

LUNCH

1 large baked potato topped with:
  $\frac{1}{2}$ cup steamed broccoli
  $\frac{1}{4}$ cup steamed grated carrots
  $\frac{1}{4}$ cup fat-free cottage cheese
  1 ounce Parmesan cheese, grated
Tossed salad:
  2 cups chopped leaf lettuce
  $\frac{1}{4}$ cup bean sprouts
  $\frac{1}{4}$ cup cooked kidney beans
  $\frac{1}{4}$ cup chopped green onions
    (optional)
  2 tablespoons French dressing
1 cup 1% low-fat milk
2 peanut butter cookies

SNACK

2 cups watermelon cubes
6 ounces lemon-flavored low-fat yogurt
Water

DINNER

Chicken fajitas:
  2 flour tortillas filled with:
  4 ounces broiled chicken breast, cut
    in strips

*Sodium will be higher if salt is added to foods.

$^1/_2$ cup yellow and red peppers, cut
   into strips and lightly steamed
$^1/_4$ cup chopped onion, steamed
   (optional)
$^1/_2$ tomato, cut into wedges
2 tablespoons fat-free sour cream
3 tablespoons salsa
1 cup cooked brown rice
Water

SNACK

1 cup raw crunchy vegetables

Daily totals: 2,691 calories; fat 25%;
protein 21%; carbohydrate 54%;
fiber 31.7 grams; salt (sodium) 3.5
grams*

*Sodium will be higher if salt is added to foods.

CHAPTER TEN

The Postpregnancy Diet: Regaining Your Figure and Eating for the Next Baby

After delivering your baby, the challenge is to nourish your body to restock your dwindling nutrient stores while you slowly regain a desirable figure. Sacrificing either optimal nutrition or a desirable weight can affect your physical and emotional health later on, not to mention the lifelong effects a poor diet can have on your baby's health if you choose to breast-feed.

As always, eating right is not an instinctive process, so you must take time to plan a healthful eating style that will suit your new, busy lifestyle while nourishing you and your baby. As with pregnancy, your goal for the first year after pregnancy, whether you choose to breast-feed or not, is to eat enough nutrient-packed foods to stay healthy, feel satisfied, and rebuild your nutritional stores.

In addition, it's never too late to start nourishing the next baby. Since some babies are planned and others are surprises, maintaining optimal nutritional status during the childbearing years is an essential part of being a mother. So if you plan to have a second baby, resume competition sports, or even survive the additional stress of juggling family, work, and home, then restocking your nutrient stores should begin immediately after the baby is born.

Having a baby is a nutritionally draining experience. Breast-feeding that baby for six months or more adds to the nutritional stress. Ideally, you should wait a year or two between babies and follow the Baby-wise Diet during that time to gear up for the next pregnancy. However, some women either intentionally or unintentionally have babies in quick succession. To reduce the nutritional risk that comes from having a large or closely spaced family, there are a few dietary guidelines worth following.

The Weighting Game

The average mother has about eight to ten pounds of extra fat tissue that is her energy bank account for breast-feeding. Whereas most women who breast-feed will lose the weight because of the added energy drain of producing milk, the nonlactating woman must cut her calories or increase her activity to achieve the same results. Keep in mind, however, that while most women can lose weight after pregnancy and many can attain a weight close to their prepregnancy weight, pregnancy may change your body shape somewhat and may even cause some weight gain that persists despite the best weight-management efforts.

Women who struggle with five or more pounds after the baby is born should be sure to avoid quick weight-loss diets, which actually work against her intentions to maintain a healthy eating plan. Researchers at the Karolinska Institute in Stockholm found that women who lost the excess postpartum weight were more likely to have gained an appropriate amount of weight during pregnancy, exercised regularly, eaten regularly, and not to have skipped meals than women who retained excess postpartum weight. In essence, a woman's weight is more a reflection of her lifestyle during pregnancy and after the baby is born than what she ate or how much she exercised before pregnancy. If she follows the Baby-wise Diet and exercises regularly, she should reach her weight goals within the first year.

A prepregnancy calorie allotment of approximately 2,000 calories from nutrient-packed foods, such as those recommended in the Baby-wise Diet, will guarantee optimal intake of nutrients while helping to lose weight. It is impossible to guarantee optimal intake of all the vitamins and minerals on a lower-calorie intake. You have just completed one of life's most strenuous feats and you have to do a lot of nutritional rebuilding and restocking. You cannot afford to cut yourself short when it comes to even one nutrient. Consequently, if you can't lose weight on 2,000 calories a day, then increase your exercise!

A few new challenges to good nutrition develop after the baby is born. For a woman who has been used to working outside the home, staying home with a baby can mean battling more than just diapers. These women are more likely to gain weight or retain the extra pounds of pregnancy, possibly because they have easy access to the refrigerator. Food can become the entertainment or stimulation that was once supplied by work.

In addition, after the baby is born a woman might spend increasing time feeding other family members, and the increased time spent tasting and preparing

30 Ways to Cut 100 Calories

1. On toast, replace 1 1/2 tablespoons of butter with 1 tablespoon all-fruit jam.

2. Replace 1/2 cup granola with 2 cups fat-free toasted oat cereal.

3. Rather than prepare 2 slices of French toast using whole milk and eggs, use nonfat milk and egg whites.

4. Choose an orange and a banana rather than a chocolate candy bar.

5. Munch on 35 pretzel sticks in place of 1 ounce of dry-roasted peanuts.

6. Select 1 cup of homestyle baked beans rather than an equal serving of baked beans with franks.

7. Replace 2 biscuits with 2 dinner rolls.

8. Replace 1/2 cup of frozen broccoli in cheese sauce with 1/2 cup steamed fresh broccoli.

9. Instead of eating 5 chocolate chip cookies, savor the taste of 2.

10. Replace 2 fried chicken drumsticks with 2 roasted drumsticks and 1 cup of peas and carrots.

11. Switch from 1 cup of whole-milk hot chocolate to 1 cup of steamed, almond-flavored 1% milk.

12. Grill a cheese sandwich using nonstick spray instead of margarine.

13. Replace 1 cup of chocolate ice cream with 2/3 cup of nonfat chocolate frozen yogurt.

14. Accompany your hamburger with a large apple rather than a side order of fries.

15. Order a sandwich on cracked wheat bread instead of a croissant.

16. Don't add the 1 ounce of croutons to your salad.

17. Instead of garlic bread made with butter, spread baked garlic cloves on French bread.

18. Dip your chips in 1/2 cup salsa, rather than 1/2 cup guacamole.

19. Just say no to a 5-ounce glass of wine.

20. Replace 3 fried fishsticks with 3 ounces of grilled halibut.

21. Replace the apple muffin with a high-fiber English muffin.

22. In sandwich spreads or salads, use 3 teaspoons of Dijonnaise instead of 4 teaspoons of mayonnaise.

23. Use 2 tablespoons of light pancake syrup instead of 2 tablespoons of regular syrup on waffles and pancakes.

24. Pour 1 cup of marinara sauce on your pasta instead of 1/2 cup Alfredo sauce.

25. Cut back on sampling during cooking. The following "tastes" have 100 calories:
   4 tablespoons beef stroganoff
   3 tablespoons homemade chocolate pudding
   2 tablespoons chocolate chip cookie dough

26. Dribble 3 tablespoons of low-calorie French dressing on salads instead of 2 tablespoons blue cheese dressing.

27. Replace 8 sticks of regular gum with sugar-free gum.

28. Eat a papaya rather than a bag of M&Ms for a midafternoon snack.

29. Have a turkey sandwich instead of a chicken salad sandwich.

30. Have a single-scoop ice cream cone instead of a double-scoop.

---

food can put on the pounds. Finally, the changed self-image a woman might experience as she makes the transition from seeing herself as a young woman to being someone's mother may shift her priorities from herself to the needs of others. Along with this change in self-image can come a more relaxed attitude toward weight.

Any of these factors might result in the "nibbling syndrome," whereby small bites, snacks, or tastes while cooking; frequent high-calorie snacks; or "grazing" from the refrigerator result in weight gain. Keep in mind that an extra 100 calories above what you need to maintain a desirable weight will result in a one-pound weight gain per month. That calorie allotment can be reached easily by finishing the buttered toast your husband left at breakfast, eating the leftover creamed tuna while cleaning up after dinner, or nibbling on two oatmeal cookies. (See "30 Ways to Cut 100 Calories," page 268.)

On the other hand, eating frequently can help you control hunger and overeating that can lead to weight gain, but it must be done wisely and with some planning. While skipping meals in an effort to lose weight is more likely to send you to the refrigerator during the afternoon or evening with a license to eat anything in sight, planned nutritious snacks can maintain a steady blood sugar and energy level, curb hunger, and prevent impulse eating, which almost always is high in sugar, fat, salt, and other unhealthful choices.

First, pay attention to and limit unwanted calories that creep into your diet, such as frequent tasting while preparing food or finishing the leftovers after a meal. Second, plan several snacks throughout your day, especially during your most crave-prone periods, such as late afternoon or after dinner. Use these snacks to meet your quota for vegetables, fruits, and grains. Cut vegetables ahead of time and have them on hand. Bring crackers, dried fruit, boxed fruit juices, or other nutritious foods with you and stash them in your glove compartment, desk drawer at work, or in your purse. As long as you choose low-fat, minimally processed fruits, vegetables, and other natural foods and stay within the

Veritable Vegetables

How can you pack more vegetables into your daily eating plan? Here are a few suggestions:

- Make shish-kabobs with more vegetables and less meat (try zucchini, crookneck squash, whole mushrooms, cherry tomatoes, eggplant chunks, baby onions, carrots, or red, green, and yellow peppers)
- Add grated carrots, celery, peas, or jicama to potato salad
- Add broccoli, spinach, or chard to lasagna
- Add zucchini, grated carrots, green peppers, chopped plum tomatoes, or mushrooms to spaghetti or pizza sauce
- Add more vegetables to soups and casseroles, such as peas, carrots, mixed vegetables, beans, or corn
- Top baked potatoes with fat-free sour cream and Parmesan cheese and one or more of the following: steamed broccoli, spinach, mixed vegetables, or mushrooms
- Steam chopped spinach and mix with fat-free sour cream and seasonings to make a vegetable dip
- Top a Boboli pizza crust with sauce, cheese, and lots of vegetables, including onions, zucchini slices, artichoke hearts, mushrooms, peppers, tomato slices, and/or asparagus
- Have vegetable stir-fry dishes at least once or twice a week
- Halve a large squash such as zucchini or crookneck, bake it, then fill the center with steamed broccoli and cheese
- Stuff vegetables such as green peppers or large tomatoes with rice and ground turkey, tuna salad, or beans
- Fill tortillas or pita bread with a variety of vegetables, kidney beans, and cheese
- Snack on baby carrots

recommended servings outlined in the Baby-wise Diet, you should have no trouble nourishing your body while gradually achieving a desirable weight. (See "Veritable Vegetables," above.)

The good news is that many of the food cravings and aversions you may have lived with during pregnancy are likely to subside after the baby is born. A random sample of 463 new mothers who had experienced one or more food cravings during pregnancy found that food cravings did not continue into the postpartum period. In addition, there was no evidence to support the theory that cravings are caused by dietary deficiencies. Without the weird food cravings and aversions, you can settle into a healthful diet based on preferences and good nutrition.

When and What to Eat and Drink

Your goal after the baby is born is to consume optimal amounts of all the essential nutrients in order to maintain health and restock dwindling nutrient stores while gradually attaining a desirable weight. For the first year after the baby is born your diet should resemble the one you followed for the months prior to pregnancy, including:

> 2 servings from the Calcium-Rich Group
> 5 servings from the Vegetable Group (at least 2 of
>   these should be folic acid–rich selections)
> 3 servings from the Fruit Group (2 of these should be
>   vitamin C–rich selections)
> 6 servings from the Grains Group (at least 4 of these
>   should be whole grain or trace mineral–rich
>   selections)
> 2 servings from the Extra-Lean Meats and Legumes
>   Group, with at least 1 serving being fish or legumes
> 5 servings from the Quenchers Group (see Worksheet
>   10.1).

Eating on the Run

Whether you are a working mother or a full-time mom, other matters often interfere with the best of eating plans. However, with a little planning, there is no excuse for not eating well.

It takes as little as five minutes to fix a nutritious meal or snack. A container of yogurt, a piece of fruit, a handful of fat-free whole wheat crackers, and a few slices of low-fat luncheon meat can make a nutritious, easy, and fast lunch. Or prepare a big pot of homemade vegetable soup on Sunday and serve it with bread and cheese for several meals throughout the week. Even a ready-to-eat turkey sandwich (hold the mayonnaise), an apple, and a carton of nonfat milk fit well

---

Worksheet 10.1   My Postpregnancy Daily Checklist (for the Non-Breast-feeding Mother)

Copy this master sheet to complete daily.

FOOD GROUPS	MINIMUM SERVINGS	ACTUAL INTAKE
Calcium-rich foods	2	_____
Vegetables (at least 2 folic acid–rich choices)	5	_____
Fruits (at least 2 vitamin C–rich choices)	3	_____
Grains (at least 4 whole-grain choices)	6	_____
Extra-lean meats and legumes	2	_____
Quenchers	5	_____

Did I reach my goals? _____

What needs improvement? _____

What will I do differently next week? _____

---

into the Baby-wise Diet. Don't forget to bring snacks with you. Pack your purse, briefcase, glove compartment, baby bag, or desk drawer with nuts, dried fruit, crackers and a jar of peanut butter, individual packs of applesauce, or cartons of 100 percent orange juice. Might as well make it a habit now, because once your baby is eating solid foods you will be carrying snacks with you for many years to come.

Stockpiling Your Nutrients

If you followed the Baby-wise Diet prior to and during your pregnancy, it should take only a few months of eating well after the baby is born to return your body to optimal nutritional health. Even if you are only now beginning to eat better, following these dietary guidelines will help you restock the nutrient stores in your tissues and energize you for parenthood. However, if you entered pregnancy only marginally nourished or if morning sickness and other pregnancy-related problems were roadblocks to eating well during your pregnancy, don't be surprised if it takes a year or more of eating well to restock your nutrient stores and regain a high level of wellness.

The foremost dietary guideline to remember is to cut the fat. By reducing your fat intake you automatically consume fewer fatty meats, dairy products, oils, convenience and snack foods, and more nutrient-packed foods such as fruits, vegetables, whole grains, and legumes. A low-fat diet also helps you regain and maintain your figure while reducing your risk for diseases later in life. Also, remember to eat as many minimally processed foods as possible. That means choosing whole wheat bread instead of white bread, baked potatoes instead of potato chips, and fresh broccoli instead of frozen broccoli in cream sauce.

While fat is the most important consideration in our diets, we may not have been given the whole scoop. For one thing, the 30 percent fat-calories rule was recommended because researchers didn't think Americans could handle going any lower (we've cut fat by only a few percentage points in the past two decades and currently hover between 34 and 37 percent). According to William Connor, M.D., professor of medicine and clinical nutrition at Oregon Health Sciences University in Portland, we would be a lot better off if we aimed for about 25 percent of our calories as fat. "That recommendation fits the epidemiological evidence and allows us to eat some fat, but not much," says Dr. Connor. This goal can be met only if the diet is planned around grains, vegetables, fruits, and legumes. There is little room for fatty foods, from hamburgers and French fries to ice cream.

When fat does creep into your food, be sure it's from fish or as canola or olive oil. These fats lower, rather than raise, the risk of heart disease. But this doesn't give us a blank check to overdose on oil. "Olive oil is an acceptable fat, but the idea that pouring it on food is alright is as absurd as the belief years ago that it was good to douse everything in corn oil," says Dr. Connor. In order to reach the 25 percent fat goal, you must cut fat everywhere.

Grains and Veggies

Ideally you should be eating at least six to nine servings daily of grains (currently three out of four women average four servings or less). At least four servings should be whole grains, such as whole wheat bread, oatmeal, or barley. It is easy to meet this quota by including a bowl of oatmeal and a piece of whole wheat toast for breakfast and a sandwich made from whole-grain bread for lunch; the other servings can come from additional whole-grain selections or from a few refined grain sources, such as white rice or white bread. However, the whole-grain varieties are higher in fiber and almost all vitamins and minerals compared to their enriched or refined counterparts. For example, a slice of white bread has only 22 percent of the magnesium, 38 percent of the zinc, 28 percent of the chromium, 12 percent of the manganese, 4 percent of the vitamin E, 18 percent of the vitamin B6, and 63 percent of the folic acid of whole wheat bread.

One thing is for sure: most women need to include a lot more fresh fruits and vegetables in their daily routines. It is impossible to reach the nutritional goals without them. Take, for example, the dark green leafies, which are nature's closest thing to the "perfect" food. They provide ample amounts of the antioxidants (vitamin C and beta carotene), folic acid, iron, calcium, and numerous other minerals essential to a woman during the childbearing years—all for virtually no fat and minimal calories.

A woman gearing up for her next pregnancy should eat eight to eleven servings daily of these nutritional powerhouses. But nine out of ten women don't eat even half this recommended amount, and when they do, more often than not the vegetable is fatty French fries, not nutrient-packed broccoli. To ensure you get your fair share, include at least one fruit and vegetable at each meal and snack, and a second vegetable at both lunch and dinner.

Fatigue: A New Mother's Biggest Challenge

Fatigue tops the list when it comes to postpregnancy problems. You're home all day, but you seldom have a chance to put your feet up and then you're up half the night with a hungry or tearful baby. New mothers have less time to spend on themselves and often dream of the days when they will again have an uninterrupted night's sleep.

To help prevent exhaustion you must eat well, which means eating plenty of the right foods without overeating and gaining weight. The first concern is to eat enough iron-rich foods to help restock your iron stores. So be sure to include at least four or five iron-rich foods, such as extra-lean meat, dark green leafy vegetables, whole-grain breads and cereals, and cooked dried beans and peas, in the daily diet. In addition, cook in cast-iron pots, combine a vitamin C–rich food such as orange juice with all iron-rich foods, and take a moderate-dose iron supplement for at least the first year after the baby is born. Monitor your iron status closely by requesting a serum ferritin test from your physician at least every six months. Once your serum ferritin value rises above 20 mcg/l, you can stop taking the iron supplement unless you are planning another pregnancy, in which case you should continue the iron-rich regimen indefinitely.

Another fatigue-fighting tactic is to eat regularly or at least every four hours. Always combine a carbohydrate-rich food such as a grain, vegetable, or fruit with a protein-rich food such as a nonfat milk product, cooked dried beans and peas, or chicken to help regulate energy and blood sugar levels. Always eat breakfast, even if it is only a piece of toast and a glass of milk, and include at least two or three small snacks between meals to keep yourself energized. Finally, drink water! Often fatigue is caused by mild dehydration.

Other tactics for warding off fatigue are to take a nap when the baby is sleeping, limit social commitments for the first few months after the baby is born, concentrate on you and your baby and decrease other tasks such as housework, and remind yourself that life will regain a normal pace in time.

Your Hair

If your hair starts falling out a few weeks after your baby arrives, don't despair. Some women lose up to 40 percent of their normal hair, but in most cases the hair grows back. Although the phenomenon is poorly understood, one theory for postpartum hair loss is that the hormones that stimulate the growth of the baby also affected your hair by stimulating growth. When the hormone storms of pregnancy subside during the weeks following birth, hair completes its natural cycle and begins falling out. Another theory states that it is the physical and emotional trauma or shock of giving birth that causes the hair loss. A third theory is that marginal nutrient deficiencies of zinc, folic acid, or other B vitamins might contribute to the shedding. In the latter case, try increasing your intake of foods rich in these nutrients, such as extra-lean meats, whole grains, dark green vegetables, and cooked dried beans and peas. Or take a moderate-dose multiple vitamin and mineral supplement.

Spacing Pregnancies

Ideally, a woman should wait one to two years between babies to restock her nutrient stores and allow her body time to mend and prepare for the next pregnancy. For example, it takes approximately three months to one year to replenish iron stores after pregnancy. The stress of pregnancy and delivery also increases the body's need for other vitamins and minerals, from vitamin A to zinc. It can take months to restock these depleted tissue stores and allow the body time to heal.

Back-to-back pregnancies also can interfere with your first baby's nutrition if you are breast-feeding. Frequent cycles of reproduction increase the risk that nursing will overlap with pregnancy and shorten the duration of the recuperative time. Women who do find themselves pregnant within a few months of giving birth can give birth to a healthy baby, but they must take extra precautions. They must eat for the growing baby, for the first child who is nursing, and for their own health. They also will be battling the physical and emotional stresses of juggling family, work, and pregnancy. That means taking extra care to eat even more fresh fruits and vegetables, nonfat dairy foods, whole grains, and cooked dried beans and peas. There is little or no room for high-fat or high-sugar items.

Heart disease is another interesting connection between health and pregnancy. Cardiovascular disease is the number one cause of death and disease in postmenopausal women in the United States. The number of pregnancies a woman has during life may contribute to this risk. For example, a study conducted at the University of Pennsylvania in Philadelphia and the Center for Disease Control and Prevention in Maryland found that women who had six or more pregnancies have higher risks of coronary artery disease and cardiovascular disease than other women. However, whether the number of pregnancies or some related factor (perhaps these women don't have the time to eat well or exercise!) is unclear.

Eating for the Next Baby

Most women are very concerned about their health and diet during their first pregnancy. They want the very best for the babies growing inside them, and they take the time to revel in the baby-making process. By the time the second or third baby comes along, these same women have their hands full with toddlers, work, and other responsibilities. The baby-making process is not as special as it was the first time around and less time is devoted to taking care of themselves. The mother who religiously took her prenatal supplements during her first pregnancy might let weeks lapse before beginning supplementation. Another woman who steamed dark green vegetables every night for dinner during her first pregnancy now skips these vegetables because her toddler won't eat them.

According to Andrew Czeizel, M.D., director of the Department of Human Genetics and Teratology at the National Institute of Hygiene in Budapest, nutrition is likely to slip in these experienced mothers unless they make a concerted effort to stick with the guidelines outlined in the Baby-wise Diet as they gear up for their next pregnancies. The research supports this finding and shows that women having their first babies gain more weight than women having their second and third babies, which suggests that women are not as nutritionally conscientious the second and third times around.

Babies, unlike birthdays and Christmas, often arrive unexpectedly. While you may not have saved your nest egg, reached the pinnacle of your career, or finished remodeling the spare bedroom before your next baby arrives, you should make sure your body is well nourished in preparation for the coming addition (planned or unplanned) to your family. It is never too late—nor too early—to begin giving your next baby the best chances for a healthy life. The second or third baby also needs the same, or even more, nutrients as your first baby, especially since your body may be entering pregnancy not fully recovered from the last pregnancy.

If you conceive while nursing, you will have an increased demand for all nutrients, from protein and carbohydrate to vitamins and minerals. You will need to consume optimal amounts of all the nutrients essential to pregnancy, including folic acid and iron, plus all the nutrients needed for nursing, including calcium, zinc, and protein. In all cases, the Baby-wise Diet is the mainstay of your eating plan, with added servings from each of the food groupings to make up the difference in calories.

The abundance of nutrients in the Baby-wise Diet allows you to stockpile all of the essential vitamins and minerals that you and your baby will need. And by starting early you can build your nutritional defenses before the onset of morning sickness, heartburn, and other pregnancy-related stumbling blocks to eating perfectly.

Other lifestyle habits, including your level of exercise and alcohol consumption, and maintaining a positive mental state continue to be important contributors to your next baby's health. During the childbearing years, and especially as you gear up for your next pregnancy, avoid tobacco and ask that other people not smoke around you. Exposure to tobacco smoke could affect the future health of your baby before you even know you are pregnant, so why take the risk?

Dad's Diet

Dad's diet may have little to do with your baby's health while you are pregnant, but how your partner eats prior to pregnancy might affect whether or not you conceive and even the future health of your next baby. If he drinks heavily, eats poorly, takes drugs, or smokes cigarettes, his habits could jeopardize the number and viability of his sperm, which would make the sperm less capable of fertilizing an egg or producing a healthy baby. On the other hand, a dad-to-be who eats well and takes good care of himself is optimizing his health and potentially the health of his offspring.

For example, men who avoid vitamin C–rich foods are more likely to have "damaged" sperm that might increase the risk for birth defects, childhood illnesses, and other problems for their offspring, according to research conducted at the University of California at Berkeley. The Recommended Daily Allowance (RDA) of 60 mg is probably adequate for nonsmoking men; however, smokers should consume at least 100 mg and it wouldn't hurt to increase intake to 250 mg or more.

Better yet, tell him to quit smoking. Men who smoke during the year before their child's conception increase their offspring's risk of leukemia and certain types of cancers. In one study, babies whose dads smoked more than one pack a day were two times as likely to be born with heart defects and cleft palate as babies born to smoke-free homes. Tobacco use also may deplete tissue levels of the health-enhancing antioxidants, such as vitamin C and beta carotene. In addition, limited evidence shows that children born to smokers are more likely to have slower intellectual development.

Tell your mate also to avoid workplace radiation and chemicals that can damage sperm, which in turn lower the sperm count or cause genetic defects in children. Researchers at McGill University in Montreal report that more than fifty industrial, medical, and other chemicals can harm sperm. (Call the National Institute for Occupational Safety and Health, or NIOSH, at 800-356-4674 for more information.)

When you are gearing up for pregnancy is an ideal time to improve the eating habits of the entire family. What is good for mom also is good for everyone else. So while you are following the guidelines of the Baby-wise Diet, everyone else will benefit as well. Encourage everyone to support and join you in eating healthfully in preparation for the next member of your family.

Dad also can be a big help as you recuperate from one pregnancy and gear up for the next. Your mate can get involved in the process by:

- Encouraging your good eating habits
- Making sure there are always good foods, plenty of milk, and iron-rich snacks on hand
- Reminding you to take your supplements, eat regularly, or limit the intake of not-so-nutritious foods
- Not bringing home tempting foods, such as cookies, cakes, candy, or doughnuts (if he wants these foods, ask him to eat them outside the home and away from you!)
- Helping with household chores, cooking nutrient-packed meals, or grocery shopping
- Bringing home fresh fruits and vegetables (and an occasional bouquet of flowers)
- Encouraging you to stick with your nutrition plan even when dining out

Light Meals

Good nutrition does not have to be time-consuming and, in fact, can be simple and elegant. For example, little, light meals—simple, elegant meals that are bigger than a first course but smaller than a main course—are one way to nourish your body while feeling satisfied, not stuffed. They also can be a way to manage your weight and even spice up your marriage.

Little, light meals can be gourmet mini-meals that emphasize nutritious foods—that is, grains, vegetables, fruits, and legumes—but they do it with flair.

You can blend unusual ingredients to tantalize the taste buds and accent the sensuous side to food—its color, texture, and aromas. A little, light meal can be anything from a tabbouleh salad to lemon chicken with minted rice.

Little, light meals may be just the ticket for adding a little romance to your marriage. For example, you can share a bowl of frozen blueberries and grapes on the floor in front of the TV, some fresh strawberries and a glass of sparkling apple cider at your own private backyard picnic, or several small, tasty dishes for a cozy candlelight dinner. (See "Just Say No to Temptation," below.)

Just Say No to Temptation

At no other time in your life are you more ready to make dietary changes for your health and the health of your baby. However, even when you are your most motivated self, you may find yourself faced with the temptation to overeat, choose the wrong foods, or give in to cravings. Here are a few tips for resisting the impulse to slip from your best intentions.

1. Schedule snack times and come prepared. When you skip meals or forget to bring nutritious foods with you, you are setting yourself up for temptation.
2. At the first sign of an urge to splurge, drink two glasses of water and wait fifteen minutes. Often the water can provide instant relief from a craving.
3. The out-of-sight-out-of-mind motto holds true for cravings. The sight, aroma, and taste of a food can undermine the best of intentions, especially during your high-risk times of day such as midafternoon or after work. So keep the cookies and cake out of the house, avoid driving by the bakery, or bypass the kitchen when you arrive home from work.
4. Switch to a mood-elevating activity. A doughnut or candy bar may give you a mental lift, but so can a brisk walk, listening to your favorite music, or spending time with people who make you laugh.
5. Work with, not against, your cravings. You are likely to swing from abstinence to bingeing if you try using willpower against your chocolate cravings. So plan a small "treat" into the day. Have a chocolate Kiss or a small peanut butter cup, or dip fresh strawberries in low-fat chocolate sauce, rather than turn to a large candy bar or a pint of ice cream.

6. Reprogram your taste buds. Often cravings for sweets are cravings for carbohydrates. Identify when you are most prone to these crave attacks, then plan to eat a carbohydrate-rich bagel with all-fruit jam, toasted English muffin with marmalade, or other nutritious, starchy snack.

7. Remember that nothing is forbidden, but everything counts.

In fact, good nutrition can be a family affair if your partner or other family members help with food preparation. You may find that you have wonderful talks or laughs while preparing dinner or a snack. Try working out shared roles, so that everyone does something he or she enjoys. One person may take over the barbecuing while the other experiments with one-dish meals. Toddlers can help set the table and older children can assist with the shopping, food preparation, or cleanup. In this way everyone is part of the process of planning and gearing up for the next pregnancy.

Recipes

· STARTERS AND SIDES ·

Spinach Hummus

> 1 16-ounce can garbanzo beans (chick-peas), rinsed and drained
> 1/4 cup raw sesame tahini
> 3 to 4 tablespoons fresh lemon juice
> 2 garlic cloves
> 1/2 teaspoon light soy sauce
> Dash of ground cumin
> 1 cup fresh spinach leaves, washed and patted dry

Combine all the ingredients in a food processor and process until smooth. Add water, if needed, a tablespoon at a time until the desired consistency is reached. Serve with toasted pita bread wedges, whole-grain crackers, or as a dip for fresh vegetables. Makes 5 servings, 1/3 cup each.

Nutrition information per serving, without bread: 104 calories, 12 grams carbohydrate, 5 grams protein, 5 grams fat (39%), 1.7 mg iron, 35 mg calcium

New-Fangled Potato Skins

7 medium Russet potatoes, washed and baked until soft
2 tablespoons light margarine
Onion powder and garlic powder to taste
2 tablespoons grated Parmesan cheese

Preheat the oven to 450° F. Cut the cooled potatoes in half and remove the pulp, leaving ⅓ inch of potato in shell. (Use the pulp for mashed potatoes or for potato soup.) Cut each potato skin in half lengthwise. With skin downward, spread a thin layer of margarine on the potato, then sprinkle with onion and garlic powders and Parmesan cheese. Cut each skin in half again, widthwise. Coat a cookie sheet with nonstick vegetable spray and place skins on sheet. Bake 15 to 20 minutes. Makes 4 servings, 14 pieces each.

Nutrition information per serving: 242 calories, 51 grams carbohydrate, 5.4 grams protein, 2 grams fat (8%), 3 mg iron, 46 mg calcium, 26 mg vitamin C, 22 mcg folic acid

Naughty Nachos

1 14-ounce bag oven-baked tortilla chips
½ cup fat-free refried beans
¼ cup grated cheddar cheese
¼ cup bottled salsa

Preheat the oven to 400° F. Place tortilla chips on a large ovenproof platter. Top with beans and cheese and bake until heated through and cheese melts, about 10 minutes. Serve with salsa. Makes 4 servings.

Nutrition information per serving: 226 calories, 40 grams carbohydrate, 8 grams protein, 4 grams fat (17%), 2 mg iron, 189 mg calcium, 46 mcg folic acid, 67 mg magnesium

Spicy Black Beans

$^1/_2$ *cup finely chopped onion*
1 teaspoon olive oil
2 16-ounce cans black beans, drained (do not rinse)
1 garlic clove, minced
$^1/_4$ *teaspoon black pepper*
Dash of cayenne pepper
$^1/_2$ *teaspoon sugar*
$^1/_4$ *teaspoon ground cumin*
$^1/_4$ *teaspoon ground ginger*

In a saucepan, sauté the onion in the olive oil for 3 to 4 minutes, until soft.
Add the remaining ingredients. Bring to a boil, reduce the heat, and simmer
5 minutes to heat through and blend flavors. Use as a burrito filling, a dip
topped with salsa, or a side dish. Makes 8 servings, $^1/_2$ cup each.

Nutrition information per serving: 119 calories, 21 grams carbohydrate,
7 grams protein, 1 gram fat (7%), 2.3 mg iron, 44 mg calcium

Cucumber Toss-Up

2 medium cucumbers, peeled and thinly sliced
1 medium Walla Walla or other sweet onion, thinly sliced
1 teaspoon Mrs. Dash or other herb seasoning mix
1 teaspoon sugar
$1^1/_2$ *teaspoon dried dill*
$^3/_4$ *cup rice wine vinegar*

Mix the cucumber and onion slices in a medium bowl. Blend the other ingredients, then pour over cucumbers and onion. Chill and serve. Makes 6 servings.

Nutrition information per serving: 23 calories, 5 grams carbohydrate,
<1 gram protein, <1 gram fat (4%)

Savory Potato Salad

1½ pounds small red potatoes (approximately 12)
1½ tablespoons minced fresh chives
1½ tablespoons chopped fresh basil or dill
1 tablespoon minced fresh parsley
½ cup grated carrots
¼ cup diced celery
1 tablespoon wine vinegar
1 tablespoon olive oil
Salt and pepper to taste

Scrub the potatoes, cover with water in a medium saucepan, and gently boil until soft but firm, approximately 20 minutes. Drain the potatoes, then cool and cut into quarters. Blend the remaining ingredients in a large bowl, then add the potatoes and toss well. Serve chilled or at room temperature. Makes 6½ servings, ½ cup each.

Nutrition information per serving: 92 calories, 16 grams carbohydrate, 2.2 grams protein, 2 grams fat (21%), 1 mg iron, 14 mg calcium, 14 mcg folic acid, 12 mg vitamin C

Spicy Carrots

½ pound carrots
¼ cup canned whole jalapeño peppers with juice
⅙ cup vinegar
1 cup water
½ teaspoon black peppercorns
⅓ cup chopped onion
Pinch of dried oregano
1 small bay leaf
1 teaspoon safflower oil
1½ teaspoons salt
2 garlic cloves, minced

Wash and peel the carrots and cut into $\frac{1}{8}$-inch slices. Place carrots in a saucepan, cover with water, and bring to a low boil. Cook until tender but still crisp, about 10 minutes. Drain and let cool. Remove seeds from jalapeños and cut into $\frac{1}{8}$-inch slices. Combine the remaining ingredients. Place carrots and jalapeños in a medium bowl and pour marinade over the top. Cover and place in refrigerator for 12 to 24 hours (the longer the better to bring out the flavor). Serve with bean burritos. Makes three servings, $\frac{1}{2}$ cup each.

Nutrition information per serving: 107 calories, 11 grams carbohydrate, 1.3 grams protein, 3.5 grams fat (39%), .7 mg iron, 29 mg calcium, 39 mg vitamin C, 16 mcg folic acid, vitamin A

· MAIN DISHES ·

Beef Fajitas

$\frac{1}{2}$ cup sliced onion
$\frac{1}{2}$ medium green bell pepper, seeded, cored, and slivered
$\frac{1}{2}$ cup sliced fresh mushrooms
$\frac{1}{2}$ cup slivered zucchini
6 ounces flank steak, cut into strips
3 tablespoons bottled fajita seasoning
4 8-inch flour tortillas
1 medium tomato, chopped
1 ounce low-fat cheddar cheese, grated
$\frac{1}{2}$ cup bottled salsa

Coat a large nonstick skillet with cooking spray. Stir-fry the onion, green pepper, and mushrooms until tender-crisp, about 3 minutes. Remove vegetables and stir-fry the flank steak until browned, about 2 minutes. Stir the vegetables back into the pan and stir in the fajita seasoning. Wrap the tortillas in a paper towel and heat in a microwave oven on high for 10 seconds. Fill each tortilla with one-fourth of the beef-vegetable mixture, then sprinkle on some chopped tomato and grated cheese. Fold the tortillas over and top with salsa. Makes 2 servings, 2 fajitas per serving.

Nutrition information per serving: 436 calories, 37 grams carbohydrate, 35 grams protein, 16.5 grams fat (24%), 5.0 grams iron, 181 mg calcium

Chicken Parmesan

1¹/₂ tablespoons plain bread crumbs
1¹/₂ tablespoons freshly grated Parmesan cheese
¹/₈ teaspoon ground pepper
¹/₂ teaspoon fines herbes (see Note)
2 skinless and boneless chicken breasts, about 4 ounces each
1 egg white

Preheat the oven to 350° F. Combine the bread crumbs, cheese, pepper, and herbs in a shallow bowl. Dip the chicken breasts in egg white and roll in bread crumb mixture. Place chicken on a baking pan coated with cooking spray and bake for 20 minutes. Serve immediately. Makes 2 servings.

Nutrition information per serving: 251 calories, 5 grams carbohydrate, 34 grams protein, 9.8 grams fat (35%), 1.5 mg iron, 117 mg calcium

Note: Fines herbes is a mixture of dried herbs, especially parsley, chervil, and tarragon. It is available in most supermarkets.

Sesame Chicken in Acorn Squash

1 teaspoon grated fresh ginger
1 teaspoon toasted sesame oil
1 garlic clove, minced
¹/₂ teaspoon chili powder
¹/₄ cup dry white wine
2 tablespoons light soy sauce
1 acorn squash, halved lengthwise

2 skinless and boneless chicken breasts, about 4 ounces each, cut into strips
1 large carrot, cut into coins
10 snow peas
1 cup broccoli florets
1/2 cup frozen corn kernels
1/4 cup flour
2 tablespoons sesame seeds

Mix the ginger, sesame oil, garlic, chili powder, wine, and soy sauce in a bowl. Put the chicken in this marinade and let it sit for 30 minutes (or overnight in the refrigerator).

Preheat the oven to 350° F. Put the squash halves, cut side down, in a 9 × 13-inch baking pan. Add 1/2 inch water and bake for 30 to 40 minutes, until squash is tender. While squash is cooking, blanch the vegetables. Bring 2 cups water to a boil. Add the carrot and cook for 3 minutes. Add the snow peas and broccoli and cook an additional 2 minutes. Add the corn and cook an additional 1 minute. Drain vegetables and set aside. Mix the flour and sesame seeds on a plate. Drain the chicken, reserving the marinade, and roll the chicken strips in the flour mixture. Spray a large nonstick skillet with cooking spray, heat the skillet, and stir-fry the chicken strips until lightly browned and cooked through. Set aside.

When the squash is done, put 1/3 cup of the reserved marinade into the skillet. Add the blanched vegetables and cook just enough to heat through. Add the chicken strips and toss well. Spoon the chicken and vegetables into the squash halves, spilling over. Makes 2 servings.

Nutrition information per serving: 497 calories, 80 grams carbohydrate, 38 grams protein, 7 grams fat (12%), 6.8 mg iron, 267 mg calcium

Spinach-Stuffed Shells

¹/₂ 1-pound box jumbo shells (15–18 shells)
8 ounces fresh spinach
1 cup nonfat ricotta cheese
¹/₄ cup grated Parmesan cheese
³/₄ cup grated low-fat mozzarella cheese
1 egg white
¹/₄ teaspoon ground nutmeg
¹/₂ teaspoon dried basil
¹/₄ teaspoon salt
¹/₈ teaspoon black pepper
2 cups bottled spaghetti sauce
2 tablespoons grated Parmesan cheese, for topping

Preheat the oven to 350° F. Cook the shells according to package directions. Drain and rinse with cold water to prevent sticking. Wash, drain, and chop the spinach. Steam or microwave the spinach for 3 to 5 minutes, until tender. Drain well, pressing the spinach against a strainer to remove as much liquid as possible. In a large bowl, mix the spinach, cheeses (except Parmesan for topping), egg white, and seasonings. Pour the spaghetti sauce into a 9 × 13-inch baking pan. Stuff each shell with about 2 tablespoons spinach mixture and arrange in the baking pan. Cover with foil and bake for 25 minutes. Remove the foil, sprinkle with the remaining Parmesan cheese, and bake uncovered for 10 minutes longer. Makes 6 servings, 3 shells each.

Nutrition information per serving: 296 calories, 34 grams carbohydrate, 17 grams protein, 11 grams fat (33%), 3.6 mg iron, 352 mg calcium

· SWEET AND FRUITY ·

Berry-Banana Salad

1 pound blueberries, raspberries, and blackberries, washed
1 cup nonfat custard-style vanilla yogurt
1 medium banana
¹/₄ cup orange juice

Gently mix berries in a large bowl and divide evenly into 3 serving bowls. Combine the yogurt, banana, and orange juice in a blender. Puree until smooth and pour over berries. Chill and serve. Makes 3 servings.

Nutrition information per serving: 192 calories, 45 grams carbohydrate, 4.5 grams protein, .9 grams fat (4%), 0.5 mg iron, 125 mg calcium, 34 mg vitamin C, 30 mcg folic acid, 32 mg magnesium

Currant-Date Muffins

1 cup applesauce
¹/₂ cup granulated sugar
¹/₄ cup brown sugar
¹/₄ cup canola oil
3 egg whites
3 tablespoons 1% milk
1 cup all-purpose flour
1 cup whole wheat flour
1 teaspoon baking soda
1 teaspoon baking powder
¹/₂ teaspoon ground cinnamon
¹/₄ teaspoon ground nutmeg
¹/₂ cup dried currants or raisins
¹/₂ cup chopped pitted dates
¹/₄ cup chopped walnuts (optional)

Preheat the oven to 350° F. In a large bowl, combine the applesauce, sugars, oil, egg whites, and milk. Mix thoroughly. Add the flours, baking soda, baking powder, cinnamon, and nutmeg. Mix only until combined. Stir in the currants, dates, and walnuts, then spoon into paper-lined muffin tins (or coat tins with cooking spray). Bake for 15 minutes or until springy and lightly brown on top. Do not overbake. Makes 24 muffins, 2 muffins per serving.

Nutrition information per serving: 227 calories, 40 grams carbohydrate, 4 grams protein, 6 grams fat (24%), 1.3 mg iron, 36 mg calcium

Razz 'n Blues Muffins

1 1/2 cups all-purpose flour
3/4 cup rolled oats
1/3 cup sugar
1 tablespoon baking powder
1 teaspoon ground cinnamon
1 cup buttermilk
3 egg whites
2 1/2 tablespoons safflower oil
1 cup fresh blueberries and raspberries, washed and drained

Preheat oven to 350° F. Coat a muffin tin with spray and set aside. In a large bowl, combine the flour, oats, sugar, baking powder, and cinnamon. In a small bowl, combine the buttermilk, egg whites, and oil. Add the liquid mixture to the dry mixture and stir until just blended. (Do not overstir!) Fold in the berries and spoon batter into muffin cups. Bake for 20 to 25 minutes or until springy and golden brown on top. Makes 12 muffins, 1 muffin per serving.

Nutrition information per serving: 142 calories, 24 grams carbohydrate, 4 grams protein, 3.5 grams fat (22%), 1.2 mg iron, 80 mg calcium

Fruit Ices

For each of the following four recipes, blend all ingredients in a blender until smooth. Pour into glasses and serve immediately. Makes 4 servings each.

Blueberry Ice
2 cups frozen blueberries
1 cup nonfat milk
2 tablespoons sugar

Nutrition information per serving: 86 calories, 19 grams carbohydrate, 2.5 grams protein, <1 gram fat (4%), 80 mg calcium

Banana Ice
4 frozen bananas, sliced
1 cup nonfat plain yogurt
1 tablespoon vanilla extract
$^1/_8$ teaspoon ground nutmeg
2 tablespoons sugar

Nutrition information per serving: 173 calories, 39 grams carbohydrate, 4.6 grams protein, <1 gram fat (3%), 129 mg calcium, 29 mcg folic acid, 45 mg magnesium, .7 mg vitamin B6

Kiwi Ice
4 frozen kiwis, peeled and sliced
$^3/_4$ cup evaporated nonfat milk
2 tablespoons sugar

Nutrition information per serving: 108 calories, 22 grams carbohydrate, 4 grams protein, <1 gram fat (3%), 158 mg calcium, 21 mcg folic acid, 75 mg vitamin C, 36 mg magnesium

Orange, Pineapple, and Apricot Ice
20-ounce can crushed or cubed pineapple, frozen
3 ripe apricots, peeled, pitted, and frozen
$^3/_4$ cup evaporated nonfat milk
$^1/_4$ cup orange juice concentrate

Nutrition information per serving: 152 calories, 34 grams carbohydrate, 4.9 grams protein, <1 gram fat (2%), 167 mg calcium, 38 mg vitamin C, 41 mcg folic acid, 44 mg magnesium

Raspberry Sauce

2 cups fresh raspberries, rinsed
4 tablespoons lemon juice
1/2 cup sugar
1 teaspoon orange flavoring

Combine all the ingredients in a blender and blend until smooth. Use as a syrup for pancakes, ice cream, or angel food cake. Makes 4 servings.

Nutrition information per serving: 131 calories, 33 grams carbohydrate, <1 gram protein, <1 gram fat (2%), .4 mg iron, 15 mg calcium, 23 mg vitamin C

Fruity Spritzer

1 cup cranberry juice cocktail, chilled
1 cup orange juice, chilled
2 cups lemon- or lime-flavored mineral water, chilled
1/2 lemon, thinly sliced

Mix all the ingredients in a pitcher and serve over ice. Makes 4 servings, 1 cup each.

Nutrition information per serving: 66 calories, 16 grams carbohydrate, <1 gram protein, <1 gram fat (3%), 10 mg calcium, 57 mg vitamin C

Glossary

ABBOS: Large chunks of protein in milk that enter the bloodstream and possibly trigger an immunological response that results in the initiation of diabetes in susceptible children.

Abortion: Loss of the fetus before it can survive outside the womb.

Abruption: Premature separation of the placenta from the uterine wall, usually associated with pain.

Acid-base balance: The equilibrium between acids and bases (alkalines) in the body.

Aerobic exercise: Slow, steady, nonstop exercise, such as jogging, walking, biking, or swimming, that requires a steady intake of oxygen and that uses large muscle groups.

Aflatoxin: A potent cancer-causing chemical produced by a mold on tainted peanuts, corn, and other grains.

Amenorrhea: Absence or unusual cessation of menstruation.

Amino acids: The building blocks of protein.

Amniocentesis: Penetration of the uterus through the abdominal wall in order to obtain a sample of amniotic fluid for testing the presence or absence of Down syndrome and other disorders.

Amniotic fluid: The fluid that surrounds and bathes the developing fetus.

Anemia: A change in the size, color, or number of red blood cells that results in reduced oxygen-carrying capacity of the blood.

Anencephaly: Developmental malformation characterized by the absence of nerve tissue in the head.

Antibiotic: A medication used for the treatment of bacterial infections, such as tetracycline and erythromycin.

Antioxidant: A compound that reduces or prevents free-radical tissue damage otherwise associated with degenerative diseases, such as heart disease and cancer, and premature aging.

Anorexia nervosa: A disorder characterized by a refusal to eat, extreme weight loss, and low basal metabolism.

Apgar score: A score used for determining an infant's condition at birth and derived by evaluating the heart rate, respiratory effort, muscle tone, reflex irritability, and skin color sixty seconds after delivery.

Areola: The circular pigmented area surrounding the nipple of the breast.

Arrhythmia: Irregular heartbeat.

Aspartame: A nonnutritive sweetener composed of two amino acids—phenylalanine and aspartic acid—and methanol.

Asthma: A condition characterized by bronchospasms of the lungs and difficulty with breathing that alternates with symptom-free periods.

Acquired immune deficiency syndrome (AIDS): Disease caused by HIV infection and characterized by suppressed immunity.

Autonomy: Independent, self-governing, functioning independently of other parts.

Bacteria: Microorganisms, some of which are capable of causing infection and disease in the body.

Beta carotene: The building block for vitamin A that also functions as an antioxidant independent of its vitamin A activity and is found in dark green or orange fruits and vegetables.

Bilirubin: A pigment produced by the breakdown of hemoglobin and found in the blood.

Binge eating: A large intake of food in a short period of time, usually less than two hours.

Biotin: One of the B vitamins involved in the metabolism of amino acids, carbohydrates, and fats.

Beriberi: A disease caused by a deficiency of vitamin B1 and characterized by nerve disorders, weakness, mental disturbances, dermatitis, and heart failure.

Blastocyte: An early stage in the development of the embryo in which cells are arranged in a single layer to form a hollow ball.

Bone density: The amount of calcium imbedded into bone. A measure of bone strength and resistance to the development of osteoporosis.

Braxton Hicks: Mild, irregular contractions of the uterus that sometimes are mistaken for labor.

Bronchitis: Inflammation of the bronchi in the lungs.

Bulimia: A condition in which food binges are followed by purging by vomiting, taking laxatives, and/or using diuretics.

Caffeine: A central nervous system stimulant found in coffee, chocolate, cola drinks, and other foods and beverages.

Calorie: A measurement of energy in food. A calorie is the amount of heat energy required to raise the temperature of 1,000 grams of water 1° centigrade. Protein and carbohydrates in foods supply 4 calories per gram, fat supplies 9 calories per gram, and alcohol supplies approximately 7 calories per gram.

Carbohydrate: The starches and sugars in food.

Cardiovascular disease (CVD): Diseases of the heart and blood vessels.

Cartilage: A white elastic substance attached to bone surfaces and forming parts of the skeleton.

Cell: A fundamental unit that comprises all body tissues and organs.

Cell differentiation: A process whereby a cell changes into a more complex or specialized form.

Cerebral palsy: Partial paralysis and lack of muscle coordination that result from a defect, injury, or disease of the brain and nervous system.

Cervix: The neck or opening of the uterus.

Cesarean: Birth of a baby through a surgical incision in the abdomen.

Cholesterol: A noncaloric fatlike substance (called a sterol) found in foods of animal origin and produced by the liver. High levels of cholesterol in the blood are associated with heart disease.

Cleft lip: Congenital fissure of the lip.

Cleft palate: Congenital fissure of the palate.

Clinical deficiency: An overt nutrient deficiency that results in classic symptoms, including beriberi (a deficiency of vitamin B1), scurvy (a deficiency of vitamin C), and xerophthalmia (a deficiency of vitamin A).

Chloasma: Excessive skin pigmentation in certain areas of the body.

Chyme: Semidigested food mixed with stomach enzymes that leaves the stomach and enters the small intestine.

Colic: An umbrella term used to describe periods of intense crying that are difficult to soothe in the newborn during the first three months of life.

Collagen: A protein in connective tissue and the organic substance in teeth and bones.

Colostrum: The first liquid excreted from the breast during the few days after delivery. Colostrum is higher in protein, some nutrients, and immune-stimulating substances and lower in fat and carbohydrate than is mature breast milk.

Complex carbohydrate: The nutrient-rich starches and fibers present in vegetables, some fruits, and cereals.

Conception: The moment when the male sperm fertilizes the female egg, making the beginning of a new organism.

Congenital: Present at and persisting after the time of birth.

Constipation: A condition characterized by infrequent and difficult evacuation of feces.

Core temperature: Internal body temperature.

Cornea: The exposed and transparent portion of the eyeball.

Cretinism: A deformity that occurs during development in the uterus and caused by deficient thyroid activity that usually result from insufficient iodine intake during pregnancy. It is characterized by poor physical and mental development, dry skin, and a low metabolic rate.

Cystic fibrosis: A fatal disease in young children characterized by general dysfunction of the exocrine glands, the pancreas, respiratory system, salivary glands, digestive tract, and other systems.

Critical period: Stages in fetal development when specific organs or tissues are developing.

Dehydration: An inadequate amount of water in the tissues.

Diabetes: A disease characterized by an inability to regulate blood sugar levels so that blood and urine levels of glucose rise in the presence of an absolute or relative deficiency of insulin.

Diastolic blood pressure: The lower of two readings that make up a blood pressure test. Diastolic pressure corresponds to the least amount of pressure in the cardiovascular system at any one time and reflects the pressure inherent in the heart and blood vessels when the heart relaxes between beats (contractions).

Dietitian: An individual with at least a bachelor's degree in nutrition or dietetics from an accredited college, who has completed the equivalent of a one-year internship in dietetics, who has successfully completed a nationally recognized exam, and who is expected to maintain the R.D. credential by completing each year several units of continuing education in a nutrition-related subject.

Dioxin: A by-product of chemical manufacturing, most commonly remembered as the contaminant in Agent Orange, the defoliant used in Vietnam.

Diuretic: Medications that promote fluid loss by increasing urinary secretion.

DNA: Deoxyribonucleic acid. The helix structure that carries the genetic information in the nucleus of all cells.

Down syndrome: A congenital condition characterized by mental retardation and abnormal facial features, including a flattened nose.

Early fetal period: The first twenty weeks of gestation.

Eclampsia: The combination of edema, high blood pressure, and protein in the urine that can occur in late pregnancy and can progress to convulsions and coma if left untreated.

Ectoderm: The outermost layer of the three primitive cell layers in the embryo.

Ectopic pregnancy: Pregnancy in which the fertilized egg becomes implanted outside the uterus.

Eczema: A skin disease with itching and redness.

Efface: A thinning and softening of the cervix in preparation for labor and delivery.

Embryo: The earliest stage of development of the baby.

Embryonic stage: The first seven to nine weeks of pregnancy.

Endoderm: The innermost layer of the three primitive cell layers of the embryo.

Endometriosis: The presence of endometrial tissue in abnormal places, such as outside the uterus in the abdominal cavity.

Enriched: The addition to processed foods of a few nutrients to bring the level back to the original vitamin or mineral content. Only four nutrients—vitamin B1, vitamin B2, niacin, and iron—are added back during enrichment, while many more nutrients are lost in processing.

Enzyme: A compound that acts as a catalyst in starting chemical reactions in the body.

Epidemiologic study: The investigation of the factors that influence the frequency and distribution of disease in humans by studying disease incidence in various countries.

Epilepsy: A disease of the nervous system characterized by convulsive seizures caused by temporary disturbances in nerve impulses.

Esophagus: The passageway or tube from the throat to the stomach.

Essential hypertension: High blood pressure not caused by a tumor on the kidneys or other diseases.

Estrogen: A family of related female sex hormones, including estradiol, estrone, and estriol, that are produced by maturing follicles in the ovary, placenta, and adrenal cortex. Estrogens are responsible for the development and growth of female sex organs, many of the physiological changes in pregnancy, and calcium metabolism.

Failure to thrive: A term used to describe infants with growth failure usually caused by poor maternal diet, excessive nutrient and calorie losses from excessive vomiting or diarrhea, or unusually high energy requirements.

Fallopian tubes: The channels that the egg travels down on its way from the ovaries to the uterus.

Fatigue: Feelings of physical or mental weariness, tiredness, or weakness.

Fatty acid: Fat fragments. A fat-soluble molecule that consists of a long chain of carbon atoms with hydrogen attached. Three fatty acids linked to a glycerol molecule constitute a triglyceride. An example is linoleic acid.

Fetal alcohol syndrome (FAS): A combination of physical deformities in the infant, including facial deformities, that result from exposure to alcohol in utero.

Fetus: The developing baby in the uterus. A term applied especially from the seventh to the ninth week of gestation until birth.

Fiber: The indigestible residue in food, composed of the carbohydrates cellulose, pectin, and hemicellulose; vegetable gums; and the noncarbohydrate lignin.

Fibrous: Composed of fibers.

Flatulence: Intestinal gas.

Flavonoids: A group of more than 200 compounds found in citrus fruits, leafy vegetables, red onions, and soybeans that may have antioxidant capability in protecting against free radical damage to tissues.

Folic acid: A B vitamin essential for cell replication.

Food and Drug Administration (FDA): An agency of the government that monitors the safety of foods, drugs, and cosmetics.

Fortified: The addition of vitamins or minerals to a processed food to levels greater than naturally found. Milk is fortified with vitamin D.

Four food groups: Outdated eating plan based on designated servings of grains, fruits and vegetables, meat, and milk products.

Fructose: A sugar found in fruits and honey. Also called fruit sugar.

Gangrene: Death of tissue usually caused by diminished blood supply and followed by bacterial infection.

Gastric: Pertaining to the stomach.

Gestation: The development of a baby within the uterus from conception to birth.

Gestational diabetes: Diabetes that develops as a result of pregnancy and usually disappears after the baby is born.

Gingivitis: Inflammation of the gums.

Glucose: The carbohydrate that makes up sugar, blood sugar, and the building blocks of starch.

Glucose tolerance: A measure of how well the body handles and regulates blood sugar levels.

Glutathione peroxidase: An antioxidant enzyme that includes selenium.

Gram (gm): A unit of weight. Twenty-eight grams equal an ounce.

Hair follicle: The organ that surrounds and nourishes the growing hair shaft.

HDL (high-density lipoprotein) cholesterol: A type of carrier of cholesterol in the blood. High levels are associated with a reduced risk of heart disease.

Head circumference: A measurement of the size of the head in an infant as measured at the forehead.

Heartburn: A burning chest pain caused by overeating, spicy food, or alcohol intake.

Hematocrit: A test for anemia that measures the percent volume of red blood cells in the blood.

Hemoglobin: The iron-rich protein in red blood cells that transports oxygen. A hemoglobin test measures the percentage of hemoglobin in the blood.

Hormone: A chemical substance secreted by an endocrine gland, such as the adrenals, the pancreas, or the pituitary, that travels in the blood to other parts of the body to help regulate function.

Hemorrhoid: An enlarged vein in the mucus membrane inside or just outside the rectum.

Human chorionic gonadotropin: A gonad-simulating substance in human urine during pregnancy, commonly abbreviated HCG.

Human immunodeficiency virus (HIV): Virus responsible for the development of AIDS.

Hydrogenated fats: Polyunsaturated vegetable oils that have been treated with hydrogen, a process called hydrogenation, to form more saturated fats and to convert a liquid oil into a solid fat. Examples include margarine and shortening.

Hyperactivity: Excessive activity.

Hyperemesis gravidarum: Severe nausea and vomiting during pregnancy.

Hyperglycemia: High blood sugar.

Hypertension: High blood pressure.

Hypoglycemia: Low blood sugar.

Immune system: The body's intricate defense system, composed of organs, tissues, and cells, that fight against disease and infection.

Infancy: From birth to the first birthday.

Infertility: The inability to conceive after twelve months or more of intercourse.

Insoluble fiber: Fiber in food that is not soluble in water and that is associated with a reduced risk for colon cancer. Examples include wheat bran.

Insomnia: Inability to fall or stay asleep.

Insulin: A hormone secreted by the pancreas that helps regulate blood sugar levels by facilitating sugar into the cells when blood sugar levels rise above normal.

International Unit (IU): An arbitrary measurement used for the fat-soluble vitamins A, D, and E. These units standardize the potency of the vitamin rather than measure it by weight. IUs can be converted to weight measurements; for example, 3.33 IU of vitamin A are equivalent to 1 mcg.

Intrauterine device (IUD): A small substance implanted within the uterus as a method of birth control.

Intrauterine growth retardation (IUGR): Small for gestational age fetus.

IQ (Intelligence Quotient): A number representing a person's level of intelligence. It is the mental age, as assessed by an intelligence test, multiplied by 100 and divided by the person's chronological age.

Iron-deficiency anemia: Insufficient red blood cell count resulting from inadequate amounts of iron to produce hemoglobin for red blood cells.

Jaundice: Yellowish discoloration of skin caused by excess accumulation of bile pigments in the blood, either from a poorly functioning liver or from increased production of the pigments from hemoglobin.

Kegels: Exercises to tone and strengthen the muscles lining the vaginal and urinary tract walls.

Lactase: The digestive enzyme that breaks down milk sugar (lactose) during digestion.

Lactobacillus acidophilus: Bacteria found in some yogurts that might assist in lactose digestion and maintain a healthy environment in the digestive tract and vagina. Also called *L. acidophilus* or *acidophilus.*

Lactobacillus bulgarius: Bacteria found in yogurt that assist in lactose digestion.

Lactose: Milk sugar.

Lactose intolerance: The inability to digest the milk sugar lactose. The condition is characterized by abdominal bloating, cramping, intestinal gas, and diarrhea.

Lanugo: A downy coat that covers the developing fetus in the second trimester and disappears prior to delivery.

Late fetal period: The second twenty weeks of gestation.

Laxative: An agent that acts mildly to promote defecation.

LDL (low-density lipoprotein) cholesterol: A type of carrier of cholesterol in the blood. High levels are associated with heart disease.

Legumes: Dried beans and peas, such as kidney or black beans, lentils, or split peas.

Lethargy: Tiredness, sluggishness, or fatigue.

Ligament: A tough band connecting bone or supporting tissues.

Lightening: A term to describe the reposition of the baby into a head-down position at the lower base of the uterus in preparation for delivery.

Linoleic acid: An essential polyunsaturated fatty acid found in safflower oil, soybean oil, and other vegetable oils. A deficiency of this fatty acid results in infantile eczema.

Listeriosis: An infection caused by an organism of the genus *Listeria.*

Low birth weight: An infant born weighing less than 2,500 grams (5 pounds, 8 ounces). These infants may be born premature or may be born on time but are too small for their gestational age.

Lymphoma: A tumor of the lymph tissue.

Macrocytic anemia: A type of anemia usually caused by a folic acid or vitamin B12 deficiency.

Magnesium: A major mineral essential for bone development, muscle relaxation, nerve transmission, and blood sugar regulation.

Manganese: A trace mineral essential for the formation of connective tissue, fat and cholesterol metabolism, bone development, and blood clotting.

Marginal deficiency: The consumption of some, but not enough, of a nutrient so that overt clinical deficiency is avoided but more subtle physiological processes are curtailed.

Menses: Pertaining to menstruation.

Menstruation: The monthly discharge of the blood-enriched lining of the uterus. Also called menses.

Mesoderm: The middle layer of cells between the endoderm and ectoderm of the embryo.

Metabolic rate: The amount of calories expended by basic body functioning and daily activities.

Metabolism: The sum of all the chemical processes that convert food and its components to the fundamental chemicals that the body uses for energy or for repair, maintenance, and growth of tissues. Metabolism includes all the building-up processes, such as tissue growth, and all the tearing-down processes, such as breaking down glycogen for energy.

Microgram (mcg): A metric unit of weight equivalent to one one-thousandth of a milligram.

Milk ducts: Canals or passageways in the breast that allow the flow of milk to the nipple.

Milligram (mg): A metric unit of weight equivalent to one one-thousandth of a gram.

Mineral: An inorganic fundamental substance found naturally in the soil and taken up by plants and animals that has specific chemical and structural properties. Many minerals are essential nutrients for growth, maintenance, and repair of tissues.

Miscarriage: Spontaneous loss of fetus before the seventh month.

Miso: A fermented soybean product.

Monosodium glutamate (MSG): A food additive that, in some people, causes an adverse reaction called Chinese restaurant syndrome.

Montgomery's glands: Raised white areas in the areola that secrete oil to keep the nipples lubricated.

Morning sickness: The nausea and vomiting that begin in the first trimester and sometimes continue into the second or even third trimester of pregnancy. Also called hyperemesis gravidarum.

Multiple birth: Giving birth to more than one infant at a time, including twins, triplets, and quadruplets.

Myoglobin: The iron-rich compound that holds and transport oxygen within the cell.

Neonatal period: The first twenty-eight days following birth.

Nervous system: The brain and nerves that coordinate and control responses to stimuli and that condition behavior and all thinking processes.

Neural tube defect: A type of birth defect in the neural tube that becomes the spinal cord and brain whereby this tube does not close in the developing embryo. Examples of neural tube defects include spina bifida, anencephaly, and encephalocoele. These birth defects result from both genetic and environmental factors, including poor maternal intake of folic acid during pregnancy.

Neurotransmitter: Chemical that transmits messages between nerve cells or between nerve cells and organs or muscles.

Nicotine: A stimulant and addictive drug found in tobacco.

Nitrites: Food additives that are converted to carcinogenic substances, called nitrosamines, in the stomach.

Nutrient: A substance essential to the body that must be obtained from the diet. Essential nutrients include protein, linoleic acid, vitamins, mineral, and water.

Obesity: Body fat weight more than 20 percent above a desirable body weight. The body weight is excess fat, not muscle or lean tissue.

Omega-3 fatty acids: Polyunsaturated fats in fish oils, including eicosapentaenoic acid (EPA) and docosahexaenoic acid (DHA), that might reduce the risk for developing cardiovascular disease and are suspected to be essential fats in the development of normal vision in infants.

Osteoporosis: A decrease in bone density resulting in brittle, porous bones that are susceptible to fractures.

Otitis media: Inflammation of the middle ear.

Ovary: A glandular organ in the female reproductive system that produces the ovum (egg) and secretes the female hormones estrogen and progesterone. Loss of ovarian function is the deciding factor in menopause.

Over-the-counter medications (OTC): Medications that can be purchased without a prescription.

Ovulation: The maturation and discharge of a mature egg from the ovary.

Ovum: Egg. The female reproductive substance that can develop into a baby if fertilized by the male sperm.

Pallor: Paleness, absence of skin color.

Pancreas: An endocrine gland in the abdomen that secretes a variety of hormones, including blood sugar–regulating hormones such as insulin and glucagon, and digestive enzymes such as pancreative lipase.

Pantothenic acid: One of the B vitamins involved in the metabolism of amino acids, carbohydrates, and fats.

Pap smear: A routine test for cervical cancer.

Passive smoking: Inhaling other people's cigarette smoke.

Penicillamine: An amino acid derived from penicillin that is used in the treatment of disease associated with excess copper accumulation in the body.

Perinatal period: Includes the late fetal period and the neonatal period—i.e., the time immediately surrounding birth.

Peristalsis: A wavelike motion in the muscles that line the digestive tract that propels food downward.

Pernicious anemia: Anemia caused by an inadequate secretion of a digestive substance called intrinsic factor, necessary for vitamin B12 absorption.

Phenylalanine: An amino acid present in many foods.

Phenylketonuria (PKU): A genetically determined metabolic disorder associated with mental retardation.

Phytochemicals: Nonnutritive substances in plants that might help in the prevention of disease. Examples include alliin in garlic and bioflavonoids in citrus fruit.

Pica: A desire to eat nonfood substances, such as chalk or dirt.

Placebo: A medicine with no effect, given to please or humor a patient.

Placenta: The organ that links the blood supply of a mother with the developing fetus.

Placenta previa: A condition in which the placenta is attached at the lower portion of the uterus, rather than higher up in the uterus.

Polyunsaturated fat: A triglyceride in which at least two of its three fatty acids are unsaturated (i.e., has room for the addition of more hydrogen atoms). Vegetable oils and fish oils are polyunsaturated fats.

Postneonatal period: From twenty-eight days after delivery to the first birthday.

Postpartum: After delivery.

Pre-eclampsia: High blood pressure, protein in the urine, and edema occurring during the latter half of pregnancy. (See eclampsia and pregnancy-induced hypertension.)

Pregnancy-induced hypertension (PIH): Another term for pre-eclampsia.

Pregnancy tumor: Benign fingerlike growth of inflamed gum tissue between the teeth.

Prenatal: Preceding birth.

Preterm infant: An infant born under thirty-seven weeks gestation.

Preterm labor: Initiation of labor prior to a woman's due date.

Progesterone: A hormone produced by the ovaries in preparation for the reception and development of a fertilized egg in the uterus. This hormone also is produced by the placenta during pregnancy.

Progestin: A substance that has the ability of the specific hormone of the corpus luteum to prepare the lining of the uterus for implantation of the fertilized egg.

Prolactin: A hormone secreted by the pituitary in the brain, which stimulates milk secretion.

Prostaglandins: A group of hormonelike substances formed from polyunsaturated fatty acids that have a profound effect on the body, including contraction of smooth muscle and dilation or contraction of blood vessels in the regulation of blood pressure.

Protein: Compounds made up of amino acids, found in many foods.

Pulse: The impact felt in the blood vessels caused by the blood as it is forced out by a contraction of the heart.

Quickening: The fluttering feeling in the abdomen that a mother experiences in the second or third trimester as a result of the movement of the developing fetus.

Recommended Dietary Allowances (RDAs): Suggested amounts of most vitamins and minerals needed by healthy individuals to avoid clinical nutrient deficiencies, based on age, gender, and size.

Red blood cells: The iron-rich cells in the blood that are responsible for transporting oxygen to the tissues and removing and transporting carbon dioxide, a waste product from cellular metabolism, back to the lungs for exhalation.

Reference Daily Intakes (RDIs): Based on former U.S. RDAs, RDIs are standards for nutrient consumption used on food and supplement labels.

Reference person: A theoretical person with average height, weight, and activity level on which the Recommended Dietary Allowances are based.

Relaxin: A hormone released during pregnancy that helps soften the mother's ligaments in preparation for childbirth.

Rickets: Vitamin D deficiency in infancy and childhood characterized by poorly calcified bones resulting in bowed legs and deformed rib cage.

Rubella: A mild viral infection, characterized by fever and a skin rash, that can be harmful to the developing infant if a previously unexposed mother contracts the infection during pregnancy.

Saccharin: A nonnutritive sweetener.

Salt: Sodium chloride.

Saturated fat: A triglyceride with the maximum possible number of hydrogen atoms. Saturated fats are solid at room temperature, such as butter and stick margarine, and are linked to an increased risk for developing heart disease and possibly breast cancer.

Semen: The fluid discharge at ejaculation in the male that consists of sperm capable of fertilizing an egg in a female as the first step in pregnancy.

Serotonin: A nerve chemical in the brain that helps regulate sleep, pain, mood, and appetite.

Serum ferritin: The form of iron in the blood that is a sensitive indicator of tissue iron levels. A value less than 20 mcg/l indicates iron deficiency.

Scurvy: A disease caused by a deficiency of vitamin C and characterized by bleeding gums, loose teeth, small hemorrhages below the skin, and weakness.

Sidestream smoke: Smoke from both the end of a burning cigarette and that is exhaled after a smoker puffs on a cigarette.

Skeletal: Pertaining to the bones.

Small for gestational age infants: Infants born underweight at birth, whatever the gestational age.

Sodium: An electrolyte that combines with chloride to make table salt.

Sphincter: A ringlike muscle that closes a natural opening, such as the passageway from the esophagus to the stomach or from the stomach to the small intestine.

Spina bifida: A congenital deformity of the spine in which the spinal column fails to close properly.

Spinal cord: The spine or vertebral column that houses the nerve connections between the brain and the body.

Spontaneous abortion: Sudden loss of the fetus before it is able to survive outside the womb.

Starch: Complex carbohydrates found in vegetables, some fruits, and cereals.

Stillbirth: A baby that is born dead.

Strict vegetarian: A subgroup of vegetarians who avoid all foods of animal origin.

Sucrose: Table sugar. A simple carbohydrate made up of two molecules, glucose and fructose.

Sudden infant death syndrome (SIDS): Unexplained death of infants less than one year old while sleeping. The third leading cause of infant mortality.

Sugar: A sweet-tasting simple carbohydrate, such as sucrose, glucose, or fructose.

Sulfites: Additives used in wine, dried fruits, and potatoes that cause adverse allergic reactions in some asthmatic people.

Systolic blood pressure: The pressure in the blood vessels when the heart contracts.

Tendon: A fibrous cord of connective tissue continuous with the muscles and that attaches to bone or cartilage.

Teratogen: An agent of disease that causes congenital deformities or other serious disorders during fetal development.

Testosterone: The male hormone responsible for secondary male characteristics.

Tofu: A curd made from soybeans that is high in protein.

Total iron binding capacity (TIBC): A blood test for iron status.

Toxemia: A general term given to disorders of late pregnancy when there is high blood pressure, protein in the urine, and edema. Also called pre-eclampsia and eclampsia.

Toxoplasma gondii bacteria: Bacteria commonly found in cat feces that cause a potentially serious infection called toxoplasmosis, which results in blindness and mental retardation in the infant.

Trace mineral: An essential mineral found in the body in amounts less than .0005 percent of body weight.

Trans fatty acids (TFAs): Polyunsaturated fats formed during hydrogenation of vegetable oils to make margarine or shortening. The shape of these fats is different from other polyunsaturated fats, and it is suspected that they act more like saturated fats in the promotion of heart disease.

Triglyceride: The most common type of calorie-containing fat found in food, a person's fat tissues, and the blood.

Trimester: One of three general periods of pregnancy: first (weeks 1–13), second (weeks 14–27), and third (weeks 28–40) trimesters.

Tryptophan: An amino acid that also is a building block for the nerve chemical serotonin, which helps regulate sleep, pain, mood, and appetite.

Tubal pregnancy: A condition in which the fertilized egg implants in the fallopian tubes rather than in the uterus.

Umbilical cord: The tissue that acts as a passageway in connecting the baby with the placenta and that transfers all nutrients and waste products to and from the baby, respectively.

Urogenital system: The urinary tract and sexual organs.

U.S. Recommended Daily Allowances (U.S. RDA): A set of nutrient recommendations used on labels and derived from the Recommended Dietary Allowances, or RDAs.

Uterus: A hollow organ in the female in which the baby develops during gestation.

UV light: Ultraviolet rays from the sun.

Varicose veins: Enlargements of the blood vessels that return blood to the heart from the body.

Vernix caseosa: A waxy covering over the fetus that protects the delicate skin from the mineralized amniotic fluid.

Villi: Small protrusions that occur uniformly over a smooth surface that increase surface area.

Vitamin: An essential nutrient that must be obtained from the diet and is required by the body in minute amounts.

Whole grain: An unrefined grain that retains its edible outside layers (the bran) and the highly nutritious inner germ (wheat germ).

References

Introduction: Eating for Baby and Me

Allen L: The nutrition CRSP: What is marginal malnutrition, and does it affect human function? *Nutr Rev* 1993;51(9):255–267.

Barker D: Impact of diet on critical events in development: The effect of nutrition of the fetus and neonate on cardiovascular disease in adult life. *P Nutr Soc* 1992;51(2):135–144.

Brewer T: Human pregnancy nutrition: An examination of traditional assumptions. *Aust NZ J O* 1970;10:87–92.

Declercq E: Where babies are born and who attends their births: Findings from the revised 1989 United States standard certificate of live birth. *Obstet Gyn* 1993;81:997–1004.

Forrest J: Timing of reproductive life stages. *Obstet Gyn* 1993;82:105–111.

Garza C: Overview and analysis. *Am J Clin N* 1994;59(suppl):542S–545S.

Godfrey K, Forrester T, Barker D, et al: Maternal nutritional status in pregnancy and blood pressure in childhood. *Br J Obst G* 1994;101(5):398–403.

Ludman E, Kang K, Lynn L: Food beliefs and diets of pregnant Korean-American women. *J Am Diet A* 1992;92(12):1519–1520.

Olson C: Promoting positive nutritional practices during pregnancy and lactation. *Am J Clin N* 1994;59(suppl):525S–531S.

The prenatal origins of adult hypertension. *Nutr Rev* 1991;49(5):160–161.

Rahmanifar A, Kirksey A, Wachs T, et al: Diet during lactation associated with infant behavior and care-giving interaction in a semi-rural Egyptian village. *J Nutr* 1993;123:164–175.

Sigman M, McDonald M, Neumann C, et al: Prediction of cognitive competence in Kenyan children from toddler nutrition, family characteristics and abilities. *J Child Psy* 1991;32:307–320.

Suitor C, Olson C, Wilson J: Nutrition care during pregnancy and lactation: New guidelines from the Institute of Medicine. *J Am Diet A* 1993;93:478–479.

1. Preparing for Pregnancy

Abrams B, Berman C: Nutrition during pregnancy and lactation. *Prim Care* 1993;20(3): 585–597.

Adams M, Bruce F, Shulman H, et al: Pregnancy planning and pre-conception counseling. *Obstet Gyn* 1993;82:955–959.

Alexander M, Lazan K, Rasmussen K: Effect of chronic protein-energy malnutrition on fecundability, fecundity, and fertility in rats. *J Nutr* 1988;118:883–887.

American College of Obstetricians and Gynecologists: *Exercise During Pregnancy and the Prenatal Period*. ACOG, Washington, D.C., 1985.

Ames B, Motchnik P, Fraga C, et al: Antioxidant prevention of birth defects and cancer (International Conference on Male-Mediated Developmental Toxicity, September 16–19, 1992). Plenum Press, in press.

Apgar J: Zinc and reproduction: An update. *J Nutr Bioc* 1992;3(6):266–278.

Armstrong J, Weijohn T: Dietary quality and concerns about body weight of low-income pregnant women. *J Am Diet A* 1991;91(10):1280–1282.

Baer J, Taper L, Gwazdauskas F, et al: Diet, hormonal, and metabolic factors affecting bone mineral density in adolescent amenorrheic and eumenorrheic female runners. *J Sport Med* 1992; 32(1):51–58.

Bakketeig L, Jacobsen G, Hoffman H, et al: Pre-pregnancy risk factors of small-for-gestational age births among parous women in Scandinavia. *Acta Obst Sc* 1993;72:273–279.

Barrett B, Gunter E, Jenkins J, et al: Ascorbic acid concentration in amniotic fluid in late pregnancy. *Biol Neonat* 1991;60:333–335.

Bendich A: Folic acid and neural tube defects. *Ann NY Acad* 1993;678:108–111.

Bendich A: Lifestyle and environmental factors that can adversely affect maternal nutritional status and pregnancy outcomes. *Ann NY Acad* 1993;678:255–265.

Berga S: How stress can affect ovarian function. *Cont Ob/Gyn* 1993;July:87–94.

Bergman E, Massey L, Wise K, et al: Effects of dietary caffeine on renal handling of minerals in adult women. *Life Sci* 1990;47(6):557–564.

Block G, Abrams B: Vitamin and mineral status of women of childbearing potential. *Ann NY Acad* 1993;678:244–254.

Borrud L, Krebs-Smith S, Friedman L, et al: Food and nutrient intakes of pregnant and lactating women in the United States. *J Nutr Ed* 1993;25:176–185.

Bower C, Stanley F, Nicol D: Maternal folate status and the risk for neural tube defects. *Ann NY Acad* 1993;678:146–155.

Brown J: Preconceptual nutrition and reproductive outcomes. *Ann NY Acad* 1993;678:286–292.

Buchdal R, Hird M, Gamsu H, et al: Listeriosis revisited: The role of the obstetrician. *Br J Obst G* 1990;97:186–189.

Butterworth C: Folate status, women's health, pregnancy outcome, and cancer. *J Am Col N* 1993;12(4):438–441.

Caffeine during pregnancy: Grounds for concern? *J Am Med A* 1993;270(24):2973–2974.

Castro L, Allen R, Ogunyemi D, et al: Cigarette smoking during pregnancy: Acute effects on uterine flow velocity waveforms. *Obstet Gyn* 1993;81:551–555.

Centers for Disease Control: Recommendations for the use of folic acid to reduce the number of cases of spina bifida and other neural tube defects. *MMWR* 1992;41:1.

Centers for Disease Control: Use of folic acid for prevention for spina bifida and other neural tube defects—1983–1991. *MMWR* 1991;40:513.

Clapp J: Exercise and fetal health. *J Dev Physl* 1991;15:9–14.

Clapp J, Capeless E: The VO2max of recreational athletes before and after pregnancy. *Med Sci Spt* 1991;23(10):1128–1133.

Clapp J, Rokey R, Treadway J, et al: Exercise in pregnancy. *Med Sci Spt* 1992;24(6 suppl): S294–S300.

Clarren S, Smith D: The fetal alcohol syndrome. *N Eng J Med* 1978;298(19):1063–1067.

Cochrane R: Women's concerns. *Practition* 1992;236:300–305.

Cockroft D: Vitamin deficiencies and neural tube defects: Human and animal studies. *Hum Repr* 1991;6(1):148–157.

Cohen H, Green J, Crombleholme W: Peripartum cocaine use: Estimating risk of adverse pregnancy outcome. *Int J Gyn O* 1991;35:51–54.

Cook D, Whincup P, Jarvis M, et al: Passive exposure to tobacco smoke in children aged 5–7 years: Individual, family, and community factors. *Br Med J* 1994;308:384–389.

Cornelissen M, Steegers-Theunissen R, Kollee L, et al: Increased incidence of neonatal vitamin K deficiency resulting from maternal anticonvulsant therapy. *Am J Obst G* 1993;168: 923–928.

Cornelissen M, Steegers-Theunissen R, Kollee L, et al: Supplementation of vitamin K in pregnant women receiving anticonvulsant therapy prevents neonatal vitamin K deficiency. *Am J Obst G* 1993;168:884–888.

Coste J, Job-Spira N, Fernandez H: Increased risk of ectopic pregnancy with maternal cigarette smoking. *Am J Pub He* 1991;81(2):199–201.

Cramer D, Xu H, Sahi T: Adult hypolactasia, milk consumption, and age-specific fertility. *Am J Epidem* 1994;139(3):282–289.

Cumming D, Wheeler G, Harber V: Physical activity, nutrition, and reproduction. *Ann NY Acad* 1994;709:55–76.

Cunningham J, Dockery D, Speizer F: Maternal smoking during pregnancy as a predictor of lung function in children. *Am J Epidem* 1994;139:1139–1152.

Czeizel A: Prevention of congenital abnormalities by periconceptual multivitamin supplementation. *Br Med J* 1993;306:1645–1648.

Czeizel A, Kodaj I, Lenz W: Smoking during pregnancy and congenital limb deficiency. *Br Med J* 1994;308:1473–1476.

Danforth W: The management of normal pregnancy (prenatal care), in Curtis A (ed): *Obstetrics and Gynaecology*, vol 1. Philadelphia, WB Saunders Co., 1933.

Dawes G: *Foetal and Neonatal Physiology.* Chicago, Year Book Medical Publishers, Inc., 1968.

Dawson E, Harris W, Teter M, et al: Effects of ascorbic acid supplementation on the sperm quality of smokers. *Fert Steril* 1992;58:1034–1039.

Department of Health and Human Services: *Caring for our Future: The Content of Prenatal Care. A Report of the Public Health Service Expert Panel on the Content of Prenatal Care.* Washington, D.C., Public Health Service, 1989.

Devoe L, Murray C, Youssif A, et al: Maternal caffeine consumption and fetal behavior in normal third-trimester pregnancy. *Am J Obst G* 1993;168:1105–1112.

Dreosti I: Nutritional factors underlying the expression of the fetal alcohol syndrome. *Ann NY Acad* 1993;678:193–204.

Favier A: The role of zinc in reproduction: Hormonal mechanisms. *Biol Tr El* 1992;32:363.

Fenster L, Eskenazi B, Windham G, et al: Caffeine consumption during pregnancy and fetal growth. *Am J Pub He* 1991;81:458–461.

Flores-Huerta S, Hernandez-Montes H, Argote R, et al: Effects of ethanol consumption during pregnancy and lactation on the outcome and postnatal growth of the offspring. *Ann Nutr M* 1992;36:121–128.

Folate and neural tube defects: US policy evolves. *Nutr Rev* 1993;51(12):358–361.

Folate supplements prevent recurrence of neural tube defects. *Nutr Rev* 1992;50(1):22–24.

Fortier I, Marcoux S, Beaulac-Baillargeon L: Relation of caffeine intake during pregnancy to intrauterine growth retardation and preterm birth. *Am J Epidem* 1993;137(9):931–940, 955–958.

Fried P: Prenatal exposure to tobacco and marijuana: Effects during pregnancy, infancy, and early childhood. *Clin 0 Gyne* 1993;36(2):319–337.

Fried P, Watkinson B, Gray R: A follow-up study of attentional behavior in 6-year-old children exposed prenatally to marihuana, cigarettes, and alcohol. *Neurotox T* 1992;14(5):299–311.

Hanson J, Streissguth A, Smith D: The effects of moderate alcohol consumption during pregnancy on fetal growth and morphogenesis. *J Pediat* 1978;92(3):457–460.

Haste F, Brooke O, Anderson H, et al: The effect of nutritional intake on outcome of pregnancy in smokers and non-smokers. *Br J Nutr* 1991;65:347–354.

Hatch E, Bracken M: Association of delayed conception with caffeine consumption. *Am J Epidem* 1993;138:1082–1092.

Hayes C, Werler M, Mitchell A: The association between folic acid supplementation and oral clefts (meeting abstract). *J Dent Res* 1994;73:445.

He Y, Lam T, Li L, et al: Passive smoking at work as a risk factor for coronary heart disease in Chinese women who have never smoked. *Br Med J* 1994;308:380–384.

Heikklila A: Antibiotics in pregnancy: A prospective cohort study on the policy of antibiotic prescription. *Ann Med* 1993;25:467–471.

Higgins P, Frank B, Brown M: Changes in health behaviors made by pregnant women. *Health Care Women* 1994;15:149–156.

Hunt C, Johnson P, Herbel J, et al: Effects of dietary zinc depletion on seminal volume and zinc loss, serum testosterone concentrations, and sperm morphology in young men. *Am J Clin N* 1992;56:148–157.

Infante-Rivard C, Fernandez A, Gauthier R, et al: Fetal loss associated with caffeine intake before and during pregnancy. *J Am Med A* 1993;270(24):2940–2943.

Jick S, Terris B, Jick H: First trimester topical tretinoin and congenital disorders. *Lancet* 1993;341:1181–1182.

Joesoef M, Beral V, Rolfs R, et al: Are caffeinated beverages risk factors for delayed conception? *Lancet* 1990;335:136–137.

John E, Savitz D, Sandler D: Prenatal exposure to parents' smoking and childhood cancer. *Am J Epidem* 1991;133:123–132.

Kehoe P, Shoemaker W: Opioid-dependent behaviors in infant rats: Effects of prenatal exposure to ethanol. *Pharm Bio B* 1991;39:389–394.

Kemmann E, Pasquale S, Skaf R: Amenorrhea associated with carotenemia. *J Am Med A* 1983;249(7):926–929.

Klonoff-Cohen H, Edelstein S, Savitz D: Cigarette smoking and preeclampsia. *Obstet Gyn* 1993;81:541–544.

Koren G, Bologa M, Pastuszak A: How women perceive teratogenic risk and what they do about it. *Ann NY Acad* 1993;678:317–324.

Kurppa K, Holmberg P, Kuosma E, et al: Coffee consumption during pregnancy and selected congenital malformations: A nationwide case-control study. *Am J Pub He* 1983;73(12):1397–1399.

Kusin J, Kardjati S, Renqvist U: Chronic undernutrition in pregnancy and lactation. *P Nutr Soc* 1993;52:19–28.

Langhoff-Roos J, Wibell L, Gebre-Medlin M, et al: Effect of smoking on maternal glucose metabolism. *Gynecol Obs* 1993;36(1):8–11.

Larroque B, Kaminski M, Lelong N, et al: Effects on birth weight of alcohol and caffeine consumption during pregnancy. *Am J Epidem* 1993;137:941–950.

Levine B: Nutrition recommendations and practices of obstetrician-gynecologists before conception and during pregnancy. *Ann NY Acad* 1993;678:353–355.

Lin G: Effect of dietary folic acid levels and gestational ethanol consumption on tissue folate contents and rat fetal development. *Nutr Res* 1991;11:223–230.

Lobaugh N, Wigal T, Greene P, et al: Effects of prenatal ethanol exposure on learned persistence and hippocampal neuroanatomy in infant, weanling and adult rats. *Behav Br Res* 1991;44:81–86.

Lotgering F, van Doorn M, Struijk P, et al: Maximal aerobic exercise in pregnant women: Heart rate, O_2 consumption, CO_2 production, and ventilation. *J Appl Physl* 1991;70(3):1016–1023.

Loucks A, Horvath S: Athletic amenorrhea: A review. *Med Sci Spt* 1985;17(1):56–72.

Loucks A, Vaitukaitis J, Cameron J, et al: The reproductive system and exercise in women. *Med Sci Spt* 1992;24(6 Suppl):S288–S293.

Martinez-Frias M, Rodriguez-Pinilla E: Folic acid supplementation and neural tube defects. *Lancet* 1992;340(8819):620.

Massey L, Berg T: The effect of dietary caffeine on urinary excretion of calcium, magnesium, phosphorus, sodium, potassium, chloride and zinc in healthy males. *Nutr Res* 1985;5: 1281–1284.

Massey L, Wise K: Impact of gender and age on urinary water and mineral excretion responses to acute caffeine doses. *Nutr Res* 1992;12(4-5):605–612.

Mayes L, Granger R, Frank M, et al: Neurobehavioral profiles of neonates exposed to cocaine prenatally. *Pediatrics* 1993;91(4):778–783.

McCabe R, Remington J: Toxoplasmosis: The time has come. *N Eng J Med* 1988;318:131–137.

McLauchlin J: Human listeriosis in Britain 1967–1985, a summary of 722 cases. *Epidem Infe* 1990;104(2):181–189.

Mehta S, Pritchard M, Stegman C: Contribution of coffee and tea to anemia among NHANES II participants. *Nutr Res* 1992;12:209–222.

Mikode M, White A: Dietary assessment of middle-income pregnant women during the first, second, and third trimesters. *J Am Diet A* 1994;94(2):196–199.

Mills J, Holmes L, Aarons J, et al: Moderate caffeine use and the risk of spontaneous abortion and intrauterine growth retardation. *J Am Med A* 1993;269:593.

Mills J, Raymond E: Effects of recent research on recommendations for periconceptional folate supplement use. *Ann NY Acad* 1993;678:137–145.

Mills J, Tuomilehto J, Colman N, et al: Maternal vitamin levels during pregnancies producing infants with neural tube defects. *J Pediat* 1992;120:863–871.

MRC Vitamin Study Research Group: Prevention of neural tube defects: Results of the Medical Research Council Vitamin Study. *Lancet* 1991;338:131–137.

Mulinare J: Epidemiologic associations of multivitamin supplementation and occurrence of neural tube defects. *Ann NY Acad* 1993;678:130–136.

Mulinare J, Cordero J, Erickson J, et al: Periconceptual use of multivitamins and the occurrence of neural tube defects. *J Am Med A* 1988;260(21):3141–3145.

Murphy P: Periconceptual supplementation with folic acid: Does it prevent neural tube defects? *J Nurse-Mid* 1992;37(1):25–31.

Nakamoto T, Gottschalk S, Yazdani M, et al: Combined effects of caffeine and zinc in the maternal diet on fetal brains. *FASEB J* 1991;5:A1319.

Narahara H, Johnston J: Smoking and preterm labor: Effect of a cigarette smoke extract on the secretion of platelet-activating factor-acetylhydrolase by human decidual macrophages. *Am J Obst G* 1993;169:1321–1326.

Nehlig A, Debry G: Consequences on the newborn of chronic maternal consumption of coffee during gestation and lactation: A review. *J Am Col N* 1994;13(10):6–21.

Nelson M: Vitamin A, liver consumption and risk of birth defects. *Br Med J* 1990;301:1176.

Ogawa H, Tominaga S, Hori K, et al: Passive smoking by pregnant women and fetal growth. *J Epidem C* 1991;45:164–168.

Olds D, Henderson C, Tatelbaum R: Intellectual impairment in children of women who smoke cigarettes during pregnancy. *Pediatrics* 1994;93(2):221–227.

Pasquali R, Antenucci D, Casimirri F, et al: Clinical and hormonal characteristics of obese amenorrheic hyperandrogenic women before and after weight loss. *J Clin End* 1989;68(1):173–177.

Pikkarainen S, Parviainen M: Vitamin A levels in bovine and pork liver. *Int J Vit N* 1993;63: 86–88.

Pirke K, Schweiger U, Laessle R, et al: Dieting influences the menstrual cycle: Vegetarian versus nonvegetarian diet. *Fert Steril* 1986;46(6):1083–1088.

Popova E: Maternal alcohol consumption before pregnancy and ultrastructure of neurons and interneuronal connections in rat offspring. *Int J Neuros* 1993;73:37–45.

Pregnancy risks determined from birth certificate data: United States, 1989. *J Am Med A* 1992;268(14):1831–1832.

Prior J, Vigna Y, McKay D: Reproduction for the athletic woman. *Sport Med* 1992;14(3): 190–199.

Qing C, Windsor R, Hassan M: Cost differences between low birthweight attributable to smoking and low birthweight for all causes. *Prev Med* 1994;23:28–34.

Qing C, Windsor R, Perkins L, et al: The impact on infant birth weight and gestational age of cotinine-validated smoking reduction during pregnancy. *J Am Med A* 1993;269:1519.

Racine A, Joyce T, Anderson R: The association between prenatal care and birth weight among women exposed to cocaine in New York City. *J Am Med A* 1993;270:1581–1586.

Rhoads G, Mills J: Can vitamin supplements prevent neural tube defects? Current evidence and ongoing investigations. *Clin O Gyne* 1986;29(3):569–579.

Rosevear S, Holt D, Lee T, et al: Smoking and decreased fertilization rates in vitro. *Lancet* 1992;340:1195–1196.

Rush D: Periconceptual folate and neural tube defect. *Am J Clin N* 1994;59(Suppl):511S–516S.

Sastry B, Mouton S, Janson V, et al: Tobacco smoking by pregnant women. *Ann NY Acad* 1993;678:361–363.

Schaffer D: Maternal nutritional factors and congenital anomalies: A guide for epidemiologic investigation. *Ann NY Acad* 1993;678:205–214.

Schnorr T, Grajewski B, Hornung R, et al: Video display terminals and the risk of spontaneous abortion. *N Eng J Med* 1991;324:727–733.

Scholl T, Hediber M, Fischer R, et al: Anemia vs iron deficiency: Increased risk of preterm delivery in a prospective study. *Am J Clin N* 1992;55:985–988.

Sheard N: Iron deficiency and infant development. *Nutr Rev* 1994;52(4):137–140.

Sheffer R, Shohat M, Merlob P: Prolonged maternal diet imbalance and recurrent fetuses with congenital anomalies. *Am J Med G* 1993;45:398–399.

Shiono P, Klebanoff M: Invited commentary: Caffeine and birth outcomes. *Am J Epidem* 1993; 137(9):951–954.

Spohr H, Willms J, Steinhausen H: Prenatal alcohol exposure and long-term developmental consequences. *Lancet* 1993;341:907–910.

Stein Z, Susser M: Miscarriage, caffeine, and the epiphenomena of pregnancy: The causal model. *Epidem* 1991;2(3):163–167, 168–174.

Srisuphan W, Bracken M: Caffeine consumption during pregnancy and association with late spontaneous abortion. *Am J Obst G* 1986;154:14–20.

Tamura T, Goldenberg R, Freeberg L, et al: Maternal serum folate and zinc concentrations and their relationships to pregnancy outcome. *Am J Clin N* 1992;56:365–370.

Terje R, Wilcox A, Skjerven R: A population-based study of the risk of recurrence of birth defects. *N Eng J Med* 1994;331:1–4.

Tolarova M: Periconceptional supplementation with vitamins and folic acid to prevent recurrence of cleft lip (Letter). *Lancet* 1982;II(8291):217.

Uhlund A, Kwiecinski G, DeLuca H: Normalization of serum calcium restores fertility in vitamin D-deficient male rats. *J Nutr* 1992;122:1338–1344.

US Department of Health and Human Services: *Alcohol, Tobacco, and Other Drugs May Harm the Unborn.* Rockville, MD, Public Health Service, 1990.

Valbo A, Schioldborg P: Smoking in pregnancy: A follow-up study of women unwilling to quit. *Addict Beha* 1993;18:253–257.

Van Allen M, Fraser F, Dallaire L, et al: Recommendations on the use of folic acid supplementation to prevent the recurrence of neural tube defects. *Can Med A J* 1993;149(9):1239–1243.

Vavrousek-Jakuba E, Baker R, Shoemaker W: Effect of ethanol on maternal and offspring characteristics: Comparison of three liquid diet formulations fed during gestation. *Alc Clin Ex* 1991;15:129–135.

Wald N: Folic acid and the prevention of neural tube defects. *Ann NY Acad* 1993;678:112–129.

Wald N, Bower C: Folic acid, pernicious anaemia, and prevention of neural tube defects. *Lancet* 1994;343:307.

Wallace A, Boyer D, Dan A, et al: Aerobic exercise, maternal self-esteem, and physical discomforts during pregnancy. *J Nurse-Mid* 1986;31:255–262.

Wallace A, Engsrom J: The effects of aerobic exercise on the pregnant woman, fetus, and pregnancy outcome. *J Nurse-Mid* 1987;32:277–290.

Watkinson B, Fried P: Maternal caffeine use before, during, and after pregnancy and effects upon offspring. *Neurob Tox* 1985;7:9–17.

Watson W, Katz V, Hackney A, et al: Fetal responses to maximal swimming and cycling exercise during pregnancy. *Obstet Gyn* 1991;77:382–386.

Werler M, Shapiro S, Mitchell A: Periconceptual folic acid exposure and risk of concurrent neural tube defects. *J Am Med A* 1993;269:1257–1261.

Willhite C: Selenium teratogenesis: Species dependent response and influence on reproduction. *Ann NY Acad* 1993;678:169–177.

Wilcox A: Birth weight and perinatal mortality: The effect of maternal smoking. *Am J Epidem* 1993;137:1098–1104.

Wilton T, Hopkins W, Seddon R: Lifestyle advice to pregnant patients. *NZ Med J* 1993;106: 157–158.

Wolff C, Portis M, Wolff H: Birth weight and smoking practices during pregnancy among Mexican-American women. *Health Care* 1993;14:271–279.

Wood J: Maternal nutrition and reproduction: Why demographers and physiologists disagree about a fundamental relationship. *Ann NY Acad* 1994;709:101–116.

Wynn A, Crawford M, Doyle W, et al: Nutrition of women in anticipation of pregnancy. *Nutr Health* 1991;7(2):69–88.

Yazdani M, Fontenot F, Gottschalk S, et al: Relationship of prenatal caffeine exposure and zinc supplementation on fetal rat brain growth. *Dev Pharm T* 1992;18:108–115.

Zaadstra B, Seidell J, Van Noord P, et al: Fat and female fecundity: Prospective study of effect of body fat distribution on conception rates. *Br Med J* 1993;306:484–487.

2. The Baby-wise Diet

Apgar J, Everett G: Low zinc intake affects maintenance of pregnancy in guinea pigs. *J Nutr* 1991;121:192–200.

Calcium supplementation prevents hypertensive disorders of pregnancy. *Nutr Rev* 1992;50(8): 233–236.

Heston T, Simkin P: Carbohydrate loading in preparation for childbirth. *Med Hypoth* 1991;34: 97–98.

Malhotra A, Fairweather-Tait S, Wharton P, et al: Placental zinc in normal and intra-uterine growth-retarded pregnancies. *Br J Nutr* 1990;63:613–621.

McCullough A, Kirksey A, Wachs T, et al: Vitamin B6 status in Egyptian mothers: Relation to infant behavior and maternal-infant interactions. *Am J Clin N* 1990;51:1067–1074.

McGarvey S, Zinner S, Willett W, et al: Maternal prenatal dietary potassium, calcium, magnesium, and infant blood pressure. *Hypertensio* 1991;17:218–224.

Neggers Y, Cutter G, Acton R, et al: A positive association between maternal serum zinc concentration and birth weight. *Am J Clin N* 1990;51:678–684.

Villar J, Belizan J, Fischer P: Epidemiologic observations on the relationship between calcium intake and eclampsia. *Int J Gyn O* 1983;21(4):271–278.

3. The Nutrition Primer for Pregnancy

Ancri G, Morse E, Clarke R: Comparison of the nutritional status of pregnant adolescents with adult pregnant women III. Maternal protein and calorie intake and weight gain in relation to size of infant at birth. *Am J Clin N* 1977;30:568–572.

Aharoni A, Tesler B, Paltieli Y, et al: Hair chromium content of women with gestational diabetes compared with nondiabetic pregnant women. *Am J Clin N* 1992;55:104–107.

Anderson G: Developmental sensitivity of the brain to dietary n-3 fatty acids. *J Lipid Res* 1994; 35(1):105–111.

Altchuler S: Dietary protein and calcium loss: A review. *Nutr Res* 1982;2:193–200.

Anderson R, Kozlovsky A: Chromium intake, absorption and excretion of subjects consuming self-selected diets. *Am J Clin N* 1985;41:1177–1183.

Atkinson S: Calcium and phosphorus needs of premature infants. *Nutr* 1994;10(1):66–68.

Apgar J: Zinc and reproduction: An update. *J Nutr Bioc* 1992;3(6):266–278.

Apgar J, Everett G: Low zinc intake affects maintenance of pregnancy in guinea pigs. *J Nutr* 1991;121:192–200.

Baly D, Golub M, Gershwin E, et al: Studies of marginal zinc deprivation in rhesus monkeys. III. Effects on vitamin A metabolism. *Am J Clin N* 1984;40:199–207.

Beare-Rogers J, Gray L, Hollywood R: The linoleic acid and trans fatty acids of margarine. *Am J Clin N* 1979;32:1805–1809.

Bogden J, Murphy M, Fraiman M, et al: Dietary calcium and lead exposure during pregnancy interact to influence erythropoiesis (meeting abstract). *J Cell Bioc* 1994;Jan 4(S18A):24.

Bostedt H, Schramel P: The importance of selenium in the prenatal and postnatal development of calves and lambs. *Biol Tr El* 1990;24:163.

Brittin H, Nossaman C: Iron content of food cooked in iron utensils. *J Am Diet A* 1986;86: 897–901.

Bunin G, Kuijten R, Buckley J, et al: Relation between maternal diet and subsequent primitive neuroectodermal brain tumors in young children. *N Eng J Med* 1993;329(8):536–541.

Buonopane G, Kilara A, Smith J, et al: Effect of skim milk supplementation on blood cholesterol concentration, blood pressure, and triglycerides in a free-living human population. *J Am Col N* 1992;11(1):56–67.

Bourgoin B, Evans D, Cornett J, et al: Lead content of 70 brands of dietary calcium supplements. *Am J Pub He* 1993;83(8):1155–1160.

Butterworth R: Maternal thiamine deficiency. *Ann NY Acad* 1993;678:325–329.

Calcium and vitamin D intakes influence the risk of bowel cancer in men. *Nutr Rev* 1985;43(6): 170–172.

Calcium supplementation prevents hypertensive disorders of pregnancy. *Nutr Rev* 1992;50(8): 233–236.

Carlson S, Werkman S, Rhodes P, et al: Visual-acuity development in healthy preterm infants: Effect of marine-oil supplementation. *Am J Clin N* 1993;58:35–42.

Chan G, Hoffman K, McMurray M: The effect of dietary calcium supplementation on pubertal girls' growth and bone mineral status. *Clin Res* 1992;40:60A.

Connor W, Neuringer M, Reisbick S: Essential fatty acids: The importance of n-3 fatty acids in the retina and brain. *Nutr Rev* 1992;50(4):21–29.

Crawford M: The role of essential fatty acids in neural development: Implications for perinatal nutrition. *Am J Clin N* 1993;57(suppl):703S–710S.

Cruz M, Mimouni F, Tsang R, et al: Effect of chronic maternal dietary magnesium deficiency on placental calcium transport. *J Am Col N* 1992;11(1):87–92.

Dawson-Hughes B, Dallal G, Krall E, et al: Effect of vitamin D supplementation on wintertime and overall bone loss in healthy postmenopausal women. *Ann Int Med* 1991;115: 505–512.

Dumont J, Corvilain B, Contempre B: The biochemistry of endemic cretinism: Roles of iodine and selenium deficiency and goitrogens. *Mol C Endoc* 1994;100(1–2):163–166.

Dunn J: Iodine supplementation and the prevention of cretinism. *Ann NY Acad* 1993;678: 158–168.

Economides D, Ferguson J, MacKenzie I, et al: Folate and vitamin B12 concentrations in maternal and fetal blood, and amniotic fluid in second trimester pregnancies complicated by neural tube defects. *Br J Obst G* 1992;99:23–25.

Enig M, Atal S, Keeney M, et al: Isomeric trans fatty acids in the U.S. diet. *J Am Col N* 1990; 9(5):471–486.

Fairweather-Tait S, Piper Z: The effect of tea on iron and aluminum metabolism in the rat. *Br J Nutr* 1991;65:61–68.

Farkas C, leRiche W: Effect of tea and coffee consumption on non-haem iron absorption. *Hum Nutr-Cl* 1987;41C:161–163.

Favier A: The role of zinc in reproduction. *Biol Tr El* 1992;32:363.

Fredriksson A, Gardlund A, Bergman K, et al: Effects of maternal dietary supplementation with selenite on the postnatal development of rat offspring exposed to methyl mercury in utero. *Pharm Tox* 1993;72:377–382.

Freudenheim J, Johnson N, Smith E: Relationship between usual nutrient intake and bone-mineral content of women 35–65 years of age: Longitudinal and cross-sectional analysis. *Am J Clin N* 1986;44:863–876.

Friel J, Andrews W: Zinc requirement of premature infants. *Nutr* 1994;10(1):63–65.

Glenn F, Glenn W: Optimum dosage for prenatal fluoride supplementation (PNF): Part IX Prenatal Fluoride. *J Dent Chil* 1987;Nov/Dec:445–450.

Glenn F, Glenn W, Duncan R: Fluoride tablet supplementation during pregnancy for caries immunity: A study of offspring produced. *Am J Obst G* 1982;143:560.

Godel J, Pabst H, Hodges P, et al: Iron status and pregnancy in a northern Canadian population: Relationship to diet and iron supplementation. *Can J Publ* 1992;83(5):339–343.

Goldenberg R, Tamura T, Cliver S, et al: Serum folate and fetal growth retardation: A matter of compliance? *Obstet Gyn* 1992;79:719–722.

Hachey D: Benefits and risk of modifying maternal fat intake in pregnancy and lactation. *Am J Clin N* 1994;59(suppl):454S–463S.

Hallberg L, Bengtsson C, Lapidus L, et al: Screening for iron deficiency: An analysis of bone-marrow examinations and serum ferritin determinations in a population sample of women. *Br J Haem* 1993;85(4):787–798.

Hallberg L, Rossander-Hulten L: Iron requirements in menstruating women. *Am J Clin N* 1991; 54:1047–1058.

Haram K, Thordarson H, Hervig T: Calcium homeostasis in pregnancy and lactation. *Acta Obst Sc* 1993;72(7):509–513.

Hathcock J, Hattan D, Jenkins M, et al: Evaluation of vitamin A toxicity. *Am J Clin N* 1990;52: 183–202.

Heaney R: Bone mass, nutrition, and other lifestyle factors. *Am J Med* 1993;95 (suppl 5A): 29S–33S.

Hoffman D, Birch E, Birch D, et al: Effects of supplementation with w-3 long-chain polyunsaturated fatty acids on retinal and cortical development in premature infants. *Am J Clin N* 1993;57(suppl):807S–812S.

Hu J, Zhao X, Jia J, et al: Dietary calcium and bone density among middle-aged and elderly women in China. *Am J Clin N* 1993;58:219–227.

Hunt J, Mullen L, Lykken G, et al: Ascorbic acid: Effect on ongoing iron absorption and status in iron-depleted young women. *Am J Clin N* 1990;51:649–655.

Husain S, Sibley C: Magnesium and pregnancy. *Min Elect M* 1993;19(3–4):296–307.

Icke G, Nicol D: Thiamin status in pregnancy as determined by direct microbiological assay. *Int J Vit N* 1993;63:33–35.

The influence of tea on iron and aluminum bioavailability in the rat. *Nutr Rev* 1992;49(9): 287–289.

Jameson S: Zinc status in pregnancy: The effect of zinc therapy on perinatal mortality, prematurity, and placental ablation. *Ann NY Acad* 1993;678:178–192.

Johnson A, Knight E, Edwards C, et al: Dietary intakes, anthropometric measurements and pregnancy outcomes. *J Nutr* 1994;124:936S–942S.

Johnson J, Greenberg R: Protein turnover in rat placenta: Effects of maternal fasting and maternal protein restriction. *Placenta* 1992;13:141–150.

Keen C: Maternal factors affecting teratogenic response: A need for assessment. *Teratology* 1992; 46(1):15–21.

Keen C, Lonnerdal B, Golub M, et al: Effect of the severity of maternal zinc deficiency on pregnancy outcome and infant zinc status in rhesus monkeys. *Pediat Res* 1993;33:233–241.

Keen C, Taubeneck M, Daston G, et al: Primary and secondary zinc deficiency as factors underlying abnormal CNS development. *Ann NY Acad* 1993;678:37–47.

Kemp F, Czerniach M, Fraiman M, et al: Dietary calcium and lead toxicity during pregnancy (meeting abstract). *FASEB J* 1993;7(3):A68.

Killholma P, et al: The role of calcium, copper, iron, and zinc in preterm delivery and premature rupture of fetal membranes. *Gynecol Obs* 1984;17:194–201.

Kirke P, Molloy A, Daly L, et al: Maternal plasma folate and vitamin B12 are independent risk factors for neural tube defects. *Q J Med* 1993;86(11):703–708.

Kirksey A, Wasynczuk A: Morphological, biochemical, and functional consequences of vitamin B6 deficits during central nervous system development. *Ann NY Acad* 1993;678:62–80.

Kizer K, Fan A, Bankowska J, et al: Vitamin A—A pregnancy hazard alert. *West J Med* 1990; 152:78–81.

Knight K, Keith R: Calcium supplementation on normotensive and hypertensive pregnant women. *Am J Clin N* 1992;55:891–895.

Kohrs M, Harper A, Kerr G: Effects of low-protein diet during pregnancy of the rhesus monkey: I. Reproductive efficiency. *Am J Clin N* 1976;29:136–145.

Kolezko B: Trans fatty acids may impair biosynthesis of long-chain polyunsaturates and growth in man. *Acta Paed Sc* 1992;81:302–306.

Kramer M: Effects of energy and protein intakes on pregnancy outcome: An overview of the research evidence from controlled clinical trials. *Am J Clin N* 1993;58:627–635.

Kummerow F: Dietary effects of trans fatty acids. *J Env P Tox* 1986;6(3–4):123–149.

Kurzel R: Is low serum magnesium associated with premature labor? *Ann NY Acad* 1993;678: 350–352.

Lane H, Strength R, Johnson J, et al: Effect of chemical form of selenium on tissue glutathione peroxidase activity in developing rats. *J Nutr* 1991;121:80–86.

Lockkitch G, Jacobson B, Quigley G, et al: Selenium deficiency in low birth weight neonates: An unrecognized problem. *J Pediat* 1989; 114:865–870.

Maden M: Vitamin A in embryonic development. *Nutr Rev* 1994;52(2):S3–S12.

Malhotra A, Fairweather-Tait S, Wharton P, et al: Maternal zinc in normal and intra-uterine growth-retarded pregnancies. *Br J Nutr* 1990;63:613–621.

Marya R, Saini A, Jaswal T: Effect of vitamin D supplementation during pregnancy on the neonatal skeletal growth in the rat. *Ann Nutr M* 1991;35:208–212.

Mask G, Lane H: Selected measures of selenium status in full-term and preterm neonates, their mothers and nonpregnant women. *Nutr Res* 1993;13(8):901–911.

Matkovic V, Heaney R: Calcium balance during human growth: Evidence for threshold behavior. *Am J Clin N* 1992;55:992–996.

Matkovic V, Ilich J: Calcium requirements for growth: Are current recommendations adequate? *Nutr Rev* 1993;51(6):171–180.

McArdle H, Erlich R: Copper uptake and transfer to the mouse fetus during pregnancy. *J Nutr* 1991;121:208–214.

McCullough A, Kirksey A, Wachs T, et al: Vitamin B6 status in Egyptian mothers: Relation to infant behavior and maternal-infant interactions. *Am J Clin N* 1990;51:1067–1074.

McGarvey S, Zinner S, Willett W, et al: Maternal prenatal dietary potassium, calcium, magnesium, and infant blood pressure. *Hypertensio* 1991;17:218–224.

Mensink R, Zock P, Katan M, et al: Effect of dietary cis and trans fatty acids on serum lipoprotein[a] levels in humans. *J Lipid Res* 1992;33(10):1493–1501.

Miller R, Faber W, Asai M, et al: The role of the human placenta in embryonic nutrition: Impact of environmental and social factors. *Ann NY Acad* 1993;678:92–107.

Milman N, Agger A, Nielsen O: Iron status markers and serum erythropoietin in 120 mothers and newborn infants. *Acta Obst Sc* 1994;73:200–204.

Milner J, Picciano M: Selenium in maternal and infant nutrition. *Cont Nutr* 1986;11(5):1–2.

Mukherjee M, Sandstead H, Ratnaparkhi M, et al: Maternal zinc, iron, folic acid, and protein nutriture and outcome of human pregnancy. *Am J Clin N* 1984;40:496–507.

Mulhern S, Taylor G, Magruder L, et al: Deficient levels of dietary selenium suppress the antibody response in first and second generation mice. *Nutr Res* 1985;5(2):201–210.

Murphy S, Khaw K, May H, et al: Milk consumption and bone mineral density in middle-aged and elderly women. *Br J Med* 1994;308:939–941.

Murphy S, Rose D, Hudes M, et al: Demographic and economic factors associated with dietary quality for adults in the 1987–1988 Nationwide Food Consumption Survey. *J Am Diet A* 1992;92:1352–1357.

Neggers Y, Cutter G, Acton R, et al: A positive association between maternal serum zinc concentration and birth weight. *Am J Clin N* 1990;51:678–684.

Nohr S, Laurberg P, Borlum K, et al: Iodine deficiency in pregnancy in Denmark. *Acta Obst Sc* 1993;72:350–353.

Oski F: Is bovine milk a health hazard? *Pediatrics* 1985;75(1):182–186.

Panth M, Shatrugna V, Ravinder P, et al: Assessment of vitamin A status in pregnant women as reflected by in vitro destruction of vitamin A by hemolysates and urinary ammonium nitrogen to creatinine ratio. *Int J Vit N* 1993;63(3):168–172.

Pratt C: Moderate exercise and iron status in women. *Nutr Rep* 1991;9(7):48,56.

Prentice A: Maternal calcium requirements during pregnancy and lactation. *Am J Clin N* 1994;59(suppl):477S–483S.

Prentice A, Laskey M, Shaw J, et al: The calcium and phosphorus intakes of rural Gambian women during pregnancy and lactation. *Br J Nutr* 1993;69:885–896.

Pritchard J, et al: Blood volume changes in pregnancy and the puerperium. II. Red blood cell loss and changes in apparent blood volume during and following vaginal delivery, cesarian section, and cesarian section plus total hysterectomy. *Am J Obst G* 1962;84:1271–1282.

Reynolds R, Polansky M, Moser P: Analyzed vitamin B6 intakes of pregnant and postpartum lactating and nonlactating women. *J Am Diet A* 1984;84:1339–1344.

Requirements of vitamin B6 during pregnancy. *Nutr Rev* 1976;34(11):15–16.

Sandstead H: Zinc deficiency: A public health problem? *Am J Dis Ch* 1991;145:853–859.

Scholl T, Hediger M: Anemia and iron-deficiency anemia: Compilation of data on pregnancy outcome. *Am J Clin N* 1994;59(suppl):492S–501S.

Scholl T, Hediger M, Fischer R, et al: Anemia vs iron deficiency: Increased risk of preterm delivery in a prospective study. *Am J Clin N* 1992;55:985–988.

Scholl T, Hediger M, Schall J, et al: Low zinc intake during pregnancy: Its association with preterm and very preterm delivery. *Am J Epidem* 1993;137:1115–1124.

Schorah C, Habibzadeh N, Wild J, et al: Possible abnormalities of folate and vitamin B12 metabolism associated with neural tube defects. *Ann NY Acad* 1993;678:81–91.

Schrijver R, Privell O: Energetic efficiency and mitochondrial function in rats fed trans fatty acids. *J Nutr* 1984;114:1183–1191.

Sharpe S, Gamble G, Sharpe D: Cholesterol-lowering and blood pressure effects of immune milk. *Am J Clin N* 1994;59:929–934.

Shojania A: Folic acid and vitamin B12 deficiency in pregnancy and in the neonatal period. *Clin Perin* 1984;11(2):433–459.

Siegenberg D, Baynes R, Bothwell T, et al: Ascorbic acid prevents the dose-dependent inhibitory effects of polyphenols and phytates on nonheme-iron absorption. *Am J Clin N* 1991;53: 537–541.

Simmer K, Punchard N, Murphy G, et al: Prostaglandin production and zinc depletion in human pregnancy. *Pediat Res* 1985;19:697–700.

Skajaa K, Dorup I, Sandstrom B: Magnesium intake and status and pregnancy outcome in a Danish population. *Br J Obst G* 1991;98:919–928.

Sklar R: Nutritional vitamin B12 deficiency in a breast-fed infant of a vegan-diet mother. *Clin Pediat* 1986;25:219–221.

Smith M, Nagey D, Moser-Veillon P: Plasma and erythrocyte magnesium changes following a glucose challenge during pregnancy. *J Am Col N* 1992;11(4):426–431.

Somer E: Trans fatty acids and disease: Fact or fallacy? *Nutr Rep* 1991;June:42.

Sommer A: Vitamin A: Its effects on childhood sight and life. *Nutr Rev* 1994;52(2):S60–S66.

Specker B: Do North American women need supplemental vitamin D during pregnancy and lactation? *Am J Clin N* 1994;59(suppl):484S–491S.

Speich M, Bousquet B, Auget J, et al: Association between magnesium, calcium, phosphorus, copper, and zinc in umbilical cord plasma and erythrocytes, and the gestational age and growth variables of full-term newborns. *Clin Chem* 1992;38(1):141–143.

Steinmetz K, Childs M, Stimson C, et al: Effect of consumption of whole milk and skim milk on blood lipid profiles in healthy men. *Am J Clin N* 1994;59:612–618.

Stemmermann G, Nomura A, Chyou P: The influence of dairy and nondairy calcium on subsite large-bowel cancer risk. *Dis Col Rec* 1990;33:190–194.

Tamm A: Management of lactose intolerance. *Sc J Gastr* 1994;29(S202):55–63.

Taper L, et al: Zinc and copper retention in pregnant women. *Fed Proc* 1981;40:855.

Teratology Society position paper: Recommendations for vitamin A use during pregnancy. *Teratology* 1987;35(2):269–275.

Thomsen J, Prien-Larsen J, Devantier A, et al: Low dose iron supplementation does not cover the need for iron during pregnancy. *Acta Obst Sc* 1993;72:93–98.

Tilyard M, Spears G, Thomson J, et al: Treatment of postmenopausal osteoporosis with calcitriol or calcium. *N Eng J Med* 1992;326:357–362.

Tonkiss J, Galler J, Morgane P, et al: Prenatal protein malnutrition and postnatal brain function. *Ann NY Acad* 1993;678:215–227.

Toss G: Effect of calcium intake vs. other life-style factors on bone mass. *J Intern M* 1992;231: 181–186.

Troisi R, Willett W, Weiss S: Trans fatty acid intake in relation to serum lipid concentrations in adult men. *Am J Clin N* 1992;56:1019–1024.

Trumbo P, Wang J: Vitamin B6 status indices are lower in pregnant than in nonpregnant women but urinary excretion of 4-pyridoxic acid does not differ. *J Nutr* 1993;123:2137–2141.

Underwood B: Maternal vitamin A status and its importance in infancy and early childhood. *Am J Clin N* 1994;59(suppl):517S–524S.

USDA (US Department of Agriculture): *Nationwide Food Consumption Survey. Nutrient Intakes: Individuals in 48 States.* 1977–1978. Report No.1-2. Consumer Nutrition Division. Human Nutrition Information Service, US Department of Agriculture, Hyattsville, MD. 1984:439.

US Department of Health and Human Services: *Nutrition Monitoring in the United States.* DHHS Publication No (PHS) 89-1255, 1989. US Preventive Services Task Force: Routine iron supplementation during pregnancy. *J Am Med A* 1993;270(23):2848–2854.

Veena R, Narang A, Banday A, et al: Copper and zinc levels in maternal and fetal cord blood. *Int J Gyn O* 1991;35:47–49.

Villar J, Belizan J, Fischer P: Epidemiologic observations on the relationship between calcium intake and eclampsia. *Int J Gyn O* 1983;21(4):271–278.

von Mandach U, Huch R, Huch A: Maternal and cord serum vitamin E levels in normal and abnormal pregnancy. *Int J Vit N* 1993;63:26–32.

Wainwright P: Do essential fatty acids play a role in brain and behavioral development? *Neurosci B* 1992;16:193–205.

Wasowicz W, Wolkanin P, Bednarski M, et al: Plasma trace element (Se, Zn, Cu) concentrations in maternal and umbilical cord blood in Poland. *Biol Tr El* 1993;38(2):205–215.

Werkman S, Peeples J, Cooke R, et al: Effect of vitamin A supplementation of intravenous lipids on early vitamin A intake and status of premature infants. *Am J Clin N* 1994;59:586–592.

West W, Knight E, Edwards C, et al: Maternal low level lead and pregnancy outcomes. *J Nutr* 1994;124:981S–986S.

Whittaker P, Lind T, Williams J: Iron absorption during normal human pregnancy: A study using stable isotopes. *Br J Nutr* 1991;65:457–463.

Willett W, Stampfer M, Manson J, et al: Intake of trans fatty acids and risk of coronary heart disease among women. *Lancet* 1993;341(March 6):581–585.

Wood R, Kubena K, O'Brien B, et al: Effect of butter, mono- and polyunsaturated fatty acid-enriched butter, trans fatty acid margarine, and zero trans fatty acid margarine on serum lipids and lipoproteins in healthy men. *J Lipid Res* 1993;34(1):1–11.

Zempleni J, Link G, Kubler W: The transport of thiamine, riboflavin and pyridoxal 5'-phosphate by human placenta. *Int J Vit N* 1992;62(2):165–172.

Zhang J, Fortney J, Feldblum P: Pregnancy and lactation as determinants of bone mineral density in postmenopausal women (letter). *Am J Epidem* 1993;138(11):1020–1021.

Zinc and parturition. *Nutr Rev* 1977;35(10):279–280.

4. Your Changing Body: What to Expect

Bobek P, Ginter E, Jarcovicova M, et al: Cholesterol-lowering effect of the mushroom pleurotus ostreatus in hereditary hypercholesterolemic rats. *Ann Nutr M* 1991;35:191–195.

Bustan M, Coker A: Maternal attitude toward pregnancy and the risk of neonatal death. *Am J Pub He* 1994;84(3):411–414.

Cara L, Armand M, Borel P, et al: Long-term wheat germ intake beneficially affects plasma lipids and lipoproteins in hypercholesterolemic human subjects. *J Nutr* 1992;122:317–326.

Committee on Maternal Nutrition: *Maternal Nutrition and the Course of Pregnancy.* Washington D.C., National Academy of Sciences, 1970.

Helser M, Hotchkiss J, Roe D: Influence of fruits and vegetable juices on the endogenous formation of N-nitrosoproline and N-nitrotheazolidine-4-carboxylic acid in humans on controlled diets. *Carcinogene* 1992;13(12):2277–2280.

Hertog M, Feskens E, Hollman P, et al: Dietary antioxidant flavonoids and risk or coronary heart disease: The Zutphen Elderly Study. *Lancet* 1993;342:1007–1011.

Hurley L: The consequences of fetal impoverishment. *Nutr Today* 1968;December:3–10.

Kitzinger S: *The Complete Book of Pregnancy and Childbirth.* New York, Alfred A. Knopf, 1993.

Little M, Hahn P: Diet and metabolic development. *FASEB J* 1990;4:2605–2611.

Rao A, Janezic S: The role of dietary phytosterols in colon carcinogenesis. *Nutr Cancer* 1992;18: 43–52.

Susser M, Stein Z: Timing in prenatal nutrition: A reprise of the Dutch Famine Study. *Nutr Rev* 1994;52(3):84–94.

Walker J: Musculoskeletal development: A review. *Phys Ther* 1991;71:878–889.

Worthington-Roberts B, Williams S: *Nutrition in Pregnancy and Lactation, ed 4.* St. Louis, Times Mirror/Mosby, 1989.

5. Nutrition During the First Trimester

Abrams B: Prenatal weight gain and postpartum weight retention: A delicate balance. *Am J Pub He* 1993;83(8):1082–1084.

Albers J, Dawson E, McGanity W: Effect of elevated pre-natal iron supplementation on serum copper, zinc, and selenium levels. *Am J Clin N* 1986;43:673.

Anderson R, Kozlovsky A: Chromium intake, absorption and excretion of subjects consuming self-selected diets. *Am J Clin N* 1985;41:1177–1183.

Armstrong J, Weijohn T: Dietary quality and concerns about body weight of low-income pregnant women. *J Am Diet A* 1991;91(10):1280–1282.

Arnaud J, Prual A, Prezioski P, et al: Effect of iron supplementation during pregnancy on trace elements (Cu, Se, Zn) concentrations in serum and breast milk from Nigerian women. *Ann Nutr M* 1993;37(5):262–271.

Backon J: Ginger in preventing nausea and vomiting of pregnancy: A caveat due to its thromboxane synthetase activity and effect on testosterone binding (letter). *Eur J Ob Gy* 1991;42(2): 163–164.

Bapurao S, Raman L, Tulpule P: Biochemical assessment of vitamin B6 nutritional status in pregnant women with orolingual manifestations. *Am J Clin N* 1982;36:581.

Barker D, Fall C: Fetal and infant origins of cardiovascular disease. *Arch Dis Ch* 1993;68: 797–799.

Barker D, Gluckman P, Godfrey K, et al: Fetal nutrition and cardiovascular disease in adult life. *Lancet* 1993;341(8850):938–941.

Behavioral consequences of pyridoxine deficiency in mothers and infants. *Nutr Rev* 1991;49(10): 312–314.

Bergmann R, Bergmann K: Fluoride nutrition in infancy: Is there a biological role of fluoride in growth? *Tr El Nutr Ch* 1991;23:105–117.

Boyce R: Enteral nutrition in hyperemesis gravidarum: A new development. *J Am Diet A* 1992; 92:733–736.

Bowen D: Taste and food preference changes across the course of pregnancy. *Appetite* 1992;19(3): 233–242.

Boyd N, Windsor R: A meta-evaluation of nutrition education intervention research among pregnant women. *Heal Educ Q* 1993;20(3):327–345.

Burke B, Beal V, Kirkwood S, et al: The influence of nutrition during pregnancy upon the condition of the infant at birth. *J Nutr* 1943;26:569–583.

Burns J, Paterson C: Effect of iron-folate supplementation on serum copper concentrations in late pregnancy. *Acta Obst Sc* 1993;72(8):616–618.

Catalano P, Hollenbeck C: Energy requirements in pregnancy: A review. *Obstet Gyn Survey* 1992; 47(6):368–372.

Clapp J, Dickstein S: Endurance exercise and pregnancy outcome. *Med Sci Spt* 1984;16:556.

Czeizel A: Controlled studies of multivitamin supplementation on pregnancy outcome. *Ann NY Acad* 1993;678:266–275.

Czeizel A, Dudas I, Fritz G, et al: The effect of periconceptional multivitamin-mineral supplementation on vertigo, nausea, and vomiting in the first trimester of pregnancy. *Arch Gyn Ob* 1992;251:181.

deAloysio D, Penacchioni P: Morning sickness control in early pregnancy by Neiguan point acupressure. *Obstet Gyn* 1992;80:852–854.

de Groot L, Boekholt H, Spaaij C, et al: Energy balances of healthy Dutch women before and during pregnancy: Limited scope for metabolic adaptations in pregnancy. *Am J Clin N* 1994;59: 827–832.

Dundee J, McMillan C: Positive evidence for P6 acupuncture antiemesis. *Postg Med J* 1991;67: 417–422.

Dunne F, Walters B, Marshall T, et al: Pregnancy associated osteoporosis. *Clin Endocr* 1993; 39(4):487–490.

Durnin J: Energy requirements of pregnancy. *Diabetes* 1991;40(Suppl 2):152–156.

Durnin J: Energy requirements of pregnancy. *Acta Paed Sc* 1991;373(suppl):33–42.

Erick M: Battling morning (noon and night) sickness. *J Am Diet A* 1994;94:147–148.

Erick M: *No More Morning Sickness: A Survival Guide for Pregnant Women.* New York, New American Library, 1993.

Evans A, Samuels S, Marshall C, et al: Suppression of pregnancy-induced nausea and vomiting with sensory afferent stimulation. *J Repro Med* 1993;38(8):603–606.

Gadsby R, Barnie-Adshead A, Jagger C: A prospective study of nausea and vomiting during pregnancy. *Br J Gen Pr* 1993;43(371):245–248.

Gorman K, Pollitt E: Relationship between weight and body proportionality at birth, growth during the first year of life, and cognitive development at 36, 48, and 60 months. *Infant Beh* 1992;15(3):279–296.

Gosselink C, Ekwo E, Woolson R, et al: Dietary habits, prepregnancy weight, and weight gain during pregnancy. *Acta Obst Sc* 1992;71:425–438.

Hack M, Breslau N, Weissman B, et al: Effect of very low birth weight and subnormal head size on cognitive abilities at school age. *N Eng J Med* 1991;325:231–237.

Halsey C, Collin M, Anderson C: Extremely low birth weight children and their peers: A comparison of preschool performance. *Pediatrics* 1993;91:807–811.

Hediger M, Scholl T, Schall J, et al: Changes in maternal upper arm fat stores are predictors of variation in infant birth weight. *J Nutr* 1994;124(1):24–30.

Hickey C, Cliver S, Goldenberg R, et al: Prenatal weight gain, term birth weight, and fetal growth retardation among high-risk multiparous black and white women. *Obstet Gyn* 1993; 81:529–535.

Institute of Medicine: *Nutrition During Pregnancy: Weight Gain, Nutrient Supplements.* Washington, D.C., National Academy Press, 1990.

Jeans P, Smith M, Stearns G: Incidence of prematurity in relation to maternal nutrition. *J Am Diet A* 1955;31:576–581.

Keen C, Zidenberg-Cherr S: Should vitamin-mineral supplements be recommended for all women with childbearing potential? *Am J Clin N* 1994;59(suppl):532S–539S.

Keppel K, Taffel S: Pregnancy-related weight gain and retention: Implications of the 1990 Institute of Medicine guidelines. *Am J Pub He* 1993;83(8):1100–1103.

King J, Butte N, Bronstein M, et al: Energy metabolism during pregnancy: Influence of maternal energy status. *Am J Clin N* 1994;59 (suppl):439S–445S.

Kousen M: Treatment of nausea and vomiting in pregnancy. *Am Fam Phys* 1993;48(7): 1279–1283.

Lawrence M, McKillop K, Durnin J: Women who gain more fat during pregnancy may not have bigger babies: Implications for recommended weight gain during pregnancy. *Br J Obst G* 1991;98:254–259.

Lechtig A, Yarbrough C, Delgado H, et al: Influence of maternal nutrition on birth weight. *Am J Clin N* 1975;28:1223–1233.

Lederman S: Recent issues related to nutrition during pregnancy. *J Am Col N* 1993;12(2): 91–100.

Lubeck P, Tholin K, Palm R: Serum concentrations of trace elements in infants and their mothers during pregnancy. *Ann NY Acad* 1993;678:356–358.

Marya R, Saint A, Jaswal T: Effect of vitamin D supplementation during pregnancy on the neonatal skeletal growth in the rat. *Ann Nutr M* 1991;35:208–212.

Murphy S, Abrams B: Changes in energy intakes during pregnancy and lactation in a national sample of US women. *Am J Pub He* 1993;83(8):1161–1163.

Naeye R: Maternal body weight and pregnancy outcome. *Am J Clin N* 1990;52:273–279.

O'Brien B, Naber S: Nausea and vomiting during pregnancy: Effects on the quality of women's lives. *Birth* 1992;19(3):138–143.

Philipps C, Johnson N: The impact of quality of diet and other factors on birth weight in infants. *Am J Clin N* 1977;30:215–255.

Pope J, Skinner J, Carruth B: Cravings and aversions of pregnancy adolescents. *J Am Diet A* 1992; 92:1479–1482.

Powers H: Micronutrient deficiencies in the preterm neonate. *P Nutr Soc* 1993;52(2):285–291.

Prentice A: Can maternal dietary supplements help in preventing infant malnutrition? *Acta Paed Sc* 1991;374(suppl):67–77.

Reeves N, Potempa K, Gallo A: Fatigue in early pregnancy; An exploratory study. *J Nurse-Mid* 1991;36(5):303–309.

Reynolds R, Polansky M, Moser P: Analyzed vitamin B6 intakes of pregnant and postpartum lactating and nonlactating women. *J Am Diet A* 1984;84:1339–1344.

Roepke J, Kirksey A: Vitamin B6 nutriture during pregnancy and lactation: I. Vitamin B6 intake levels of the vitamin in biological fluids and condition of the infant at birth. *Am J Clin N* 1979;32:2249.

Rothstein R, Rombeau J: Intestinal malrotation during pregnancy. *Obstet Gyn* 1993;81:817–819.

Safety of some calcium supplements questioned. *Nutr Rev* 1994;52(3):95–97.

Sahakian V, Rouse D, Sipes S, et al: Vitamin B6 is effective therapy for nausea and vomiting of pregnancy: A randomized double-blind placebo-controlled study. *Obstet Gyn* 1991;78:33–36.

Seligman P, Caskey J, Frazier J, et al: Measurements of iron absorption from prenatal multi-vitamin mineral supplements. *Obstet Gyn* 1983;61(3):356–362.

Shimoshima C, Nishioka C, Takiyama K, et al: Influences of protein malnutrition on amino acid composition, trace metal elements and tensile strength of rat hairs. *J Nutr Sc V* 1988;34: 67–78.

Simmer K, Iles C, James C, et al: Are iron-folate supplements harmful? *Am J Clin N* 1987;45: 122–125.

Somer E: Can vitamin supplements prevent birth defects? *Nutr Rep* 1991;Nov:82.

Springer N, Bischoping K, Sampselle C, et al: Using early weight gain and other nutrition-related risk factors to predict pregnancy outcome. *J Am Diet A* 1992;92(2):217–219.

Suitor C: Perspectives on nutrition during pregnancy: Part I, weight gain; Part II, nutrient supplements. *J Am Diet A* 1991;91:96–98.

Susser M: Maternal weight gain, infant birth weight, and diet: Causal sequences. *Am J Clin N* 1991;53:1384–1396.

Taper L, Oliva J, Ritchey S: Zinc and copper retention during pregnancy: The adequacy of prenatal diets with and without dietary supplementation. *Am J Clin N* 1985;4:1184–1192.

Thauvin E, Fusselier M, Arnaud J, et al: Effects of a multivitamin mineral supplement on zinc and copper status during pregnancy. *Biol Tr El* 1992;32:405.

Toorians A, Drost-Driessen M, Snellen J, et al: Acute hernia of Bochdalek during pregnancy: Hyperemesis for the first time in a third pregnancy? *Acta Obst Sc* 1992;71:547–549.

Use of an antinausea drug by a pregnant woman. *Am J Hosp P* 1993;50:109–112.

Werler M, Mitchell A: Case-control study of vitamin supplementation and neural tube defects. *Ann NY Acad* 1993;678:276–283.

West L, Warren J, Cutts T: Diagnosis and management of irritable bowel syndrome, constipation, and diarrhea in pregnancy. *Gastro Clin* 1992;21(4):793–802.

Wheatley D: Treatment of pregnancy sickness. *Br J Obst G* 1977;84:444–447.

6. Nutrition During the Second Trimester

American Diabetes Association: *Diabetes in the Family.* New York, Prentice-Hall Publishing, 1982.

Baron, T, Richter J: Gastroesophageal reflux disease in pregnancy. *Gastro Clin* 1992;21(4):777–791.

Barrett B, Gunter E, Sowell A, et al: Ascorbic acid, beta carotene, and preterm rupture of fetal membranes (meeting abstract). *FASEB J* 1994;8(5):A941.

Belfort M, Saade G, Moise K: The effect of magnesium sulfate on maternal and fetal blood flow in pregnancy-induced hypertension. *Acta Obst Sc* 1993:72:526–530.

Blume E: Poisoned peaches, toxic tomatoes: Reckoning pesticide risks. *Nutr Action HealthLetter* 1987;October:8–9.

Calcium supplementation prevents hypertensive disorders of pregnancy. *Nutr Rev* 1992:50(8):233–235.

Castor W: Dietary aflatoxin, intelligence and school performance in southern Georgia. *Int J Vit N* 1986;56:291.

Catalano P, Roman N, Tyzbir E, et al: Weight gain in women with gestational diabetes. *Obstet Gyn* 1993;81;523–528.

Clapp J, Capeless E: The VO2max of recreational athletes before and after pregnancy. *Med Sci Spt* 1991;23(10):1128–1133.

Cruikshank D, Chan G, Doerrfeld D: Alterations in vitamin D and calcium metabolism with magnesium sulfate treatment of preeclampsia. *Am J Obst G* 1993;168:1170–1177.

Cousins L: Insulin sensitivity in pregnancy. *Diabetes* 1991;40(suppl 2):39–43.

D'Almeida A, Carter J, Anatol A, et al: Effects of a combination of evening primrose oil (gamma linolenic acid) and fish oil (eicosapentaenoic + docahexaenoic acid) versus magnesium, and versus placebo in preventing pre-eclampsia. *Women Health* 1992;19(2/3):117–130.

Dewey K, McCrory M: Effects of dieting and physical activity on pregnancy and lactation. *Am J Clin N* 1994;59 (suppl):446S–453S.

Environmental Protection Agency: The EBDC pesticides and EPA's proposed regulatory decision: Facts for consumers. December 4, 1989.

Fadigan A, Sealy D, Schneider E: Preeclampsia: Progress and puzzle. *Am Fam Phys* 1994;March: 849–856.

Ferris A, Reece E: Nutritional consequences of chronic maternal conditions during pregnancy and lactation: Lupus and diabetes. *Am J Clin N* 1994;59(suppl):465S–473S.

Giavini E, Airoldi L, Broccia M, et al: Effects of diets with different content in protein and fiber on embryotoxicity induced by experimental diabetes in rats. *Biol Neonat* 1993;63:353–359.

Grandjean P, Weihe P, Jorgensen P, et al: Impact of maternal seafood diet on fetal exposure to mercury, selenium, and lead. *Arch Env He* 1992;47(3):185–195.

Hatch M, Shu X, McLean D, et al: Maternal exercise during pregnancy, physical fitness, and fetal growth. *Am J Epidem* 1993;137(10):1105–1114.

Hollingsworth D, Ney D: Caloric restriction in pregnant diabetic women: A review of maternal obesity, glucose and insulin relationships as investigated at the University of California, San Diego. *J Am Col N* 1992;11(3):251–258.

Husain S, Sibley C: Magnesium and pregnancy. *Min Elect M* 1993;19(4–5):296–307.

Institute of Medicine: *Nutrition During Pregnancy: Part I. Weight Gain, Part II. Nutrient Supplements.* Washington, D. C., National Academy Press, 1990:117.

IPCS (International Programme on Chemical Safety): Methylmercury (Environmental Health Criteria 101). Geneva: World Health Organization, 1990.

Is our fish fit to eat? *Consumer Reports* 1992;February:103–114.

Jacobson J, Jacobson S, Humphrey H: Effects of in utero exposure to polycholorinated biphenyls and related contaminants on cognitive functioning in young children. *J Pediat* 1990;116(1): 38–45.

Jovanovic-Peterson L, Peterson C: Abnormal metabolism and risk for birth defects with emphasis on diabetes. *Ann NY Acad* 1993;678:228–240.

Jovanovic-Peterson L, Peterson C: Pregnancy in the diabetic woman. *End Metab C* 1992;21(2): 433–456.

Jovanovic-Peterson L, Peterson C, Reed G, et al: Maternal postprandial glucose levels and infant birth weight: The diabetes in early pregnancy study. *Am J Obst G* 1991;164:103–111.

Kincaid-Smith P: Hypertension in pregnancy. *Med J Aust* 1993;158:655.

Kline J, et al: Spontaneous abortion and the use of sugar substitutes. *Am J Obst G* 1978;130:708.

Knight K, Keith R: Calcium supplementation on normotensive and hypertensive pregnancy women. *Am J Clin N* 1992;55:891–895.

Knopp R, Magee M, Raisys V, et al: Hypocaloric diets and ketogenesis in the management of obese gestational diabetic women. *J Am Col N* 1991;10(6):649–667.

Lefferts L: Pesticides: Fact vs fantasy. *Nutr Action HealthLetter* 1989;June:8–9.

Lotgering F, van Doorn M, Struijk P, et al: Maximal aerobic exercise in pregnant women: Heart rate, O_2 consumption, CO_2 production, and ventilation. *J Appl Physl* 1991;70(3):1016–1023.

Lutale J, Justesen A, Swai A, et al: Glucose tolerance during and after pregnancy in nondiabetic women in an urban population in Tanzania. *Diabet Care* 1993;16(4):575–577.

Management of hypertension in pregnancy: Executive summary. *Med J Aust* 1993;158:700–702.

Marrero J, Goggin P, deCaestecker J, et al: Determinants of pregnancy heartburn. *Br J Obst G* 1992;99:731–734.

McMurray R, Mottola M, Wolfe L, et al: Recent advances in understanding maternal and fetal responses to exercise. *Med Sci Spt* 1993;25(12):1305–1321.

Montgomery A: America's pesticide-permeated food. Nutr Action HealthLetter 1987;June:1,4–7.

Mottola M, Mezzapelli J, Schachter C, et al: Training effects on maternal and fetal glucose uptake following acute exercise in the rat. *Med Sci Spt* 1993;25(7):841–846.

National Research Council: *Regulating Pesticides in Food: The Delaney Paradox*. Washington, D.C., National Academy Press, 1987.

Natural Resources Defense Council: *Intolerable Risk: Pesticides in Our Children's Food*. New York, Natural Resources Defense Council, February 27, 1989.

O'Brien P, Morrison R, Pipkin F: The effect of dietary supplementation with linoleic and gamma-linolenic acids on the pressor response to angiotensin. II. A possible role in pregnancy-induced hypertension. *Br J Cl Ph* 1985;19(3):335–342.

O'Neill M, Cooper K, Hunyor S, et al: Cardiorespiratory response to walking in trained and sedentary pregnant women. *J Sport Med* 1993;33:40–43.

Pass the pesticides. *Nutr Action HealthLetter* 1989;April:5–7.

Peterson C, Jovanovic-Peterson L: Percentage of carbohydrate and glycemic response to breakfast, lunch, and dinner in women with gestational diabetes. *Diabetes* 1991;40(suppl 2):172–174.

Phelps R, Metzger B: Caloric restriction in gestational diabetes mellitus: When and how much? *J Am Col N* 1992;11(3):259–262.

Phillipou G: Relationship between normal oral glucose tolerance test in women at risk for gestational diabetes and large for gestational age infants. *Diabet Care* 1991;14(11):1092–1094.

Pivarnik J, Mauer M, Ayres N, et al: Effects of chronic exercise on blood volume expansion and hematologic indices during pregnancy. *Obstet Gyn* 1994;83:265–269.

Prada J, Ross R, Clark K: Hypocalcemia and pregnancy-induced hypertension produced by maternal fasting. *Hypertensio* 1992;20:620–626.

Pratt C: Moderate exercise and iron status in women. *Nutr Rep* 1991;9(7):48,56.

Rasmussen S, Oian P: First- and second-trimester hemoglobin levels. *Acts Obst Sc* 1993;72:246–251.

Redman C, Roberts J: Management of pre-eclampsia. *Lancet* 1993;341:1451–1454.

Roberts R, Moohan J, Foo R, et al: Fetal outcome in mothers with impaired glucose tolerance in pregnancy. *Diabet Med* 1993;10:438–443.

Roberts J, Redman C: Pre-eclampsia: More than pregnancy-induced hypertension. *Lancet* 1993; 341:1447–1450.

Rothstein R, Rombeau J: Intestinal malrotation during pregnancy. *Obstet Gyn* 1993;81:817–819.

Rudnicki P, Frolich A, Fischer-Rasmussen W: Magnesium supplementation in pregnancy-induced hypertension and preeclampsia. *Acta Obst Sc* 1994;73:95–96.

Seelig M: Interrelationship of magnesium and estrogen in cardiovascular and bone disorders, eclampsia, migraine and premenstrual syndrome. *J Am Col N* 1993;12(4):442–458.

Silver H: Nutritional management of diabetes in pregnancy. *J Am Diet A* 1993;93(12): 1381–1382.

Skajaa K, Dorup I, Sandstrom B: Magnesium intake and status and pregnancy outcome in a Danish population. *Br J Obst G* 1991;98:919–928.

Smith M, Nagey D, Moser-Veillon P: Plasma and erythrocyte magnesium changes following a glucose challenge during pregnancy. *J Am Col N* 1992;11(4):426–431.

Sonstegard L: Pregnancy-induced hypertension: Prenatal nursing concerns. *Am J Mat-Ch Nurs* 1979;4:90–95.

Sparks S, Jovanovic-Peterson L, Peterson C: Blood glucose rise following prenatal vitamins in gestational diabetes. *J Am Col N* 1993;12(5):543–546.

Stowers J, Ewen S: Health implications of nutrient-gene interactions: Possible dietary factors in the induction of diabetes and its inheritance in man, with studies in mice. *P Nutr Soc* 1991; 50:287–298.

Suchecki D, Neto J: Prenatal stress and emotional response of adult offspring. *Physl Behav* 1991;49:423–426.

Villar J, Belizan J, Fischer P: Epidemiologic observations on the relationship between calcium intake and eclampsia. *Int J Gyn O* 1983;21(4):271–278.

Wang Y, Kay H, Killam A: Decreased levels of polyunsaturated fatty acids in preeclampsia. *Am J Obst G* 1991;164:812–818.

Watson W, Katz V, Hackney A, et al: Fetal response to maximal swimming and cycling exercise during pregnancy. *Obstet Gyn* 1991;77:382–386.

West L, Warren J, Cutts T: Diagnosis and management of irritable bowel syndrome, constipation, and diarrhea in pregnancy. *Gastro Clin* 1992;21(4):793–802.

Worthington-Roberts B, Williams S: *Nutrition in Pregnancy and Lactation, ed.4.* St. Louis, Times Mirror/Mosby College Publishing. 1989:33–35.

7. Nutrition During the Third Trimester

Abrams S, Yergey A, Schanler R, et al: Hypercalciuria in premature infants receiving high mineral-containing diets. *J Ped Gastr* 1994;18(1):20–24.

Agren M, Stromberg H, Rindby A, et al: Selenium, zinc, iron, and copper levels in serum of patients with arterial and venous leg ulcers. *Acta Der-Ven* 1986;66:237–240.

Bieri J, Corash L, Hubbard V: Medical uses of vitamin E. *N Eng J Med* 1983;308(18):1063–1071.

Black M, Medeiros D, Brunett E, et al. Zinc supplements and serum lipids in young adult white males. *Am J Clin N* 1988;47:970–975.

Blum I, Vered Y, Graff E, et al: The influence of meal composition on plasma serotonin and norepinephrine concentrations. *Metabolism* 1992;41(2):137–140.

Boosalis M, Solem L, Cerra F, et al: Increased urinary zinc excretion after thermal injury. *J La Cl Med* 1991;118:538–545.

Brown Z, Benedetti J, Ashley R, et al: Neonatal herpes simplex virus infection in relation to asymptomatic maternal infection at the time of labor. *N End J Med* 1991;324:1247–1252.

Cheraskin E: The prevalence of hypovitaminosis C. *J Am Med A* 1985;254:2894.

Christensen L: The roles of caffeine and sugar in depression. *Nutr Rep* 1991;9(3):16,24.

Christensen L, Burrows R: Dietary treatment of depression. *Behav Ther* 1990;21:183–193.

Christensen L, Krietsch K, White B, et al: Impact of a dietary change on emotional distress. *J Abn Psych* 1985;94(4):565–579.

Dumoulin J, Foulkes J: Ketonuria during labor (commentary). *Br J Obst G* 1984;91:97–98.

Ershow A, Brown L, Cantor K: Intake of tapwater and total water by pregnant and lactating women. *Am J Pub He* 1991;81:328–334.

Felig P, Kim Y, Lynch V, et al: Amino acid metabolism during starvation and pregnancy. *J Clin Inv* 1972;51:1195–1202.

Fitzgerald S, Gibson R, deSerrano J, et al: Trace element intakes and dietary phytate/Zn and Ca X phytate/Zn millimolar ratios of periurban Guatemalan women during the third trimester of pregnancy. *Am J Clin N* 1993;57:195–201.

Gibson R: Trace element deficiencies in humans. *Can Med A J* 1991;145:231.

Gjerdingen D, Chaloner K: The relationship of women's postpartum mental health to employment, childbirth, and social support. *J Fam Pract* 1994;38(5):465–472.

Goldstein R, Augustine A, Purucker E, et al: Effect of vitamin E and allopurinol on lipid peroxide and glutathione level in acute skin grafts. *J Inves Der* 1990;95:470.

Growdon J, Wurtman R: Nutrients and neurotransmitters. *Cont Nutr* 1979;4(12):1–2.

Hazle N: Hydration in labor: Is routine intravenous hydration necessary? *J Nurse-Mid* 1986;31:171–176.

Heston T, Simkin P: Carbohydrate loading in preparation for childbirth. *Med Hypoth* 1991;34:97–98.

Institute of Medicine: *Nutrition During Pregnancy: Part I. Weight Gain. Part II.* Nutrient Supplements. Washington, D.C., National Academy Press, 1990:192–198.

Jackson R, Jackson F, Yu S: The relationship between third trimester maternal weight gain, hematologic status and infant birthweight in Liberian mothers. *Ecol Food N* 1993;30(3–4): 309–319.

Josten B, Johnson T, Nelson J: Umbilical cord pH and Apgar scores as an index of neonatal health. *Am J Obst G* 1987;157:843–888.

Kurolwa K, Nelson J, Boyce S, et al: Metabolic and immune effect of vitamin E supplementation after burn. *J Parent En* 1991;15:22–26.

Kusin J, Kardjati S, Houtkooper J, et al: Energy supplementation during pregnancy and postnatal growth. *Lancet* 1992;340(8820):623–626.

Lee K, DeJoseph J: Sleep disturbances, vitality, and fatigue among a select group of employed childbearing women. *Birth* 1992;19(4):208–213.

Lieberman H, Corkin S, Spring B, et al: Mood, performance, and pain sensitivity: Changes induced by food constituents. *J Psych Res* 1982/1983:17:135–145.

Ludka L, Roberts C: Eating and drinking in labor: A literature review. *J Nurse-Mid* 1993;38(4): 199–207.

Lukashi H, Siders W, Nielsen E, et al: Total body water in pregnancy: Assessment by using bioelectrical impedance. *Am J Clin N* 1994;59:578–585.

National Academy of Sciences: *Drinking Water and Health.* Washington, D.C., National Academy of Sciences, 1987.

Olson S, Sorensen J, Secher N, et al: Randomized controlled trial of effect of fish oil supplementation on pregnancy duration. *Lancet* 1992;339:1003–1007.

O'Reilly S, Hoyer P, Walsh E: Low-risk mothers: Oral intake and emesis in labor. *J Nurse-Mid* 1993;38(4):228–235.

Padh H: Vitamin C: Newer insights into its biochemical functions. *Nutr Rev* 1991;49:65–70.

Sandstead H: Zinc deficiency: A public health problem? *Am J Dis Ch* 1991;145:853–859.

Sharp K, Brindle P, Brown M, et al: Memory loss during pregnancy. *Br J Obst G* 1993;100:209.

Sosa R, Kennell J, Klaus M, et al: The effect of a supportive companion on perinatal problems, length of labor, and mother-infant interaction. *N Eng J Med* 1980;303:597–600.

Sozman M: Fasting during the last 3 months of pregnancy and effect on birth weight. *J Trop Pedi* 1993;39:116–117.

Steer R, Scholl T, Hediger M, et al: Self-reported depression and negative pregnancy outcomes. *J Clin Epid* 1992;45(10):1093–1099.

Sugden P, Fuller S: Regulation of protein-turnover in skeletal and cardiac-muscle (review). *Biochem J* 1991;273:21–37.

Susser M, Stein Z: Timing in prenatal nutrition: A reprise of the Dutch Famine Study. *Nutr Rev* 1994;52(3):84–94.

Tucker D, Penland J, Sandstead H, et al: Nutrition status and brain function in aging. *Am J Clin N* 1990;52:93–102.

Vaxman F, Chalkiadakis G, Maldonade H, et al: Pantothenic acid and wound healing process: Strength improvements in colonic anastomosis. *Dig Dis Sci* 1986;31:469S.

Wurtman J: Recent evidence from human studies linking central serotoninergic function with carbohydrate intake. *Appetite* 1987;8(3):211–213.

Wurtman J: The involvement of brain serotonin in excessive carbohydrate snacking by obese carbohydrate cravers. *J Am Diet A* 1984;84(9):1004–1007.

Wurtman R: Introduction. *J Psych Res* 1982/1983;17(2):103–105.

Wurtman R, Wurtman J: Carbohydrates and depression. *Sci Am* 1989;January;68–75.

8. Nutrition and High-Risk Pregnancies

Backe B: Maternal smoking and age: Effect on birthweight and risk for small-for-gestational age births. *Acta Obst Sc* 1993;72:172–176.

Baird P, Sadovnick A, Yee I: Maternal age and birth defects: A population study. *Lancet* 1991; 337:527–530.

Beard J: Iron deficiency: Assessment during pregnancy and its importance in pregnant adolescents. *Am J. Clin N* 1994;59(suppl):502S–510S.

Bendich A: Lifestyle and environmental factors that can adversely affect maternal nutritional status and pregnancy outcome. *Ann NY Acad* 1993;678(Mar):255–265.

Berger D, Rivera M, Perez G, et al: Risk assessment for human immunodeficiency virus among pregnant Hispanic adolescents. *Adolescence* 1993;28(111):597–607.

Biggar R, Rosenberg P: HIV infection/AIDS in the United States during the 1990s. *Clin Inf Dis* 1993;17(suppl 1):S219–S223.

Brierley J: HIV and AIDS in childbirth. *Midwives Chron Nurs Notes* 1993;September:317–325.

Brown J, Schloesser P: Prepregnancy weight status, prenatal weight gain, and the outcome of term twin gestations. *Am J Obst G* 1990;162:182–186.

Cardiac considerations related to pregnancy. *J Intern M* 1994;235:383–385.

Carruth B: Adolescent pregnancy and nutrition. *Cont Nutr* 1980;5(10):1–2.

Cetrulo C, Ingardia C, Sbarra A: Management of multiple gestation. *Clin O Gyne* 1980;23: 533–548.

Cherry F, Sandstead P, Rojas L, et al: Adolescent pregnancy: Association between body weight, zinc nutriture and pregnancy outcome. *Am J Clin N* 1989;50:945–954.

Cherry F, Sandstead H, Wickremasinghe A: Adolescent pregnancy: Zinc supplementation and iron effects. *Ann NY Acad* 1993;678:330–333.

Cherry F, Sandstead H, Wickremasinghe A: Adolescent pregnancy: Weight and zinc supplementation effects. *Ann NY Acad* 1993;678:334–337.

Committee on Adolescence: Adolescent pregnancy. *Pediatrics* 1989;83:133.

Dietary Intake Source Data, United States 1976–1980. Data from the National Health Survey, Series 11, no. 231. DHHS Publication No. (PHS) 83–1681, March 1983.

Dubois S, Dougherty C, Duquette M, et al: Twin pregnancy: The impact of the Higgins

Nutrition Intervention Program on maternal and neonatal outcomes. *Am J Clin N* 1991;53: 1397–1403.

Edge V, Laros R: Pregnancy outcome in nulliparous women aged 35 and older. *Am J Obst G* 1993;168:1881–1885.

Elster A, Bleyl J, Craven T: Birth weight standards for triplets under modern obstetric care in the United States, 1984–1989. *Obstet Gyn* 1991;77:387.

Farahati M, Bozorgi N, Luke B: Influence of maternal age, birth-to-conception intervals and prior perinatal factors on perinatal outcomes. *J Repro Med* 1993;38(10):751–756.

Fenton T, Thirsk J: Twin pregnancy: The distribution of maternal weight gain of non-smoking normal weight women. *Can J Publ* 1994;85(1):37–40.

Gadowsky S, Wolfe J, Jory D, et al: Laboratory folate and iron indices of pregnancy adolescents accessed through the public health system in southern Ontario. *FASEB J* 1992;6: A1959.

Goldberg D, Carruth B, Skinner J: Television viewing and dietary intake of pregnant adolescents. *Nutr Res* 1993;13(6):621–632.

Guinee V, Olsson H, Moller T, et al: Effect of pregnancy on prognosis for young women with breast cancer. *Lancet* 1994;343:1587–1589.

Hediger M, Scholl T, Belsky D, et al: Patterns of weight gain in adolescent pregnancy: Effects on birth weight and preterm delivery. *Obstet Gyn* 1989;74:6–12.

Johnson C, Kandell L: Prepregnancy weight and rate of maternal weight gain in adolescents and young adults. *J Am Diet A* 1992;92(12):1515–1517.

Kiely J: The epidemiology of perinatal mortality in multiple births. *B NY Ac Med* 1990;66: 618–637.

Koonin L, Ellerbrock T, Atrash K, et al: Pregnancy associated deaths due to AIDS in the United States. *J Am Med A* 1989;261:1306–1309.

Lambe M, Hseih C, Trichopoulos D, et al: Transient increase in the risk of breast cancer after giving birth. *N Eng J Med* 1994;331:5–9.

Lauritsen J: Aetiology of spontaneous abortion: A cytogenetic and epidemiological study of 288 abortuses and their parents. *Acta Obst Sc* 1975;54:261.

Lenz W: Epidemiology of congenital malformations. *Ann NY Acad* 1965;123:228.

Leonard C, Piecuch R, Ballard R, et al: Outcome of very low birth weight infants: Multiple gestation versus singletons. *Pediatrics* 1994;93(4):611–615.

Liu H, Momotani N, Yoshimura J, et al: Maternal hypothyroidism during early pregnancy and intellectual development of the progeny. *Arch In Med* 1994;154:785–787.

Loris P, Dewey K, Poirier-Brode K: Weight gain and dietary intake of pregnant teenagers. *J Am Diet A* 1985;85;1296–1302.

Luke B: Twin births: Influence of maternal weight gain on intrauterine growth and prematurity. *Fed Proc* 1987;46:1015.

Luke B, Johnson T, Petrie R: *Clinical Maternal-Fetal Nutrition.* Boston, Little, Brown & Company, 1993.

Luke B, Keith L: The contribution of singletons, twins, and triplets to low birth weight, infant mortality, and handicap in the United States. *J Repro Med* 1992;37:661–666.

Luke B, Witter F, Abbey H, et al: Gestational age-specific birthweights of twins versus singletons. *Acta Genet M* 1991;40:69–76.

Magenis R, Chamberlain J: Paternal origin of non-dysfunction, in de la Crus F, Gerald P (eds): *Trisomy 21 Down's Syndrome. NICHD-Mental Retardation Research Center Series.* Baltimore, University Park Press, 1981.

Maroulis G: Fertility, pregnancy, and the older woman. *Cont Ob/Gyn* 1993;May:101–122.

Milner M, Barry-Kinsella C, Unwin A, et al: The impact of maternal age on pregnancy and its outcome. *Int J Gyn O* 1992;38:281–286.

Naeye R: Teenaged and pre-teenaged pregnancies: Consequences of the fetal-maternal competition for nutrients. *Pediatrics* 1981;67:146.

Nair P, Alger L, Hines S: Maternal and neonatal characteristics associated with HIV infection in infants of seropositive women. *J AIDS* 1993;6:298–302.

National Center for Health Statistics: *Advance report of final natality statistics, 1989.* Hyattsville, Maryland: US Public Health Service, 1991. Monthly vital statistics report 40(8); supplement.

Neri A, Sabah G, Samra Z: Bacterial vaginosis in pregnancy treated with yoghurt. *Acta Obst Sc* 1993;72:17–19.

Newton E: Antepartum care in multiple gestation. *Sem Perinat* 1986;10:19–29.

Novik F, Berns D, Stricof R, et al: HIV sero prevalence in newborns in New York State. *J Am Med A* 1989;261:1745–1750.

The Office of Disease Prevention and Health Promotion: *Disease Prevention/Health Promotion.* Palo Alto, Bull Publishing, 1988:2–29;129–146.

Overturf C, Smith A, Engelbert-Fenton K, et al: Potential role of energy and nutrient intakes in decreasing the incidence of genitourinary tract infections in pregnant adolescents. *J Am Diet A* 1992;92(12):1513–1515.

Pao E, Mickle S: Problem nutrients in the United States. *Food Tech* 1981;September:58–69.

Pederson A, Worthington-Roberts B, Hickok D: Weight gain patterns during twin gestation. *J Am Diet A* 1989;89:642–646.

Pellicer A, Meri M, de los Santos M, et al: Effects of aging on the human ovary: The secretion of immunoreactive alpha-inhibin and progesterone. *Fert Steril* 1994;61:663–668.

Perry P: The iron epidemic. *Am Health* 1984;October:41–43.

Pitt J: Perinatal human immunodeficiency virus infection. *Clin Perin* 1991;18(2):227–239.

Position of the American Dietetic Association: Nutrition care for pregnant adolescents. *J Am Diet A* 1994;94(4):449–450.

Powers W, Kiely J: The risks of confronting twins: A national perspective. *Am J Obst G* 1994; 170:456–461.

Rees J: Nutrition in adolescence, in Krause M, Mahan K: *Food, Nutrition, and Diet Therapy,* ed 7. Philadelphia, WB Saunders Co., 1984:309.

The role of calcium in health. *Dairy Council Digest* 1984;55:1–8.

Rossi P, Moschese V: Mother-to-child transmission of human immunodeficiency virus. *FASEB J* 1991;5:2419–2426.

Ryder R, Nsa W, Hassig S, et al: Perinatal transmission of the human immunodeficiency virus type I to infants of seropositive women in Zaire. *N Eng J Med* 1989;320:1637–1642.

Sauer M, Paulson R, Lobo R: Pregnancy after age 50: Application of oocyte donation to women after natural menopause. *Lancet* 1993;341(8841):321–323.

Sauer M, Paulson R, Lobo R: Reversing the natural decline in human infertility. *J Am Med A* 1992;268:1275–1279.

Schenker J, Yarkoni S, Granat M: Multiple pregnancies following induction of ovulation. *Fert Steril* 1981;35:105.

Scholl T, Hediger M: A review of the epidemiology of nutrition and adolescent pregnancy: Maternal growth during pregnancy and its effect on the fetus. *J Am Col N* 1993;12(2): 101–107.

Scholl T, Hediger M, Ances I, et al: Weight gain during pregnancy in adolescence: Predictive ability of early weight gain. *Obstet Gyn* 1990;75:948–953.

Scholl, T, Hediger M, Cronk C, et al: Maternal growth during pregnancy and lactation. *Hormone Res* 1993;39(S3):59–67.

Scholl T, Hediger M, Khoo C, et al: Maternal weight gain, diet and infant birth weight: Correlations during adolescent pregnancy. *J Clin Epid* 1991;44(4/5):423–428.

Semba R, Miotti P, Chiphangwi J, et al: Maternal vitamin A deficiency and mother-to-child transmission of HIV-1. *Lancet* 1994;343:1593–1597.

Science and Education Administration, Nationwide Food Consumption Survey, 1977–1978, Preliminary Report No. 2, Food and Nutrient Intakes of Individuals on One Day in the United States, Spring 1977, USDA, Washington, D.C., September 1980.

Skinner J, Carruth B: Dietary quality of pregnant and nonpregnant adolescents. *J Am Diet A* 1991;91(6):718–720.

Skinner J, Carruth B, Pope J, et al: Food and nutrient intake of white, pregnant adolescents. *J Am Diet A* 1992;92(9):1127–1129.

Stevens-Simon C, Kaplan D, McAnarney E: Factors associated with preterm delivery among pregnant adolescents. *J Adoles H* 1993;14(4):340–342.

Stevens-Simon C, McAnarney E: Skeletal maturity and growth of adolescent mothers: Relationship to pregnancy outcome. *J Adoles H* 1993;14(6):428–432.

Stevens-Simon C, McAnarney E: Determinants of weight gain in pregnant adolescents. *J Am Diet A* 1992;92:1348–1351.

Stevens-Simon C, McAnarney E, Roghmann K: Adolescent gestational weight gain and birth weight. *Pediatrics* 1993;92(6):805–809.

Stevens-Simon C, Nakashima I, Andrews D: Weight gain attitudes among pregnant adolescents. *J Adoles H* 1993;14(5):369–372.

Story M, Alton I: Nutrition issues and adolescent pregnancy. *Cont Nutr* 1987;12(1):1–2.

Sule-Odu A: Maternal perinatal HIV 1 transmission. *Int J Gyn O* 1993;42:265–267.

Wolfe S, Gibson R, Gadowsky S, et al: Zinc status of a group of pregnant adolescents at 36 weeks gestation living in southern Ontario. *J Am Col N* 1994;13(2):154–164.

9. Nutrition and Nursing Your Baby

Abrams B, Berman C: Nutrition during pregnancy and lactation. *Prim Care* 1993;20(3): 585–597.

Acheson L: Postpartum care and breast-feeding. *Prim Care* 1993;20(3):729–747.

ACOG Technical Bulletin: Nutrition during pregnancy. *Int J Gyn O* 1993;43:67–74.

Adair L, Popkin B: Prolonged lactation contributes to depletion of maternal energy reserves in Filipino women. *J Nutr* 1992;122:1643–1655.

Anderson R, Bryden N, Patterson K, et al: Breast milk chromium and its association with chromium intake, chromium excretion, and serum chromium. *Am J Clin N* 1993;57: 519–523.

Andrews W: Nutrition and development in premature infants. Overview. *Nutr* 1994;10(1):62.

Aniansson G, Andersson B, Hakansson A, et al: A prospective cohort study on breast-feeding and otitis media in Swedish infants. *Pediat Inf* 1994;13(3):183–188.

Arnold L, Larson E: Immunological benefits of breast milk in relation to human milk banking. *Am J Infect* 1993;21(5):235–242.

Birch E, Birch D, Hoffman D, et al: Breast-feeding and optimal visual development. *J Pediat Op* 1993;30(1):33–38.

Bjorksten B: Does breast feeding prevent the development of allergy? *Immunol Tod* 1983;4(8): 215–217.

Bjorksten B, Kjellman N: Does breast-feeding prevent food allergy? *Allergy P* 1991;12(4): 233–237.

Boersma E, Offringa P, Muskiet F, et al: Vitamin E, lipid fractions, and fatty acid composition of colostrum, transitional milk and mature milk: An international comparative study. *Am J Clin N* 1991;53:1197–1204.

Bonnin F: Cortisol levels in saliva and mood changes in early postpartum. *J Affect D* 1992;26(4): 231–239.

Breastfeeding and HIV. *Lancet* 1993;342:1437–1438.

Breast feeding prevents otitis media. *Nutr Rev* 1983;41(8):241–242.

Breast milk and subsequent intelligence quotient in children born preterm. *Nutr Rev* 1992;50 (11):334–335.

Brinsmead M, Smith R, Singh B, et al: Peripartum concentration of beta endorphin and cortisol and maternal mood states. *Aust NZ J O* 1985;25(3):194–197.

Butte N, Jensen C, Moon J, et al: Sleep organization and energy expenditure of breast-fed and formula-fed infants. *Pediat Res* 1992;32(5):514–519.

Byczkowski J, Gearhart J, Fisher J: "Occupational" exposure of infants to toxic chemicals via breast milk. *Nutr* 1994;10(1):43–48.

Calvo E, Celindo A, Aspres N: Iron status in exclusively breast-fed infants. *Pediatrics* 1992;90: 375–379.

Carlson S, Cooke R, Rhodes P, et al: Effect of vegetable and marine oils in preterm infant formulas on blood arachidonic and docohexaenoic acids. *J Pediat* 1992;120(4 pt 2):S159–S167.

Carrion N, Itriago A, Murilla M, et al: Determination of calcium, potassium, magnesium, iron, copper and zinc in maternal milk by inductively-coupled plasma-atomic emission-spectrometry. *J Anal Atom* 1994;9(3):205–207.

Cerebral Cortex Docosahexaenoic acid is lower in formula-fed than in breast-fed infants. *Nutr Rev* 1993;51(8):238–240.

Clemens J, Rao M, Ahmed F, et al: Breastfeeding and the risk of life-threatening retrovirus diarrhea: Prevention or postponement? *Pediatrics* 1993;93(5):680–685.

Clyne P, Kulcycki A: Human breast milk contains bovine IgG: Relationship to infant colic? *Pediatrics* 1991;87(4):439–444.

Committee on Drugs: The transfer of drugs and other chemicals into human milk. *Pediatrics* 1994;93(1):137.

Connor W, Neuringer M, Reisbick S: Essential fatty acids: The importance of n-3 fatty acids in the retina and brain. *Nutr Rev* 1992;50(4):21–29.

Cooper P, Murray L, Stein A: Psychosocial factors associated with the early termination of breastfeeding. *J Psychosom* 1993;37(2):171–176.

Croucher C, Azzopardi D: Compliance with recommendations for giving vitamin K to newborn infants. *Br Med J* 1994;308:894–895.

Cumming F, Fardy J, Woodward D: Selenium and human lactation in Australia: Milk and blood selenium levels in lactating women, and selenium intakes of their breast-fed infants. *Acta Paed Sc* 1992;81(4):292–295.

Cumming R, Klineberg R: Breastfeeding and other reproductive factors and the risk of hip fractures in elderly women. *Int J Epid* 1993;22(4):684–691.

Cunningham A: Otitis and breast-feeding (letter). *J Pediat* 1985;105(5): 854–855.

Davidson L: Minerals and trace elements in infant nutrition. *Acta Paediat* 1994;83(S395): 38–42.

Dewey K, Lovelady C, Nonmsen-Rivers N, et al: A randomized study of the effects of aerobic exercise on lactating women on breast-milk volume and composition. *N Eng J Med* 1994; 330:449–453.

Dewey K, McCrory M: Effects of dieting and physical activity on pregnancy and lactation. *Am J Clin N* 1994;59(suppl):446S–453S.

Dewey K, Heinig M, Nommsen L, et al: Breast-fed infants are leaner than formula-fed infants at 1 y of age: The DARLING study. *Am J Clin N* 1993;57:140–145.

Dewey K, Heinig M, Nommsen L: Maternal weight-loss patterns during prolonged lactation. *Am J Clin N* 1993;58:162–166.

Dotson K, Picciano J, Jerrell J, et al: Maternal selenium (Se) nutrition affects both milk Se and lipid patterns (meeting abstract). *FASEB J* 1991;5(5):A917.

Duncan B, Holberg C, Wright A, et al: Exclusive breast-feeding for at least 4 months protects against otitis media. *Pediatrics* 1993;91(5):867–872.

Dusdieker P, et al: Prolonged maternal fluid supplementation in breastfeeding. *Pediatrics* 1990; 86:737–740.

Dusdieker L, Hemingway D, Stumbo P: Is milk production impaired by dieting during lactation? *Am J Clin N* 1994;59:833–840.

Eckhert C: Isolation of a protein from human milk that enhances zinc absorption in humans. *Bioc Biop R* 1985;130:264–269.

Edwards D, Porter S, Stein G: A pilot study of postnatal depression following caesarean section using two retrospective self-rating instruments. *J Psychosom* 1994;38(2):111–117.

Eidelman A, Hoffmann N, Kaitz M: Cognitive deficits in women after childbirth. *Obstet Gyn* 1993;81:764–767.

Extended lactation and loss of bone. *Nutr Rev* 1994;52(1):26–28.

Ferris A, Heubauer S, Bendel R, et al: Perinatal lactation protocol and outcome in mothers with and without insulin-dependent diabetes mellitus. *Am J Clin N* 1993;58:43–48.

Ferris A, Reece E: Nutritional consequences of chronic maternal conditions during pregnancy and lactation: Lupus and diabetes. *Am J Clin N* 1994, 59(suppl):465S–473S.

Ford R, Taylor B, Mitchell E, et al: Breastfeeding and the risk of sudden infant death syndrome. *Int J Epid* 1993;22(5):885–890.

Friggens N, Hay D, Oldham J: Interactions between major nutrients in the diet and the lactational performance of rats. *Br J Nutr* 1993;69:59–71.

Gardner D: Fatigue in postpartum women. *Appl Nurs Res* 1991;4(2):57–62.

Giugliani E, Caiaffa W, Vogelhut J, et al: Factors influencing the duration of breastfeeding in a cohort of mothers in Baltimore (meeting abstract). *Pediat Res* 1994;35(4):A113.

Gjerdingen D, Froberg D, Kochevar L: Changes in women's mental and physical health from pregnancy through six months postpartum. *J Fam Pract* 1991;32(2):161–166.

Grazioso C, Buescher E: Mature human milk shares the antioxidant and enzyme inhibitory effects of human colostrum (meeting abstract). *Pediat Res* 1994;35(4):A127.

Gruber H, Stover S: Maternal and weanling bone: The influence of lowered calcium intake and maternal dietary history. *Bone* 1994;15(2):167–176.

Grummer-Strawn L: Does prolonged breast-feeding impair child growth? A critical review. *Pediatrics* 1993;91(4):766–771.

Gupta A, Gupta A: Zinc absorption from human milk: Need for zinc supplementation. *Am J Dis Ch* 1984;138:989–990.

Hachey D: Benefits and risks of modifying maternal fat intake in pregnancy and lactation. *Am J Clin N* 1994;59(suppl):454S–464S.

Hall B: Changing composition of human milk and early development of an appetite control. *Lancet* 1975;April 5, 779–781.

Hannah P, Adams D, Lee A, et al: Links between early post-partum mood and post-natal depression. *Br J Psych* 192;160:777–780.

Harfouche J: The importance of breast-feeding. *J Trop Pedi* 1970; September:135–175.

Harris B, Lovett L, Newcombe R, et al: Maternity blues and major endocrine changes: Cardiff puerperal mood and hormone study II. *Br Med J* 1994;308:949–953.

Heck H, deCastro J: The caloric demand of lactation does not alter spontaneous meal patterns, nutrient intakes, or moods of women. *Physl Behav* 1993;54(4):641–648.

Hill P, Aldag J: Insufficient milk supply among black and white breast-feeding mothers. *Res Nurs H* 1993;16(3):203–211.

Hills-Boncyk S, Avery M, Savik K, et al: Women's experiences with combining breast-feeding and employment. *J Nurse-Mid* 1993;38(5):257–266.

Hino S, Katamine S, Miyamoto T, et al: Maternal anti-HTLV-1 ENV antibody titer as a marker of mother-to-child transmission: Differential risk in bottle fed and breast fed children (meeting abstract). *AIDS Res H* 1994;10(4):453.

Howard F, Howard C, Weitzman M: The physician as advertiser: The unintentional discouragement of breastfeeding. *Obstet Gyn* 1993;81(6):1048–1051.

Ito S, Blajchmana A, Stephenson M, et al: Prospective follow-up of adverse reactions in breast-fed infants exposed to maternal medication. *Am J Obst G* 1993;168:1393–1399.

Jakobsson I, Lindberg T: Cow's milk proteins cause infantile colic in breastfed infants. *Pediatrics* 1983;71(2):268.

Jelliffe D, Jelliffe E: Breast feeding is best for infants everywhere. *Nutr Today* 1978;May/June: 12–16.

Kang-Yoon S, Kirksey A, Giacoia G, et al: Vitamin B6 status of breast-fed neonates: Influence of pyridoxine supplementation on mothers and neonates. *Am J Clin N* 1992;56:548–558.

Kirubakaran C: Exclusive breast feeding and weight gain in preterm infants. *Pediat Res* 1994; 35(2):275.

Knight R, Thirkettle J: The relationship between expectations of pregnancy and birth, and transient depression in the immediate post-partum period. *J Psychosom* 1987;31(3):351–357.

Kramer F, Stunkard A, Marshall K, et al: Breast-feeding reduces maternal lower-body fat. *J Am Diet A* 1993;93:429–433.

Kritz-Silverstein D, Barrett-Connor E, Hollenbach K: Pregnancy and lactation as determinants of bone mineral density in postmenopausal women. *Am J Epidem* 1992;136(9):1052–1059.

Kumpulainen J, Salmenpera L, Siimes M, et al: Selenium status of exclusively breast-fed infants as influenced by maternal organic or inorganic selenium supplementation. *Am J Clin N* 1985; 42:829–835.

Kurz K, Habicht J, Rasmussen K, et al: Effects of maternal nutritional status and maternal energy supplementation on length of postpartum amenorrhea among Guatemalan women. *Am J Clin N* 1993;58:636–640.

Lederman S: The effect of pregnancy weight gain on later obesity. *Obstet Gyn* 1993;82(1): 148–155.

Lilja G, Dannaeus A, Foucard T, et al: Effects of maternal diet during late pregnancy and lactation on the development of IgE and egg- and milk-specific IgE and IgG antibodies in infants. *Clin Exp Al* 1991;21:195–202.

Little R, et al: Maternal alcohol use during breastfeeding and infant mental and motor development at one year. *N Eng J Med* 1989;321:425–430.

Littman H, Medendorp S, Goldfarb J: The decision to breastfeed: The importance of father's approval. *Clin Pediat* 1994;33(4):214–219.

Locklin M, Naber S: Does breastfeeding empower women? Insights from a select group of educated low-income, minority women. *Birth* 1993;20(1):30–35.

Lonnerdal B, Hernell O: Iron, zinc, copper and selenium status of breast-fed infants and infants fed trace element fortified milk-based infant formula. *Acta Paediat* 1994;83(4):367–373.

Lovelady C, Lonnerdal B, Dewey K: Lactation performance of exercising women. *Am J Clin N* 1990;52:103–109.

Lucas A: Does early diet program future outcome? *Acta Paed Sc* 1990;365:58–67.

Lucas A, Morley R, Cole T, et al: Breast milk and subsequent intelligence quotient in children born preterm. *Lancet* 1992;339:261–264.

MacIntyre U, Walker A: Lactation: How important is it? *J Roy S Hea* 1994;114(1):20–28.

Maehr J, Lizarraga J, Wingard D, et al: A comparative study of adolescent and adult mothers who intend to breastfeed. *J Adoles H* 1993;14(6):453–457.

Martin J, Bougnoux P, Fignon A, et al: Dependence of human milk essential fatty acids on adipose stores during lactation. *Am J Clin N* 1993;58:653–659.

McCullough A, Kirksey A, Wachs T, et al: Vitamin B6 status of Egyptian mothers: Relation to infant behavior and maternal-infant interactions. *Am J Clin N* 1990;51:1067–1074.

McGuire M, Burgert S, Milner J, et al: Selenium status of infants is influenced by supplementation of formula or maternal diets. *Am J Clin N* 1993;58:643–648.

McGuire M, Burgert S, Milner J, et al: Selenium status of lactating women is affected by the form of selenium consumed. *Am J Clin N* 1993;58:649–652.

McNeilly A: Lactational amenorrhea. *End Metab C* 1993;22(1):59–73.

Medina J, Pena C, Piva M, et al: Benzodiazepine-like molecules in human milk. *Lancet* 1990; 336(6727):1379.

Mehta S: Bone loss, contraception, and lactation. *Acta Obst Sc* 1993;72(3):148–156.

Mennella J, Beauchamp G: The effects of repeated exposure to garlic-flavored milk on the nursling's behavior. *Pediat Res* 1993;34(6):805–808.

Mennella J, Beauchamp G: Beer, breast feeding, and folklore. *Devel Psych* 1993;26(8):459–466.

Mennella J, Beauchamp G: The transfer of alcohol to human milk. *N Eng J Med* 1991;325: 981–985.

Michaelsen K, Larsen P, Thomsen B, et al: The Copenhagen Cohort Study on infant nutrition and growth: Breast-milk intake, human milk macronutrient content, and influencing factors. *Am J Clin N* 1994;59:600–611.

Miller R: Factors influencing lactation: Part I. Maternal. *Arch Dis Ch* 1952;27:187–204.

Mitchell M, Snyder E: Dietary carnitine effects on carnitine concentrations in urine and milk in lactating women. *Am J Clin N* 1991;54:814–820.

Moser-Veillon P, Reynolds R: A longitudinal study of pyridoxine and zinc supplementation of lactating women. *Am J Clin N* 1990;52:135–141.

Motil K, Sheng H, Montandon C: Case report: Failure to thrive in a breast-fed infant is associated with maternal dietary protein and energy restriction. *J Am Col N* 1994;13(2):203–208.

Murphy S, Abrams B: Changes in energy intakes during pregnancy and lactation in a national sample of US women. *Am J Pub He* 1993;83(8):1161–1163.

Nehlig A, Debry G: Consequences on the newborn of chronic maternal consumption of coffee during gestation and lactation: A review. *J Am Col N* 1994;13(1):6–21.

Neubauer S, Ferris A, Chase C, et al: Delayed lactogenesis in women with insulin-dependent diabetes mellitus. *Am J Clin N* 1993;58:58–60.

Newcomb P, Storer B, Longnecker M, et al: Lactation and a reduced risk of premenopausal breast cancer. *N Eng J Med* 1994;330(2):81–87.

Ohlin A, Rossner S: Maternal body weight development after pregnancy. *Int J Obes* 1990;14:159–173.

Ohlin A, Rossner S: Development of body weight during and after pregnancy, in Obesity in Europe 88: *Proceedings of the First European Congress on Obesity.* Stockholm, Sweden, John Libby and Co., 1989.

Ohtake M, Tamura T: Changes in zinc and copper concentrations in breast milk and blood of Japanese women during lactation. *J Nutr Sc V* 1993;39(2):189–200.

Orzalesi M: Do breast and bottle fed babies require vitamin supplements? *Acta Paed Sc* 1982;299 (suppl):77.

Ostrom K, Ferris A: Prolactin concentrations in serum and milk of mothers with and without insulin-dependent diabetes mellitus. *Am J Clin N* 1993;58:49–53.

Parker J, Abrams B: Differences in postpartum weight retention between black and white mothers. *Obstet Gyn* 1993;81(5):768–774.

Pedersen C, Stern R, Pate J, et al: Thyroid and adrenal measures during late pregnancy and the puerperium in women who have been major depressed or who become dysphoric postpartum. *J Affect D* 1993;29:201–211.

Perez-Escamilla R, Pollitt E, Lonnerdal B, et al: Infant feeding policies in maternity wards and their effect on breast-feeding success: An analytical overview. *Am J Pub He* 1994;84(1):89–97.

Picciano M, Guthrie H: Copper, iron, and zinc contents of mature human milk. *Am J Clin N* 1976;29:242–254.

Pizacane A, Impagliazzo N, Russo M, et al: Breast feeding and multiple sclerosis. *Br Med J* 1994; 308:1411–1412.

Pop V, Essed G, De Geus C, et al: Prevalence of post partum depression. *Acta Obst Sc* 1993;72:354–358.

Position of the American Dietetic Association: Promotion and support of breast-feeding. *J Am Diet A* 1993;93(4):467–469.

Potteiger J, Welch H, Byrne J: From parturition to marathon: A 16-week study of an elite runner. *Med Sci Spt* 1993;25(6):673–677.

Prentice A: Maternal calcium requirements during pregnancy and lactation. *Am J Clin N* 1994; 59(suppl):477S–483S.

Quadagno D, Dixon L, Denny N, et al: Postpartum moods in men and women. *Am J Obst G* 1986;154(5):1018–1023.

Rahmanifar A, Kirksey A, Wachs T, et al: Diets during lactation associated with infant behavior and caregiver-infant interaction in a semirural Egyptian village. *J Nutr* 1993;123(2):164–175.

Resman B, Blumenthal H, Jusko W: Breastmilk distribution of theobromine from chocolate. *J Pediat* 1977;91(3):477–480.

Righard L, Flodmark C, Lothe L, et al: Breastfeeding patterns: Comparing the effects on infant behavior and maternal satisfaction of using one or two breasts. *Birth* 1993;20(4):182–185.

Rogan W, Gladen B: Breast-feeding and cognitive development. *Ear Hum Dev* 1993;31(3): 181–193.

Rogan W, et al: Polychlorinated biphenyls and dichlorodiphenyl dichloroethene in human milk: Effects on growth, morbidity and duration of lactation. *Am J Pub He* 1987;77:1294–1297.

Rookus M, Rokebrand P, Burema J, et al: The effect of pregnancy on the body mass index 9 months postpartum in 49 women. *Int J Obes* 1987;11:609–618.

Ruff A, Halsey N, Coberly J, et al: Breast-feeding and maternal-infant transmission of human immunodeficiency virus type 1. *J Pediat* 1992;121(2):325–329.

Ryan A, Rush D, Krieger F, et al: Recent declines in breast-feeding in the United Sates, 1984 through 1989. *Pediatrics* 1991;88(4):719–727.

Salmenpera L, Perheentupa J, Nanto V, et al: Low zinc intake during exclusive breast-feeding does not impair growth. *J Ped Gastr* 1994;18(3):361–370.

Schauberger C, Rooney B, Brimer L: Factors that influence weight loss in the puerperium. *Obstet Gyn* 1992;79:424–429.

Sheard N: Breast-feeding protects against otitis media. *Nutr Rev* 1993;51(9):275–277.

Sichel D, Cohen L, Rosenbaum J, et al: Postpartum onset of obsessive-compulsive disorder. *Psychosomat* 1993;34(3):277–279.

Simmons B, Andrews W, Friel J, et al: Infant nutrition and visual acuity (meeting abstract). *Pediat Res* 1994;35(4):A77.

Smith D, Lewis C, Caveny J, et al: Longitudinal changes in adiposity associated with pregnancy: The Cardia study. *J Am Med A* 1994;271(22):1747–1751.

Sosa R, Klaus M, Urrutia J: Feed the nursing mother, thereby the infant. *J Pediat* 1976;88(4): 668–670.

Spaaij C, van Raaij J, de Groot L, et al: Effect of lactation on resting metabolic rate and on diet- and work-induced thermogenesis. *Am J Clin N* 1994;59:42–47.

Specker B: Do North American women need supplemental vitamin during pregnancy and lactation? *Am J Clin N* 1994;59(suppl):484S–491S.

Stumbo P, et al: Water intakes of lactating women. *Am J Clin N* 1985;42:870–876.

Temboury M, Otero A, Polanco I, et al: Influence of breast-feeding on the infant's intellectual development. *J Ped Gastr* 1994;18(1):32–36.

Tsukasaki M, Ohta Y, Oishi K, et al: Types and characteristics of short-term course of depression after delivery: Using Zung's Self-Rating Depression Scale. *Jpn J Psy N* 1991;45(3):565–576.

Tyrala E, Dodson W: Caffeine secretion into breastmilk. *Arch Dis Ch* 1979;54:787–800.

Uauy R, Hoffman D, Birch E, et al: Safety and efficacy of omega-3 fatty acids in the nutrition of very low birth weight infants: Soy oil and marine oil supplementation of formula. *J Pediat* 1994;124(4):612–620.

United Kingdom National Case-Control Study Group: Breast feeding and risk of breast cancer in young women. *Br Med J* 1993;307:17–20.

US Department of Health and Human Services: Lead in wine. September 9, 1991, press release.

Valentine C, Hurst N, Schanler R: Hindmilk improves weight gain in low-birth-weight infants fed human milk. *J Ped Gastr* 1994;18(4):474–477.

van Beusekom C, Zeegers T, Martini I, et al: Milk of patients with tightly controlled insulin-dependent diabetes mellitus has normal macronutrient and fatty acid composition. *Am J Clin N* 1993;57:938–943.

van de Perre P, Simonon A, Hitimana D, et al: Infective and anti-infective properties of breast-milk from HIV-1 infected women. *Lancet* 1993;341:914–918.

van Raaij J, Schonk C, Vermaat-Miedema S, et al: Energy cost of lactation, and energy balances of well-nourished Dutch lactating women: Reappraisal of the extra energy requirements of lactation. *Am J Clin N* 1991;53:612–619.

Vestermark V, Hogdall C, Plenov G, et al: Postpartum amenorrhoea and breast-feeding in a Danish sample. *J Biosoc Sc* 1994;26(1):1–7.

Waldenstrom U, Swenson A: Rooming-in at night in the postpartum ward. *Midwifery* 1991;7(2):82–89.

Walravens P, Chakar A, Mokni R, et al: Zinc supplements in breastfed infants. *Lancet* 1992;340(8821):683–685.

Wang I, Fraser I: Reproductive function and contraception in the postpartum period. *Obstet Gyn Surv* 1994;49(1):56–63.

West K, Kirksey A: Influence of vitamin B6 intake on the content of the vitamin in human milk. *Am J Clin N* 1976;29:961–966.

Williams A: Human milk and the preterm baby. *Br Med J* 1993;306:628–629.

Wolman W, Chalmers B, Hofmeyr J, et al: Postpartum depression and companionship in the clinical birth environment: A randomized, controlled study. *Am J Obst G* 1993;168:1388–1393.

Worthington-Roberts B, Little R, Lambert M, et al: Dietary cravings and aversions in the postpartum period. *J Am Diet A* 1989;89:647–651.

Wright P, Deary I: Breastfeeding and intelligence. *Lancet* 1992;339:612–614.

Wylie J, Verber I: Why women fail to breast-feed: A prospective study from booking to 28 days post-partum. *J Hum Nu D* 1994;7:115–120.

Yang C, Weiss N, Band P, et al: History of lactation and breast cancer risk. *Am J Epidem* 1993; 138:1050–1056.

10. The Postpregnancy Diet

ACOG Technical Bulletin: Nutrition during pregnancy. *Int J Gyn O* 1993;43:67–74.

Cumming D, Wheeler G, Harber V: Physical activity, nutrition, and reproduction. *Ann NY Acad* 1994;709:55–76.

General session. *Am J Clin N* 1994;59(suppl):474S–476S.

Huffman S, Martin L: Child nutrition, birth spacing, and child mortality. *Ann NY Acad* 1994; 709:236–248.

Johnson J, Walker P: Zinc and iron utilization in young women consuming a beef-based diet. *J Am Diet A* 1992;92:1474–1478.

Kahn A, Growasser J, Sottiaux M, et al: Prenatal exposure to cigarettes in infants with obstructive sleep apneas. *Pediatrics* 1994;93(5):778–783.

Lawless J, Latham M, Stephenson L, et al: Iron supplementation improves appetite and growth in anemic Kenyan primary school children. *J Nutr* 1994;124(5):645–654.

Merchant K, Martorell R, Haas J: Consequences for maternal nutrition of reproductive stress across consecutive pregnancies. *Am J Clin N* 1990;52(4):616–620.

Monsen E, Breskin M, Worthington-Roberts B: Iron status of women and its relation to habitual dietary sources of protein. *Fed Proc* 1986;45(4):978.

Ness R, Harris T, Cobb J, et al: Number of pregnancies and the subsequent risk of cardiovascular disease. *N Eng J Med* 1993;328:1528–1533.

Ohlin A, Rossner S: Trends in eating patterns, physical activity and socio-demographic factors in relation to postpartum body weight development. *Br J Nutr* 1994;71:457–470.

Ohlin A, Rossner S: Maternal body weight development after pregnancy. *Int J Obes* 1990;14: 159–173.

Rookus M, Rokebrand P, Burema J, et al: The effect of pregnancy on the body mass index 9 months postpartum in 49 women. *Int J Obes* 1987;11:609–618.

Smith D, Lewis C, Caveny J, et al: Longitudinal changes in adiposity associated with pregnancy. *J Am Med A* 1994;271(22):1747–1751.

Springer N, Bogue E, Arnold M, et al: Nutrition locus of control and dietary behaviors of pregnant women. *Ap Nurs Res* 1994;7(1):28–31.

Susser M, Stein Z: Timing in prenatal nutrition: A reprise of the Dutch Famine Study. *Nutr Rev* 1994;52(3):84–94.

Ulbricht T, Southgate D: Coronary heart disease: Seven dietary factors. *Lancet* 1991;338: 985–992.

US Department of Agriculture. *Provisional Table on the Nutrient Content of Bakery Goods and Related Items.* May 1981.

Wood J: Maternal nutrition and reproduction: Why demographers and physiologists disagree about a fundamental relationship. *Ann NY Acad* 1994;709:101–116.

Worthington-Roberts B, Little R, Lambert M, et al: Dietary cravings and aversions in the post-partum period. *J Am Diet A* 1989;89:647–651.

Index

Entries in **boldface** refer to charts, quizzes, tables, and worksheets. Entries in *italics* refer to recipes.

AAR-2995

UNION COUNTY COLLEGE

3 9354 00131834 0

618.24So53

Somer, Elizabeth.

Nutrition for a healthy
pregnancy : the
1995.

ELIZABETH

UNION COUNTY COLLEGE LIBRARIES
CRANFORD, N.J. 07016